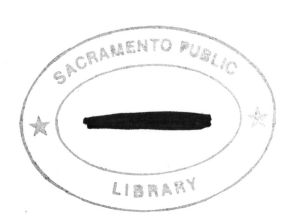

ALSO BY THE AUTHOR

Strikes in France, 1830–1968, with Charles Tilly, co-author (1974)

The Making of the Modern Family (1975)

A History of Women's Bodies (1982)

BEDSIDE MANNERS

The Troubled History of Doctors and Patients

by

EDWARD SHORTER

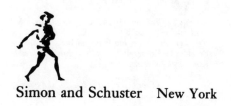

Simon and Schuster   New York

Published by Simon and Schuster
A Division of Simon & Schuster, Inc.
Simon & Schuster Building
Rockefeller Center
1230 Avenue of the Americas
New York, New York 10020
SIMON AND SCHUSTER and colophon are regis-
tered trademarks of Simon & Schuster, Inc.
Designed by Irving Perkins Associates
Manufactured in the United States of America
10   9   8   7   6   5   4   3   2   1
Library of Congress Cataloging in Publication Data
Shorter, Edward.
   Bedside manners.

   Bibliography: p.
   Includes index.
   1. Physician and patient—United States—History.
2. Physician and patient—England—History.   3. Medical
care—United States—History.   4. Medical care—
England—History.   I. Title.
R727.3.S49   1985   610.69'52   85-14619
ISBN: 0-671-53254-5

Grateful acknowledgment is made to the following societies, companies, authors, publications, publishing houses, and museums for permission to print the materials mentioned:

Academy of Medicine, Toronto
Courtesy the History of Medicine Museum:
Plates 1, 2, and 3.
   American Medical Association and Family
Media, Inc.
Reprinted from Hygeia, May 1929, p. 513; copy-
right 1929, American Medical Association,

Family Media, Inc. All rights reserved:
Plate 12.
   Annals of Internal Medicine, Philadelphia, PA
Published in Howard G. Bruenn, "Clinical
Notes on the Illness and Death of President
Franklin D. Roosevelt," Annals of Internal Med-
icine 72 (1970): Plate 17.

(Continued at the back of the book)

To my dear wife,
Anne Marie Shorter, M.D.

CONTENTS

Contents

ABBREVIATIONS USED IN THE NOTES

BMJ
British Medical Journal
JAMA
Journal of the American Medical Association
NEJM
New England Journal of Medicine

In references, the name of the publisher has been omitted from books published before 1940.

LIST OF FIGURES AND TABLES

PREFACE

I WAS having lunch with some medical students just before the beginning of classes in the first year. I was a "special" med student, intent upon learning how things worked on the inside.

One of them threw the anatomy textbook on the table, a thick volume of almost three hundred pages. "You'll end up memorizing every line of this," he said.

I laughed. On each page there were dense masses of detail about where muscles ran and the names of the nerves and arteries that supplied them. But he was right. I ended up memorizing almost every detail. And I took the various courses and passed them, surprising myself, a humanist, with my love for the subject matter.

At the end of several years of study, I thought I understood what medicine was all about: learning the scientific facts so that when you saw what was wrong inside patients with your physician's X-ray vision, a knowledge of the facts would permit you to heal them. In fact, this is what many doctors—and most of the public—believe about medicine as well.

The point of this book is to demonstrate that that view is quite wrong. I later realized as much, and so do many doctors. But it's the doctors and patients who don't realize it who today are so unhappy with each other. This book is written for angry patients and puzzled doctors who want to understand why there is so much ill feeling around the subject of "bedside manners."

It is a historian's book, even though the last third of it is about our own time. My personal conviction is that you can understand problems only by going back and examining their roots. So I tried to figure out, as a historian, how doctors and patients in times past were able to avoid the antagonistic stance that characterizes so much of what happens today in the doctor's office.

When it came to understanding bedside manners today, my books and archives were of little use. I returned to the clinic, this time as an observer of doctors and patients as they met. I wanted to figure out what went on in the head of the typical "family doctor" and what was on patients' minds.

The doctors I have worked with have been enormously kind and generous. They have given freely of their time. Taking the risk that I might be preparing some antidoctor hatchet job, they have been thoroughly professional, in the knowledge that they had nothing to conceal. And indeed, this is not a hatchet job. I would not hesitate to entrust myself to the care of any of the practitioners I have encountered.

The fact that they and their patients are increasingly at loggerheads has nothing to do with character faults. The doctors are not "brutal" or "grasping." The patients are not "silly" or "hysterical." The conflict has to do with deeper historical forces of which most doctors and patients are scarcely aware. That is why I wrote this book.

Although they will remain nameless, I should like to acknowledge the sympathetic cooperation I received from the many physicians who permitted me to observe their encounters with their patients. I may, however, express my thanks to Dr. Henry Shykoff, Dr. Ruth Skye-Shykoff, and Dr. Anne Marie Shorter, all of whom read the manuscript, engaged me in spirited debate, and rectified several factual errors. Bianca Roberts, too, went over an earlier draft, and the pleasure she took in it provided me with much encouragement.

The staffs of the Toronto Academy of Medicine Library and the Science and Medicine Library of the University of Toronto have, as always, been wonderfully helpful. John Glover and Louise Yick kindly assisted with photographs. And Kate Hamilton typed the manuscript.

Finally, let me say what a pleasure it has been to work with Robert Asahina and Ruth Kozodoy of Simon & Schuster. It would be hard to imagine more pleasant or quick-witted editorial guidance.

Edward Shorter
Toronto, Canada
August 1984

CHAPTER ONE
Introduction

*I*N JUNE of 1979 Dr. David Rabin, director of Endocrinology at Vanderbilt Medical Center, started to have feelings of restlessness in his legs. By that autumn he was walking with a limp, and a year later he was scarcely able to walk at all. He had contracted a crippling affliction called *Lou Gehrig's disease*. The disease would have been bad enough, but Dr. Rabin was further horrified by the reactions of his medical colleagues.

"One day, while crossing the little courtyard outside the emergency room, I fell. A longtime colleague was walking by. He turned, and our eyes met as I lay sprawled on the ground. He quickly averted his eyes, pretended not to see me, and continued walking."

Dr. Rabin sought medical help, traveling to a "prestigious medical center" to consult a neurologist. The man was able to diagnose Dr. Rabin's condition without difficulty, but what surprised Rabin was the neurologist's "impersonal manner." "He exhibited no interest in me as a person and did not even make a perfunctory inquiry about my work." The neurologist made no suggestions about specific daily activities; nor did he give psychological advice about mustering "the emotional strength to cope with a progressive degenerative disease."[1]

After hearing of this tragic story, one listener responded, "I marvel at Dr. Rabin's naiveté. His account of his experiences . . . indicates that he has simply found himself on the unfamiliar side of the typical physician-patient relationship." Ordinary people have come to expect this kind of treatment from doctors, she pointed out. Other doctors behaved impersonally with Dr. Rabin, not because they were embarrassed at weakness in a fellow physician, but just because Dr. Rabin "had the misfortune to become a patient."[2]

I am observing in a "family medicine" clinic. A woman, thirty-one, comes in complaining of deep, constant chest pain, night and day. It's not relieved by bending forward or lying down. She has other aches about the neck as well, plus a feeling of tiredness so great that she's had to stop jogging entirely this week and only went out a few times last week. Stress? Apparently none. Her work is going fine. She says nothing about her personal life. "This chest pain is the major problem in my life right now."

She has already had a chest X-ray, complete blood tests, electrocardiogram, a barium swallow, and a sigmoidoscopy (examination of her colon with a long viewing tube). She is exasperated at the length of time it takes for the results to come back.

In addition, someone forgot her appointment today and let her cool her heels for an hour and a half in the waiting room. She believes the doctor has lost interest in her case and, as someone in a fast-track career who is accustomed to having things happening, wants very much for them to start happening around her *now*.

While she's talking, unbeknown to her, things really are happening. Two senior doctors whom the resident has summoned are phoning around the hospital for the results of the X-ray and tests. The tests show anemia. In other words, she's losing blood somewhere, probably from the digestive tract. An intense discussion is going on over whether it's an ulcer.

None of this activity is apparent to her. The resident soothes her. "You can be sure we're taking your problems very seriously." The resident wants her to come back for another barium swallow. She is irritated and asks whether it is absolutely necessary. She is tired of being "fucked around" by the system.

As a historian, I am well aware that a hundred years ago her problem would have been diagnosed as "hysteria," and the investigation terminated. In contrast, these postmodern doctors—those trained in a certain style since the 1950s—are intent upon finding out exactly what's wrong and fixing it. But she, as patients often do, sees only delays, bureaucratic foul-ups, and impassive clinical expressions.

Something is wrong with the practice of medicine today. Although this young woman is receiving far better medical attention than she would have at any other time in history, she is quite possibly feeling worse. Medical knowledge has rapidly expanded in recent years, but medical *care* has in certain crucial ways deteriorated. For a whole complex of reasons, doctors and patients eye each other with mistrust. A medical encounter today is very likely to produce an explosion of mutual resentment and frustration. And this tension has quite a direct bearing on whether or not the treatment is clinically successful. In other words, medicine is currently in crisis.

My intention, in writing this book, has been to trace the history of doctor-patient relations as they have evolved alongside the science of medicine. It is in this history, especially that of the last century and up to our own time, that we can discover the roots of the present crisis. I believe we will also find, in following that story, significant insights into what the shortcomings of present-day medical practice actually are.

Doctor bashing would be easy in a book like this: lining up the horrible anecdotes and concluding that doctors have become a lot of heartless brutes. But in recounting the story of the present crisis in doctor-patient relations I want to make sure the doctors tell their side as well. You are a doctor practicing in the pain program of the Mayo Clinic in Rochester, Minnesota. Many patients who have intractable pain you are able to help, with drugs, psychotherapy, or surgery. But some you are not. Their pains are agonizing and unendurable but seem to have no organic cause. What's more, these patients are constantly firing off letters of complaint about how wretchedly they're being treated and threatening to sue. One, for example, is a forty-four-year-old woman, separated from her husband, whose pain—which nobody has been able to diagnose—has been going on for about ten years. She has had "many falls, operations, treatment failures, and marital problems." This time in the clinic she says she "stumbled over some physical therapy equipment," hurting her arm. Nothing appears on X-ray. She develops many other new problems as well, and complains of "anxiety and depression." When she leaves the hospital, she secretly takes the X-rays with her, has her new doctor send his bills to the Mayo Clinic, and threatens to sue.[3]

It's easy for doctors to be unsympathetic to this woman. Even though she feels genuine pain and believes herself to be physically ill, they see her as suffering from a psychiatric disorder. Most doctors would dismiss her as a "crock," a pain in the neck, and even the psychiatrists who treated her in Rochester would not have admitted her again to their pain clinic. Doctors officially call it "pain of psychological origin," but her real problem is the "white knuckle syndrome": not that the patient's knuckles are white, but that the doctor's are, every time a patient like this comes through the door.

Thus, for both sides, harsh judgments of the other come easily. But let us for a moment suspend moral judgments. In the 1980s more than a billion encounters between doctors and patients occur annually in the United States. Three-fourths of all Americans see a doctor at least once a year, and the average person has about five contacts a year with a physician.[4] Many of these contacts end with anger and frustration on both sides.

What is this consultation like that it so frequently produces anger? One British study shows the main features of a typical encounter. You walk in the door and the doctor asks, "What is wrong with you today?" "What's hurting today, and where is it?" Then occur the actual history taking, the physical exam, the forming of a diagnosis and organizing of a plan of treatment: these procedures will occupy us in considerable detail in this book. Then the consultation ends, a common way being the physician's "symbolically tearing off a piece of paper and offering no explanation, only a set of instructions." Patients often find these highly directed consultations unsatisfactory, because the doctor is so intent upon dealing with the main symptom, or "chief complaint," that patients don't have a chance to express what is really on their minds.[5]

Consider this young woman whose "chief complaint" is painful diarrhea. The doctor asks her a number of questions about her attacks and where she feels pain. Each question is precise:

DOCTOR: Any particular sort of foods upset you?
PATIENT: At one time I did knock off the fats; fatty foods, you know.
DOCTOR: Does it make any difference when you have them?
PATIENT: No, not really. Well, I put a bit of margarine on and scrape it off again. . . .
DOCTOR: Do you get any other trouble, apart from the pain and sickness?
PATIENT: Well, I don't know whether this has anything to do with it. . . . (She begins to cry. The telephone rings.)
DOCTOR (after finishing the phone call): You were telling me you've had this [vaginal] discharge. How long have you had that?
PATIENT (talking rapidly, still crying): I've had a D and C [an operation to scrape out the uterus] and I thought . . . and there it was . . . . He said I should have told you. . . .
(The doctor obviously does not want to hear any more about the D and C or why she's so upset about the discharge. Even though she is still trying to blurt it out, he changes the subject back to her diarrhea.)
DOCTOR: I see. Do you get any indigestion, wind or any of that sort of stuff . . .?[6]

Many doctor-patient encounters of this nature add up to a crisis: frustrated patients, unable to express what is really troubling them, and doctors irritated by what they see as an avalanche of trivial symptoms, both blindly caroming off each other to end up later at cocktail parties, venting their anger with amusing stories.

As I shall demonstrate, consultations of this nature were quite unusual in the days before postmodern medicine. We shall follow the story of the massive breakdown in doctor-patient relations from the side of both the doctor and the patient.

The doctor's transformation began in 1945, with the diffusion of mass-produced penicillin to the civilian population, just after

World War II. In the next decade a whole series of antibiotics became available, effective mainly against bacterial infections. It is difficult for us to recall now how dramatically these "wonder drugs" transformed our encounter with disease: pneumonias that had previously swung the balance of life and death were now whisked away; rheumatic fevers that earlier had left patients with permanently damaged hearts now vanished with a few pills; gonorrheas, which once young men gave to their wives at marriage, cursing the couple to a lifetime of infertility, could now be cured with a course of tablets. And the antibiotics were just the beginning. In the 1950s and 1960s came other drugs: medicines for preventing inflammation in the joints and the kidneys, making the arteries larger in fighting high blood pressure or making the blood vessels smaller in fighting shock, causing the heart to beat more slowly or more rapidly, composing the mind, and thinning the blood. Never before had medicine possessed—with a few exceptions we shall read about—drugs that could actually *cure* disease. After this incredible leap forward in drug therapy, one could more easily list the diseases that couldn't be cured than those that could, so numerous had the latter become. (Granted, viral infections have remained untreatable, as have a number of diseases that affect relatively small numbers of patients.) Even some cancers, with the exception of those caused by smoking, have in the 1970s and 1980s acquired favorable prognoses (chances for recovery) as a result of this incredible therapeutic revolution.

These stunning changes were not confined to drugs. Becoming disoriented and confused? We'll clean out the arteries that supply blood to your brain with a scraper. Blood in the stool? We'll find out what's wrong with an endoscope. Feeling tired and run down? By the 1980s entire new *sciences*, such as immunology and clinical biochemistry, have a good chance of figuring out why. Most practicing doctors before World War II had only the vaguest notions of what the chemistry of the body entailed.

The upshot of all these changes was to fill doctors with an aggressive new confidence about their ability to diagnose and cure disease. Postmodern medicine is characterized not only by its ability to diagnose with near certainty what's wrong with you, *but to cure it as well.* This is the revolutionary feature: the ability to cure disease, an ability that doctors had never before possessed.

The medical profession now bristles with new self-confidence. I asked a young family doctor, once you succeed in making the diagnosis, do you think you can cure whatever the patient has?

"Oh, absolutely," she replied.

This is wonderful, right, the ability to cure disease? Indeed it is. But this new medical enthusiasm has had a transforming effect upon the doctor-patient relationship, causing the doctor to be much more disease-oriented and less patient-oriented. Being *disease-oriented* means that you, the doctor, basically believe the patient has some kind of physical disease, the result perhaps of the invasion of a microorganism (such as a cold) or of a degenerative process (such as osteoarthritis), and that you believe your job as a doctor is to diagnose and appropriately treat that disease. Therefore, encounters with disease-oriented doctors are likely to lack, for the patient, a certain human dimension. Such doctors tend to be perfunctory in history taking (not believing the "history of the illness" to be all that revealing); to be concerned principally with gathering diagnostic data and interpreting it with specialists; and to evidence little personal interest in the patient. It is not that they are *un*interested in patients and their personal problems. It is just that there is no medical need to *show* interest.

But so what? As long as the doctor diagnoses and fixes what's wrong with you, does it matter whether there's a little heartburn? The mechanic that fixes your car may be gruff, but at the end the thing runs, and who needs a blabby mechanic? But it does matter, because patients are different from cars: about a quarter to a third of the symptoms that a family doctor sees are not the result of well-defined disease processes. Instead they are of psychological origin. They arise in the mind and spread to the body, from "stress" perhaps or from some disorder of the mind, but not from the usual causes of disease that one learns about in medical school. And disease-oriented doctors are unable to do much for these "psychosomatic" or "psychoneurotic" conditions, because these doctors lack the sympathetic relationship to the patients that is a *precondition of their cure.*

It is my belief that doctors before World War II focused more strongly on the person than on the disease. Because of this sympathy for the patient, they had far better results treating so-called psychosomatic disease and psychoneuroses than doctors do today.

Two preconditions are necessary for the cure of disease of psychological origin: (1) the opportunity for the patient to explain the symptoms and their presumed origin thoroughly in a relaxed conversation with the doctor; (2) the patient's implicit belief in the powers of modern medicine, and thus in the doctor's ability to effect a cure, whatever the doctor does. All of this brings us to the second half of our story, the patient's track.

In the years since 1960 several aspects of the world of the patient have changed. There has been an enormous increase in the number of symptoms for which patients seek relief. Presumably patients in the 1920s, or in the fourteenth century, felt an itching ankle or a stomach pain as acutely as people do today. What has changed is the patient's willingness to define bodily symptoms as an illness and to seek help for this illness. Patients in the 1980s are far more willing to rest up or consult a doctor than ever before. And the glut of illnesses created by this willingness has swamped not only the medical profession but the pharmacies and "alternative healers" as well.

In addition, patients have begun to abandon their reverential faith in the doctor's powers. This is of particular relevance to diseases of psychological origin. How ironical that people should stop believing in "Rex Morgan, M.D.," just as he begins to acquire his powers!

Why these changes have occurred, in both doctor and patient is the subject of this book. The effect of these developments has been to poison the consultation and encourage doctors and patients to take an adversarial stand toward each other—and thus to deny the doctor the possibility of treating effectively just those disorders that in family practice are the most frequently seen of all.

My discussion starts with the traditional doctor of the eighteenth century, although the book's center of gravity is the 1970s and 1980s. One of the heroes will be the *modern doctor:* that is, the kind of physician who started to be "scientifically" trained by medical schools in the 1870s and 1880s and who eventually gave way to the postmodern doctor trained in the 1950s and 1960s. This modern doctor was quite distinctive. Unlike the traditional doctor preceding him, he could diagnose successfully most of the diseases he saw in general practice, although he was able to do little about curing them. Partly as a result of his new scientific abilities at diagnosis and "prognosis," he acquired a new esteem in the eyes of his patients. It is this curious esteem, so different from the fear in which the traditional doctor was held and the anger and irritation that greet the postmodern doctor, that made the modern doctor a singular figure.

The book's center of gravity is the 1970s and 1980s. My intention is to explain the transition from modern to postmodern doctor, and from modern to postmodern patient. I will begin by describing the world of the traditional doctor and patient. Then we shall watch the modern doctor and the modern patient emerge after the 1870s and flourish deep into the twentieth century, as a long series of advances in the basic medical sciences starts to pay off in bedside medicine. Then we shall observe the shattering of the sympathetic alliance between modern doctor and patient under the hammer blows of the 1970s and 1980s.

CHAPTER TWO
The Traditional Doctor

*C*ALLING THE years between 1750 and 1850 *traditional* does not mean that medicine had remained unchanged since the ancient Greeks; certainly there was an evolution of medical ideas over that millennium and a half. But pre-1850 medicine was very different from what would come later. Our point of departure is an examination of these traditional practitioners, doctors who were often ruinously incompetent and aggressively meddlesome.

An English Elite

Lowly though the average doctor was before the late nineteenth century, he could to some extent bask in the reflected light of quite a brilliant corner of medicine, that occupied by the physicians and surgeons of the Royal Colleges in London. It is not that American medicine was any more "back-

26

ward" in the eighteenth century than that practiced by the average British surgeon-apothecary (later called *GP*). Indeed, later on, American doctors would be thought more scientific than British ones. But American medicine in those years was a small tail wagged by a big British dog. Without the existence of this British medical elite, the average American practitioner would have seemed little different from a carpenter or bricklayer. To the extent that the typical American doctor could call himself a "gentleman" in the years before 1870, it was assuming the borrowed mantle of the handful of consultants in the Royal Colleges.

The most prestigious of these medical bodies, the Royal College of Physicians in London, had received its royal charter in 1518. By the early nineteenth century its only remaining power was to license those who had formal M.D.'s, mainly from Oxford and Cambridge, to practice around London. But its prestige was immense. It is touching to read, in the autobiographies of rough-hewn frontier physicians, of the excitement they felt, on what would be their only trip to Europe, at being received at the Royal College of Physicians. Always a mark of cachet in medical publishing were the letters *FRCP* (Fellow of the Royal College of Physicians of London) after an author's name, although men all over the British Isles and beyond could be invited to join. Armed with Doctor of Medicine diplomas, after perhaps fourteen years of study at Oxford or Cambridge, these men knew the ancients, such as Galen, by heart. They were the doctors of the rich in London and provincial English cities and were summoned as "consultants" in cases of special difficulty. Called *physicians* because they had presumably learned in medical school how to prescribe *physic*, or drugs, many of them amassed great fortunes and lived in lovely townhouses in the West End of London.

After the middle of the nineteenth century, the surgeons vaulted past the physicians. But earlier on they were somewhat less prestigious, since one didn't require a university education or a medical degree to become a surgeon, just a completed apprenticeship. The surgeons of London had formed a Royal College only in 1800, having organized previously in various associations resembling guilds. In 1843 the organization came to be national, becoming the Royal College of Surgeons of England. The distinction between surgeons and physicians applied only at the highest levels. Of the eight thousand members of the RCS in 1834, for example, only about two hundred made a full-time living in surgery.[1] The others were, in effect, general practitioners (GPs).

The point is that medicine did have a rich historical pedigree, entitling its practitioners to the status of gentlemen, as members of the learned professions, alongside law and the clergy.

Upper-class American doctors, such as the Philadelphia neurologist Silas Weir Mitchell, later made themselves positively ludicrous in their efforts to identify with that tradition. At dinner with a "distinguished Englishman," Mitchell offered such pronouncements as "There are three things worthwhile in life—to rise to a foremost position in the profession one has chosen—to write a good novel and to catch a salmon in the summer"![2] The study in Mitchell's Walnut Street home was dominated by a copy of Joshua Reynolds's *Hunter*, which hangs in the Royal College of Surgeons in London, and a copy of Cornelius Janssen's *Harvey*, which hangs in the Royal College of Physicians.[3] (William Harvey, a seventeenth-century London physician, discovered the circulation of the blood; John Hunter, an eighteenth-century London surgeon, was famous for a number of discoveries, including his work on inflammation.)

These exalted members of the Royal Colleges also provided the classical model of arrogance in relations between doctors and patients. The reformist Edinburgh physician John Gregory wrote in 1770 that after a physician has been in practice for a while, "he becomes haughty, rapacious, careless, and often somewhat brutal in his manners. Conscious of the ascendancy he has acquired, he acts a despotic part."[4] And why not? They had come from the country gentry of English society, attended university in an era that permitted a bachelor's degree only to men of independent wealth, and had acquired all the snobbishness of their class, adopting, according to Gregory, "an affectation of knowledge, inscrutable to all . . . an air of perfect confidence in their own skill and abilities; and a demeanor solemn, contemptuous, and highly expressive of self-sufficiency."[5] This was the world of the bewigged doctor, or the doctor outfitted with top hat and cane, and spending as much time in the coffee houses of London as in the practice of medicine. It was a world miles away from that of the ordinary doctor. I mention it to make clear that the undoubted social prestige these men possessed came from the social class into which they had been born, and not from their medical knowledge.

THE DOCTOR AS THREAT TO HIS PATIENTS

The typical American doctor of the eighteenth and early nineteenth centuries was as unlike the Fellow of the Royal College as night is from day. Of the estimated thirty-five hundred doctors in the American colonies in 1776, there were probably "not ... 400 who had received medical degrees." "The colonists at first, it would seem, rather preferred to patronize the medical man who was also minister, farmer, merchant, or mechanic, in addition to being a physician."[6] With the exception of the handful of degreed men, most of whom had trained in Europe (especially Edinburgh), American doctors had little going for them: no books, no libraries, no medical societies, no hospitals to "walk the wards" of.

As might be expected, these early American doctors were horrible, a menace to their patients. "When I first arrived in New-England," wrote the Boston physician William Douglass in 1755, "I asked G.P., a noted facetious [sic] practitioner, what was their general method of practice; he told me their practice was very uniform, bleeding, vomiting, blistering, purging. ... Nature was never to be consulted or allowed to have any concern in the affair."[7] Douglass was writing at a time when British opinion, under the influence of the Enlightenment, was starting to argue that much disease could be left to nature. "In general, the physical practice in our colonies is so perniciously bad, that excepting in surgery and some very acute cases, it is better to let nature ... take her course. ... Our American practitioners are so rash and officious," he continued, that the Biblical saying could be applied to them, " 'He that sinneth before his maker, let him fall into the hands of the physician.' Frequently there is more danger from the physician than from the distemper."[8]

When Illinois passed its first medical practice law in 1878, it granted licenses to men who had already been practicing for ten years or more solely because of their "years of practice"; hence the phrase *Y. of P. men.* Dr. Thomas Shastid, a quite competent physician who practiced in a small town in Illinois, recalled one such Y. of P. man, called "Dr. Dictionary" because he "so often boasted that he knew the 'Devil's Dictionary' by heart and that he could swear rapidly for thirty-five minutes and never repeat himself once."

Dr. Dictionary was called to see a woman who had severed one of the arteries in her forearm (radial artery) with a piece of glass. He had apparently never learned how to deal with this problem. One is supposed to tie both ends, but Dr. Dictionary "merely sprinkled tannic acid on the wound and told the patient to lie very quiet and that soon all would be well. The patient, after the doctor's departure, did lie very quiet. She lay very quiet for a very long time—until, in fact, her son, becoming suspicious, investigated her quietness and found she was going to be quiet from that time on."[9]

Why were these traditional doctors so bad? It was partly due to the theories of medicine they held, partly to their inadequate medical educations.

There was nothing illogical about traditional medical theories. All, in fact, were rigorously logical as abstract systems of reasoning. But rather than being based on observed facts they were more or less spun out of the air and thus were of no use in understanding how the body actually worked. These theories would be of interest mainly to historians of ideas, were it not that programs of therapy were based upon them, and millions of people systematically poisoned, dehydrated, and exsanguinated as their medical attendants applied theory to practice.

To give the reader a sense of one of these many competing systems, let us take that of Hermann Boerhaave, a famous theorist who taught around 1700 at the University of Leyden, then perhaps the foremost medical center in the world. Boerhaave said the body consisted of two main components: the solids, and the blood and humors. What could go wrong with the solids? Here we see the classifying mind at work: they could be either too weak or too rigid. Weak fibers were caused, logically enough, by bad digestion, and so you gave iron and prescribed plenty of exercise and a sound diet, especially milk, for such diseases of weak fibers as tuberculosis. On the other hand, aging, or too much exercise, might cause rigid fibers. Then you would have to give thin gruel to soften them up again, thus curing diseases caused by overly rigid blood vessels, such as blood clots. Similarly, things can go wrong with the blood and other bodily fluids ("the humors"). The patient can drink too much water, for example, causing the tissues to swell ("dropsy"), or take too much salt, making the fluids "acrid." What's wrong with acrid fluids? They can cause belching, heartburn, and flatus or cause the small arteries to narrow in size. What happens if the arteries are too narrow? Obstructions develop, which in turn cause inflammation. Finally we have reached a familiar concept: inflammation, when the affected tissues hurt, swell, turn red, and feel hot. Boerhaave's therapy? Dissolve the obstruction by giving "diluents"; soften the diet to relax the blood vessels; and remove blood from the body to reduce its velocity.[10]

The diagnoses that flowed from these larger systems of pathophysiology (as medical systems are called nowadays) seemed relatively straightforward. Thus the Edinburgh physician William Buchan: "In childhood the fibers are lax and soft, the nerves are extremely irritable, and the fluids thin; whereas in old age the fibers are rigid, the nerves become almost insensible, and many of the vessels are almost imperviable." Accordingly, the diseases of the young and old "must require a different method of treatment."[11]

What therapy would you as a physician undertake to make the fibers less rigid or the nerves less irritable? To reduce blood volume and velocity, the causes of inflammation, you perform bleeding and purging (giving powerful laxatives). Or if local congestion of the blood is causing inflammation, you divert the blood by raising blood blisters with cupping glasses, by making the skin red with mustard plasters, or by giving warm baths to bring the blood to the surface.

Thus we have a medical program: bleeding and purging. Edward Baynard, an M.D. who evidently had trained with Boerhaave at Leyden before settling into a London practice, commemorated bleeding in 1719:

Bleed only when you find the blood
Abound, or stagnate; then 'tis good;
Which you may very eas'ly guess,
By heavy stiff unwieldiness,
Short breath, high pulse, et cetera:
Then quickly take some blood away;
But more especially in stitches,
Pleuritic pains and pungent twitches;
Then out of hand without delay,
Take a good quantity away.[12]

Other system builders would add refinements: get the corrupt humors out by sweating, vomiting, urinating. The underlying logic of these theories was clear: the disease is caused by excesses or by things turning putrid inside the body. We get those bad humors and those excess fluids out by evacuating fluids from as many channels as possible: excess salivation, massive bowel movements, venesection (removing blood by opening a vein), kidney stimulation to produce a urine flow, or heating of the room to make sweat pour off the patient. Whatever system you subscribed to, the therapeutic regimen would be pretty much the same. If, for example, the patient had an inflammation in the colon, John Howship, member of the Royal College of Surgeons of London, would try to produce the following evacuations:

1. *Stool: Give some purgatives, senna perhaps or castor oil; maybe a "large and gently laxative enema."*
2. *Urine: "With a view to moderate arterial action, it may also be expedient to direct, at intervals some of the saline diuretics."*
3. *Blood: "If the patient be young, and the symptoms strongly marked, with much pain and local tenderness, the practitioner will require all his discernment in determining the moment for having recourse to the lancet. . . ."*[13] (Note: *A lancet was a little knife for opening a vein, hence the title of a major British medical weekly,* The Lancet.)

However complex and disparate the medical theories of the time, therapy boiled down to the following, in Baynard's words:

> For in ten words the whole Art is comprised;
> For some of the ten are always advised.
> Piss, Spew, and Spit,
> Perspiration and Sweat;
> Purge, Bleed, and Blister,
> Issues and Clyster. . . .
>
> Most other specifics
> Have no visible effects,
> But the getting of fees,
> For a promise of ease;
> (Much like the South S———).[14]

(*Note:* "Issues" are discharges from the skin; "clysters" are enemas.) "South S———" is a reference to an eighteenth-century stock fraud, the "South Sea Bubble.")

It was not among the Fellows of the Royal Colleges, but with the backwoods doctors of the United States, that the passion for bleeding and blistering, purging and peeing, reached its nineteenth-century high point: It was called "heroic medicine." Particularly as a result of the writings of the Philadelphia physician Benjamin Rush, there was a surge in the popularity of the purgative mercurous chloride (calomel), a heavy, white, odorless powder that in addition to producing massive evacuations also induced the classical signs of mercury poisoning, including rich salivation: all to the good, according to the logic of the time.[15]

Oliver Wendell Holmes, a Boston physician and essayist (and father of the Supreme Court Justice), believed there was a unique American attraction to this horrible dosing:

> How could a people which . . . has contrived the Bowie-knife and the revolver, which has chewed the juice out of all the superlatives in the language in Fourth of July orations, . . . which insists in sending out yachts and horses and boys to out-sail, out-run, out-fight, and checkmate all the rest of creation; how could such a people be content with any but "heroic" practice? What wonder

33

that the stars and stripes wave over doses of ninety grains of sulphate of quinine, and that the American eagle screams with delight
to see three drachms of calomel given at a single mouthful?[16]

Another Boston physician, Jacob Bigelow, mocked in 1844 the
backwoods doctors for getting into "the blind routine of always
thinking that you must make your patients worse before they can
be better." Much of the current hostility to doctors, Bigelow continued, "is sustained in places where practice has previously been
over-heroic, and because mankind are gratified to find that they
and their families can get well without the lancet, the vomit, and
the blister. . . ."[17] If we find traditional patients to be sullen and
hostile toward doctors and willing to consult them only in ex-
tremis, we will begin to understand why.

Traditional doctors were saddled with a second handicap: inadequate medical training. They imperfectly understood even the
correct information that, by 1800, centuries of medical learning
had accumulated. Before the early eighteenth century there were
no "medical schools," in the sense of courses of lectures one could
attend while acquiring experience at the bedside. At Oxford and
Cambridge one could get an M.D., but without the necessity of
actually seeing and learning from sick patients. And even though
in London several medical schools attached to the large hospitals
appeared in the eighteenth century, the normal route to becoming
a doctor would remain apprenticeship for many years.

In Britain, the average medical student would be apprenticed
to a surgeon or an "apothecary" rather than to a degreed physician. Indeed, one of the peculiarities of the British system is that
the vast majority of medical men were really surgeon-apothecaries rather than physicians. In practice the distinction is meaningless, since no surgeon outside London could live full-time from
surgery, and "apothecaries" were really GPs who charged for the
medicines they prescribed and dispensed, rather than for the
house call itself.[18]

Similarly in the United States, most traditional doctors would
start their training as apprentices, paying the *preceptor* who had
taken them on a hundred or so dollars a year for three years, living in the doctor's house, helping him compound his prescriptions and wrap his bandages, and accompanying him on house

calls. When in 1822 Samuel Gross, a Pennsylvania Dutch farm-boy, decided at the age of seventeen to become a doctor, he signed on with one "country physician; but he afforded me no aid, and I therefore soon quit him and tried another, with no better luck. They had none but old, if not obsolete books; they were constantly from home, never examined me, or gave me any encouragement . . . and I at length gave up in despair." So Gross entered high school, Wilkesbarre Academy, to learn "Latin, English, grammar, mathematics, and Greek" and then at nineteen tried apprenticing himself again, this time to Dr. Joseph Swift of Easton, Pennsylvania,

> a practitioner of some note, with considerable pretention to scientific knowledge. . . . His library was small, and its contents of little value. He had no apparatus of any kind, plates or diagrams, no specimens in materia medica [drugs], or anatomical preparations; nothing, in short, but a skeleton, and this, with the aid of Wistar's *Anatomy* was the first thing I set about to master.

Swift would examine the young apprentice every Saturday for an hour and a half, and thus Gross made his way through surgery, internal medicine, and midwifery. Well, sort of. Because "my preceptor was not popular, and few of his patients could be visited by an 'unfledged doctor,' " Gross saw little bedside medicine. Finally, in 1826 he enrolled at Jefferson Medical College in Philadelphia.[19]

It was in the mid-1870s that Franklin Martin, a Wisconsin farmboy, decided to become a doctor. So he wrote to his Aunt Mary to ask whether Dr. Spaulding would take him on as an apprentice. Dr. Spaulding said yes, if he would "tend the fires and care for [the] office in the Winter." When Martin arrived at Dr. Spaulding's office, he found

> a large table . . . covered with half-filled ink bottles and ink-stained pen holders; several rickety chairs stood about . . . in the center of the room, a large, bulging cast-iron stove, set in a sand-box several feet square which was well decorated with cigar stubs and other refuse. There were a few large tin spittoons about; the floor was bare and had the appearance of the backyard of a third-class tenement. Of course there were layers of dust and dirt everywhere.

Dr. Spaulding "went to the book case and after a long search in the confusion brought out an old Wilson's *Anatomy* that had re-

35

ceived hard usage, blew the dust off the yellow cover, handed it to me and said, 'All right, you learn what is in that, and occasionally I will quiz you.' "[20]

Who became apprentices? Highly motivated young scientists? In 1832 Daniel Drake described the way that future doctors were selected. "A neighbouring physician wants a student to reside in his office; or one son of the family is thought too weakly to labour on the farm . . . ; he is indolent and averse to bodily exertion; or addicted to study, but too stupid for the Bar, or too immoral for the pulpit; the parents wish to have a gentleman in the family, *and a doctor is a gentleman.*"[21]

The apprentice doctor would then polish off his training in medical school. What were those schools like? The first one founded in America was a medical college tacked on to the College of Philadelphia in 1765; then Columbia, Harvard, and Dartmouth all acquired rudimentary courses of medical lectures before 1800. The College of Philadelphia inflated its medical degree from a bachelor's to a doctorate in 1789, and by the War of 1812 all American medical colleges were granting the degree "doctor of medicine," though of course one didn't require a previous undergraduate degree to acquire this "doctorate" (nor does one in many medical schools today).[22]

The United States saw a huge explosion in medical education in the nineteenth century: by 1860 there were forty-seven medical schools, which had turned out about seventeen thousand graduates.[23] Most were little "proprietary" schools, founded by a few doctors, who lived from the students' fees. These three or four doctors did all the lecturing, requiring attendance at two courses of lectures of perhaps five months each for a degree, and repeating the same lectures both years. There were no laboratories, little dissection, and few chances to see patients. Arthur Hertzler, a Kansas country doctor, remembered some of the stories from those days. "For instance, a lecturer on anatomy held at arm's length a bone from a skull. In a high-pitched oratorical voice he delivered himself of the following: 'Gentlemen, this is a sphenoid bone. Damn the sphenoid bone.' Having thus expressed his opinion of the value of a knowledge of this particular bone, he threw it back into the box."[24] Attendance was often optional, the final exams easy, and the classroom riotous: medical autobiographies from these years are full of tales of students' throwing shoes and bouncing one another around the classroom.

Why were conditions so slack? Because these proprietary schools were desperate for students. Since their owners lived from the fees, there was seldom a question of expelling anyone; they would take all comers, not even insisting on certification of a previous apprenticeship.

Even at the larger medical colleges, the level of education was poor. The Alabama surgeon James Marion Sims wrote that when he graduated in 1835 from Philadelphia's Jefferson Medical College, he felt "absolutely incompetent to assume the duties of a practitioner."[25] Daniel Drake, who in 1832 was teaching at the Medical College of Ohio in Cincinnati, wrote in fury that not only would these American doctors never "contribute a single new fact to the archives" of medicine, but they could not even spell. "I am constrained to say that even at this late period the profession abounds in students and practitioners who are radically defective in spelling, grammar, etymology, descriptive geography, arithmetic, and, I might add, book-keeping." (I myself, in the 1980s, have watched so many physicians at medical seminars spell *inflammation* with one *m*, or disarray the *m*'s and *r*'s in *hemorrhage*, that I conclude that spelling is probably not synonymous with scientific accomplishment.) Yet in Drake's judgment, "The ranks of the profession are in a great degree filled up with recruits, deficient either in abilities or acquirements . . . who thus doom it to a mediocrity."[26]

The traditional medical education in the United Kingdom was much superior, since it proceeded within the great teaching hospitals of London, Edinburgh, and Dublin, and students had to pass fairly rigorous exams. But even so, the standards, by comparison with what was to come later, were abysmal. Candidates were "hopeless specimens of dulness and danger," the London surgeon Walter Rivington wrote of the years before 1858 (when a considerable tightening up occurred). "Candidates there were who did not know that 'scabies' was the Latin for itch—who recommended immediate amputation for a wounded artery . . . candidates who, after four years' study, had not seen a case of strangulated hernia, or a case of retention of urine."[27]

Turning these young medical graduates loose upon patients

was like unleashing the pest upon them. J. Marion Sims returned in 1835 from Philadelphia, his freshly minted diploma in hand, to practice medicine in Lancaster, Alabama, where he had grown up. This twenty-two-year-old doctor now saw his first patient, "a child about eighteen months old, very much emaciated, who had what we would call the summer complaint, or chronic diarrhea." So the doctor went to work: he took out his lancet and "cut the gums down to the teeth." But then Sims didn't know what to do next, for "when it came to making up a prescription, I had no more idea of what ailed the child, or what to do for it, than if I had never studied medicine." Thus he hurried back to his office, took out "Eberle," a pediatrics textbook, and selected a prescription at random. "I do not remember whether it was a powder or a mixture. There was chalk in it." The infant failed to improve on this regimen, however.

Now Sims "turned to Eberle again, and to a new leaf. I gave the baby a prescription from the next chapter. Suffice it to say, that I changed leaves and prescriptions as often as once or twice a day. The baby continued to grow weaker."

So as he sat one night feeling the baby's pulse "and watching it carefully," an "old nurse" whom the family had engaged asked, "Doctor, don't you think that this baby is going to die?"

"No, madam, I do not think so, not at all," Sims replied. "Presently the child stopped breathing, and I thought it a case of syncope [fainting].... So I jerked the baby from the bed, and held its head down, and shook it, and blew into its mouth, and tried to bring it to."

Then the old nurse laid her hand on his shoulder and said, "No use shakin' that baby any more, doctor, for that baby's dead!"[28]

The reader will therefore not be surprised to encounter massive patient distrust of the traditional doctor.

THE TRADITIONAL DOCTOR SEES HIS PATIENTS

Until the 1920s in the United States, and perhaps a bit later in Britain, doctors saw most of their patients in house calls. We therefore shall understand little of the traditional doctor's life unless we recall that he was on the road constantly. Here are some entries for 1750 from the diary of Doctor Richard Kay, who had apprenticed with his father before going down to London to spend a year at Guy's Hospital. Dr. Kay lived in Baldingstone, a village in Lancashire.

7 June. He was at home in the morning, made house calls ("visits") in the afternoon, not returning home until 1:00 A.M., having been "detained on account of reducing a shoulder that has been dislocated a month of Robert Schofield's at Mill-hill in Hapton."

12 June. House calls in the afternoon.

13 June. House calls, then a "long visit" to some patient. "My return home this evening was very late."

14 June. Church (chapel). He apparently saw fellow church member Joseph Baron, who had "a pain in his right hip and belly" plus gout. The Baron children all had small-pox.

15 June. He and another Doctor Kay from Manchester went to see Mr. Joseph Pilkington in Bolton.

16 June. A number of house calls, but several omitted as well because "Brother Baron's illness, he having made no water for some days past, has prevented me."

On and on. Dr. Kay himself died the following year, at age thirty-five, of a "spotted fever," probably typhus.[29]

These entries are of interest from several viewpoints. One, Doctor Kay spent so much time on the road that he couldn't have seen very many patients, especially since he usually devoted mornings to his private affairs. Therefore, his practice could not have been very lucrative. Second, once Dr. Kay arrived at a patient's house, he evidently passed quite a bit of time there. Some of his patients, like the Baron family, he knew well indeed. I emphasize this because doctors of the 1920s and 1930s, whom we shall observe later, were not alone in devoting considerable time to each patient. It's just the manner in which they *inspired* their patients that differed.

Traditional doctors with urban practices were much busier than village doctors and for obvious reasons wasted less time to-ing and fro-ing. Thus Richard Arnold, a popular physician in antebellum Savannah, Georgia, would see thirty to forty private patients a day, "and to get through these, as you know," he wrote to his daughter in 1849, "I am going the round from sunrise to nine or ten o'clock at night. The frequent changes in our fevers render it necessary to see a patient oftener than in the diseases of the North. Hence it is frequently necessary to see a patient three or four times a day."[30] A doctor in Reading, England, calculated in 1842 that for his 1,349 patients, the average duration of each case was about three weeks.[31] Thus, whether in countryside or city, the traditional doctor saw his patients often and knew their lives well. Intimacy, as such, was not the creation of the modern doctor. It was the therapeutic use to which modern doctors would apply this age-old intimacy that counted.

How did a consultation proceed? Let's divide what a doctor does with a given patient into four stages: history taking, physical examination, making the diagnosis, and treatment. These traditional doctors were fair at history taking, spectacular at treatment (by their standards), poor in making a concrete diagnosis, and zero in physical examination.

HISTORY

In thinking that emphasized diet and "constitution" so much, it was possible to classify a patient as "bilious" or "choleric" solely on the basis of the history. For example, John Woodward, a distinguished fellow of the Royal College of Physicians, took notes on his patients that often followed the history back into childhood, paying meticulous attention to the location and intensity of the pain, so as to form an estimation of how relaxed were the fibers, or how irritable the nerves, depending on which system a particular doctor embraced. (Whatever theoretical system he may have subscribed to, in practice Woodward vomited and purged and bled like all the others, so the exact system made little real difference.) Here we have Mr. Edward Butlin, forty-three, whom Woodward saw in 1710 and 1711. "His parents were both healthy and strong till they had attained to old age." Butlin himself had had the measles and small pox "very young," then at age twelve a "violent pain in his head for about two hours." This is the level of detail these men thought essential, and Mr. Butlin's case, which we shall not go into, extended for three pages.[32]

PHYSICAL EXAMINATION

Indeed, doctors needed to take careful histories, because that was all they had to go on, given their almost complete lack of interest in physical exam or in "lab findings" (aside from the color of the urine or the nature of the crust on coagulated blood). The curse that clung to traditional medicine was its indifference to the physicality of the human body. Many doctors felt themselves perfectly able to make a diagnosis without seeing the patient at all.

When the Scottish physician and novelist Tobias Smollett traveled in France in 1763, he stopped at Montpellier to consult the celebrated Professor Antoine Fizes about his health. Smollett dispatched a long account of his symptoms, written in Latin, via his *valet de place* to Fizes's home, along with a gold *louis* (coin): "The patient's age is forty-three; his constitution moist, gross, abounding with phlegm, and very subject to rheums ...," et cetera. Appetite, skin, and nature of the expectorant (Smollett apparently had tuberculosis) were described in minute detail. He expected Fizes to make a diagnosis. Smollett tells us, "The professor's eyes sparkled at the sight of the fee; and he desired the servant to call next morning for his opinion of the case. ..." The professor wrote a long-winded reply, the gist of which was that Smollett probably had TB. Elaborate medications and a special diet were prescribed. Smollett was furious (1) that Fizes had responded in French rather than Latin, and (2) that Fizes's "remedies savour strongly of the old woman" (thus quackery). "I observe that physicians in this country," he noted of France, "pay no regard to the state of the solids in chronical disorders; that exercise and the cold bath are never prescribed. ..." Indeed, Smollett was to become steadily more enraged as he continued his famous progress across France, but the point here is that *it occurred to neither man that a physical examination would be of value.*[33]

When a physical examination actually occurred, it would be

limited to the pulse and the tongue. One can, in fact, learn several interesting things from the condition of the tongue, such as whether the patient is anemic (pale tongue) or dehydrated (furrowing); the tongue is dry and brown in the later stage of any acute illness, and this is useful information. But doctors also attached great significance to whether the tongue was furred or "black and hairy," neither of which means much of anything. However, to patients all these symptoms were of great significance, and they expected their doctors routinely to examine the tongue.

Similarly, one may learn from the pulse: by pressing their fingers against the radial artery at the wrist, doctors could measure the pulse rate (fast in infections). Was it "full" (high blood pressure)? Was it weak (shock or progressive decline of circulation to the arms and legs)? Did it collapse suddenly after a full pulse (a history of rheumatic heart disease, perhaps, with a damaged aortic valve)? Indeed, the cardiologist can derive all kinds of information from the arterial and venous pulses, but because there was little progress in cardiology until the midnineteenth century these traditional doctors were able to determine little more than whether the patient had an acute infection or was experiencing heart failure or shock.

That was the extent of the physical exam: no palpation of the abdomen, no careful inspection of the veins in the neck, no checking of the cranial nerves, no listening to the body's sounds, no rectal or vaginal exams. Arthur Hertzler described a previous generation of old-time doctors making a house call. "The usual procedure for a doctor when he reached the patient's house was to greet the grandmother and aunts effusively and pat all the kids on the head before approaching the bedside. He greeted the patient with a grave look and a pleasant joke. He felt the pulse and inspected the tongue, and asked where it hurt. This done, he was ready to deliver an opinion and prescribe his pet remedy."[34] Even in 1885, when bedside medicine was in full transformation, the Baltimore physician Daniel Cathell rather cynically counseled his readers to keep the exam short. "The laity expect you to examine your patient at every visit. Never neglect the following five cardinal duties: to feel the pulse, to examine the tongue, to inquire about the appetite, the sleep and the bowels. No difference what your case is, be sure to attend to these ... at every visit."[35]

Nor was there anything especially private about the examination. "Most of the doctors of that day," recalled Hertzler of his Kansas boyhood, "had drugstores and wore whiskers and examined patients as they were seated beside the counter in view of other customers, and loafers. That is to say, the patients' tongues were looked at, and the more thorough, if they had a watch, counted their pulses; then medicines were handed out from the stock on the shelves." Hertzler's father had taken him to such a doctor-druggist "when I had repeated attacks of severe pains in my back which radiated to my groin. . . . After the doctor heard the story he stroked his long gray beard, looked at me for a moment over his glasses and, turning to my father, delivered himself of the following: 'Dan, he yust grow too fast.' " In fact, Hertzler had a kidney stone, which he passed several months later.[36]

DIAGNOSIS

The physical exam complete, the doctor could now make a diagnosis. This was relatively uncomplicated, as the diagnosis was simply the name of the main symptom, modified by whatever other symptoms the patient had. Thus if the patient had a hot, flushed face, racing pulse, and furrowed tongue, the diagnosis would be "fever," and if jaundice (yellowed skin and yellowed whites of eyes) was present as well, "bilious fever." If the fever were accompanied by diarrhea, "malignant fever." Or if the fever spiked every third day (as for example in malaria), "tertian fever"; every fourth day, "quartan fever."[37] You see how simple it was. Of course one could debate endlessly about how some particular symptom was to be classified: did red sores on the tongue mean an "adynamic" or a "putrid inflammatory fever"? The impact on medicine of those endless classifications of symptoms as separate diseases is felt even today: in *Dorland's Illustrated Medical Dictionary*, 1981 edition, *fever* covers four pages, over three hundred separate kinds and synonyms being mentioned.[38]

It need only be added that most of these traditional "symptomatic" diagnoses were useless. They gave no clue as to the underlying process producing the symptoms. (Most fevers, for example, are the result of infection, and only in the 1880s was the "germ theory" of disease elaborated.) They gave little indication of "prognosis," for the patient might as easily recover as not. And the diagnoses gave few guidelines for "rational," specific therapy, because the therapy for all fevers, as indeed for most diseases, was virtually the same.

TREATMENT

It was in therapy that traditional medicine showed its most dismal face. Treatment was oriented toward evacuation, and there were two ways of getting those evacuations going: "surgical," opening a vein with a lancet and letting a pint of blood drain out, and "medical," giving purgatives, diuretics, and potions to make one defecate, sweat, and salivate.

What main drugs did the doctor have in his bag? Many fit the notion of some kind of all-purpose tonic that patients called simply "a dose of medicine." For example, surgeon-apothecary Richard Smith of Bristol dispensed large amounts of "powders" to the patients he saw at the Royal Infirmary in the 1790s. "The powders," he writes, "were chiefly rhubarb [a purgative] and prepared chalk with two or three grains of pulvis antimonalis [an emetic].... To grandees, or where a costly charge might be made, a drop or two of cinnamon oil was added and rubbed up and then the packet was six or seven shillings [instead of four]."[39] The outpatient department of St. Bartholomew's Hospital in London, which saw approximately 190,000 patients a year, giving each an average of a minute and a quarter, dispensed the standard tonic out of "a big brown jug" for all complaints. It consisted "essentially of purgatives, a mixture of iron, sulphate of magnesia and quassia [a bitter-tasting medicine to combat worms], and cod-liver oil...."[40]

Both doctors and patients had an abiding confidence in alcohol against respiratory conditions and other diseases, so it would be the main ingredient in commercial preparations like "Lydia Pinkham's Compound." In 1866 Bellevue Hospital in New York City made enormous purchases of it, "including 1637 gallons best whiskey, 161 gallons common whiskey, 40 gallons brandy, 260 sherry, 68 port, 20 gin, 134 barrels of ale, 85 cases tarragona wine."[41] Joseph Mathews, a Kentucky doctor who had learned his medicine in the 1860s, listed the essentials a doctor should have with him at all times:[42]

- *Calomel (mercurous chloride), for purging, and so on, as described previously.*
- *Quinine, for fever, discussed further on page 95.*
- *Buchu, the dried leaves of the* Barosma *genus of plants, which irritates kidneys (and is thus "diuretic") and has the "diaphoretic" effect of causing sweating.*
- *Ipecac, large doses of which cause vomiting.*
- *"Dover's powder," a mixture of ipecac and opium, used among other things to "forestall" colds, on the grounds that a "chill" may produce "congestion" of internal organs, which in turn could lead to inflammation, colds, pneumonia, and so on. Small doses of ipecac were supposed to stimulate secretion in the airways, thus relieving the "excess dryness" associated with airway infections.*

The therapeutic virtues attributed to all these drugs were, except for quinine imaginary. We now know that you make people worse, not better, by causing them to urinate, defecate, and sweat. This entire logic of treating colds, although still widely believed today, is completely erroneous. (And opium "cured" nothing except diarrhea, while addicting hundreds of thousands of people.)

It is astonishing to run one's eye over the traditional pharmacopoeia and note what a small possibility it offered of "curing" anything. For one thing, perhaps a third of the drugs it contained were inactive, having not even a physiological effect on the body.[43] One opens the 1834 *Pharmacopoeia* of the London Royal College of Physicians to "Infusions." It contains pages of instructions: infusion of chamomile, infusion of horseradish, infusion of orange peel, infusion of cloves, infusion of cascarilla, infusion of cinchona (used not for malaria but for indigestion, the ancestor of "quinine water," as in gin-and-tonic), infusion of gentian, infusion of linseed, and so on.[44] Some of these would have been nasty, some pleasant-tasting; some would have produced powerful bowel movements; some would have done nothing. *None* is used medically today, and not because we have somehow forgotten about our rich "herbal heritage." The traditional pharmacopoeia passed away because (with a couple of exceptions to be mentioned in Chapter 4) its contents didn't work. It was rejected toward the end of the nineteenth century. Oliver Wendell Holmes wrote in 1860, precisely of the kinds of drugs found in the London *Pharmacopoeia*, "I firmly believe that if the whole materia medica, *as now used,* could be sunk to the bottom of the sea, it would be all the better for mankind,—and all the worse for the fishes." The best proof of the fact that the community is "overdosed," he said, "is that no families take so little medicine as those of doctors, except those of apothecaries. . . ."[45]

Here a somewhat unpleasant note must be struck. I have no wish to join that whole school that attacks doctors by attributing to them sinister, mercenary motives. But it is clear that what kept many physicians afloat before 1900 was the drugs they compounded and dispensed themselves. One scholar writes of England that the GP was a "general practitioner in medicine, surgery, midwifery, and pharmacy, but in the first half of the nineteenth century the practice of pharmacy was, for the large majority, their main source of income."[46] If they didn't dispense medicines, they wouldn't make any money. Thomas Shastid, an apprentice to his own doctor father in Pittsfield, Illinois, in the 1870s, remembers patients saying, "I been to Wrexham and bought medicine off of him [a doctor-druggist] fer my wife, an' it ain't done 'er no good. I been to Casal and bought medicine off of *him* and it ain't done no good. An' then I been to Dublin, that high an' mighty feller, an' he sold me some pills all done up in silver leaf and gold packages, an' *they* ain't done 'er no good. Now I'm goin' to buy some medicine off of your pappy. . . ." The truth was, as Shastid observed, "Large numbers of doctors *were in fact* druggists, or, to put it more properly perhaps, large numbers of druggists had medical licenses and, so, quite incidentally, were doctors."[47]

The second kind of treatment would be "surgical," which in those preanesthetic, pre-germ-theory days meant little more than the "dressing of minor injuries, sores, and ulcers, opening abscesses, extracting teeth, and occasionally setting fractures and reducing dislocations." Arthur Hertzler remembers his predecessors on the Great Plains as able to cure little more than malaria and "the itch" and "to set bones, sew up cuts and open boils on small boys."[48] There was one more surgical procedure they were able to do: open up a vein with a lancet and let the blood run out, and as far as the doctors of the time were concerned, this was perhaps their most efficacious remedy.

In September 1840, Dr. Sims, who was eking out a living in Mount Meigs, Alabama, fell sick with what seems to have been malaria, feeling after his rounds "a little shiver run down my back. I made my way to the overseer's house [he had been treating plantation slaves], and soon I had a heavier chill, and half an hour later a raging fever with delirium." The next day Dr. Lucas went to see him. "Looking around, [Lucas] saw a little mulatto girl, Anarcha, in the room, and he said, 'Bring me a string, and a little cotton, and a bowl; I am going to draw a little blood from the doctor.' "

Sims said, "My dear, good doctor, you are not going to bleed me, are you?"

The doctor said, "Yes, sir, old fellow, I'm going to bleed you." Sims pleaded with him not to.

"Well," Doctor Lucas replied, "that is just as you please; but you ought to be bled. I had an idea that you were a d———d contrary fellow, and now I know it."

Sims concludes, "If I had been bled I should never have got well nor been here to tell you this story."[49]

These doctors bled for everything: typhoid, malaria, yellow fever, tuberculosis. In Mount Meigs, when Miss Ashurst, "a very beautiful woman in the last stages of consumption," was approaching the end, she once again called Dr. Childers to her. She was by this time "nothing but a skeleton, and certainly had but a few days to live." But Dr. Childers believed in bleeding patients when *any* signs of fever were present: "Miss Ashurst, I believe, as you have a good deal of fever, I will have to draw a little blood from you." He said this, Sims tells us, "in the sweetest, mildest, most gentlemanly tones possible. So he took from his pocket a cord, and drew it over the little skeleton arm above the elbow. Presently the blood came trickling down from the elbow, and, when a tablespoonful had run, the poor little woman fainted and fell over."

"Ah," said Dr. Childers, "that is just what I wanted. Now she will be better." She died soon thereafter. Sims concludes, "The practice at that time was heroic; it was murderous."[50]

A CASE IN POINT: CONGESTIVE HEART FAILURE

Most people today don't die of yellow fever or TB. So let's take a disease they *do* die of, and see how traditional doctors went about treating it. In conditions such as high blood pressure, coronary artery disease, or advanced syphilis, the ability of the heart to supply the body with blood (or indeed to supply itself with blood) is threatened. At first it simply pumps more powerfully, but then it must find other mechanisms of getting out the blood. So the heart beats faster or grows larger. Finally the heart runs out of new ways to keep up the output of blood.

At this point "heart failure" begins. Blood starts to back up in the venous circulation because the heart is faltering in pumping it onward. The individual's consciousness starts to diminish as less blood reaches the brain; the kidneys liberate a substance that further increases arterial resistance to the tired heart. Also, the kidneys stop making urine, thus increasing the amount of fluid the heart must pump.

The patient goes into a downward spiral. Finally the backup of blood on the venous side becomes so bad that venous blood starts oozing from the capillaries of the lung into the spaces where oxygen and carbon dioxide are exchanged. The patient, who has started out short of breath, is now coughing. A pink foam begins to appear in the mouth because the lungs have become so congested with blood. No more oxygen comes in, and the patient dies. Before the rise of modern medicine this would have been considered "lung failure," and not the failure of the heart, which has congested the lungs (hence the phrase "congestive heart failure").

Before 1900, what the heart was doing was often a great mystery to doctors. In the 1840s, how puzzled was Dr. Worthington Hooker, of Norwich, Connecticut, at a patient's heart attack. "A gentleman, while quietly sitting in his counting-room, was attacked as suddenly as if it were from a blow with a great sense of oppression in the region of the heart, almost arresting the action of this organ and at once prostrating his strength. . . ." He concluded that "it is sometimes impossible to detect the immediate cause of an attack of sickness. . . ."[51]

In the late 1880s when Dr. William Macartney was a surgical intern at New York's Bellevue Hospital, the elevator was so slow that he would "commonly run up the nine flights without stopping." One morning Professor John Gouley stopped him as he was running up the stairs.

"Don't do that, doctor," said Gouley.

"Do what?"

"Run up stairs like that," answered Gouley. "You will ruin your heart. You will not live three years if you continue doing it."

Macartney laughed and "slowed down until he was out of sight."[52]

Professor Gouley's confusion about what was good and bad for the heart was common in his day. The mechanism of heart failure in particular was poorly understood, and doctors called it "dropsy" or "hydrops" (which mean the same thing). Dropsy is indeed one of the symptoms of chronic heart failure: As the blood backs up, blood serum starts to exudate from the vessels and to accumulate in the tissues. The legs and wrists become swollen (edema) and a little "pit," or depression, is left when, for example, you poke your finger against the shin bone. The abdomen starts to swell out (ascites) as water accumulates there. The appearance of dropsy, therefore, is a sign that the heart is slowly failing. (Liver and kidney failures may cause dropsy, too.)

Given the universality of conditions such as hardening of the arteries and high blood pressure, and the high incidence of syphilis in those days, congestive heart failure was often seen. "There is no disease," said Edinburgh professor of medicine Francis Home in 1780, "which affords hospitals more numerous patients than the different species of hydrops, and none of which fewer are cured." A patient of Home's named John Farquhar, age sixty, had first consulted Howe at the beginning of January with "a pain in the region of the liver, especially on being pressed. His belly began to swell about the middle of the month." In February his legs started to swell up and now, on 4 March, "he can scarcely lie horizontally in bed, and starts, for fear of suffocation, when going to sleep." Mr. Farquhar, moreover, was short of breath, had a dry cough, and was putting out "urine of deep colour, diminished in quantity." Pulse was 110 (normal would be 60–70).

Mr. Farquhar was in heart failure. He started gasping for breath when he lay down because blood that otherwise would have pooled in his legs was now added to the burden his heart had to pump. His kidneys were shutting down, hence his dark, scanty urine. And the blood on the venous side was damming up in his lungs, causing his cough, weariness, and fear of suffocation.

How did Dr. Home treat Mr. Farquhar? He applied the same remedies used for everything else in traditional medicine and so gave cream of tartar as a purgative. The man's urine increased briefly, probably because the cream of tartar was irritating his kidneys, and he died four days later, the cavities of his lungs and abdomen full of "lymph."[53]

Thus the medical profession of Home's day had no inkling that failure of the heart was involved in dropsy and chose spectacularly inappropriate means of treating it. When Dr. Richard Brookes, an early-eighteenth-century textbook writer who practiced in London, saw dropsy patients, he treated them as follows:

- First, he gave purgatives, an ounce of "syrup of buckthorn will be sufficient." Or try elaterium, derived from the juice of the squirting cucumber. But attention: "all cathartics [laxatives] that work slowly are rather hurtful than beneficial; therefore a purge had better be too strong than too weak." Get those poisons out of there.
- Second, if you're dealing with a patient "of a weak constitution, or women subject to vapours," give a diuretic, something like squills or mercury. Now this does make sense, especially squills, which are the fleshy bulb of the sea onion plant; squill had been used on and off since antiquity for dropsy. It does have an action upon the heart, similar to digitalis, but the doctors of the day used it in such weak doses that its salutary effects were lost from view.
- Finally, after purging, give wines and "steel" (iron in some form).[54]

No wonder the heart failure patients of the day slid so inevitably to their end; they were purged and diuresed to get that fluid off, but nothing was done for their hearts.

Then in 1785 William Withering published his famous book about use of the foxglove plant, from which the drug digitalis is derived (digoxin is its active ingredient), in treating dropsy. One would think this might have revolutionized medicine, for digitalis strengthened the heart, thus slowing its rate and making it possible for the kidneys to begin dumping water. But digitalis enjoyed a vogue of only a few years, peaking around 1800. Thereafter it fell into disuse because doctors became so excited about its success that they tried applying it to everything imaginable, for example, tuberculosis, and when it failed with these other diseases they gradually forgot about it.[55] It was only much later that digitalis would be rediscovered, when enough knowledge had been accumulated of how the heart worked for it to be used rationally. In the meantime, doctors would remain meddlers.

THE DOCTOR NOT YET A GENTLEMAN

It will not surprise us that society did not reward these meddlers with great social prestige. Being largely uneducated, hopelessly overnumerous, and saddled with an almost maniacally perverse therapeutic philosophy, most doctors were not, in fact, the gentlemen that Daniel Drake had hoped.[56]

For one thing, they made little money. Here is an 1806 fee schedule for doctors in Portsmouth, New Hampshire:[57]

- *Visit in ordinary cases with advice, recipe or one dose of medicine*   *$0.75*
- *Visit and bleeding at the patient's house*   *1.00*
- *Visit and amputating toes and fingers ...*   *2.00*
- *Amputating, trepanning ... and amputating cancerous breast*   *30.00*

Still, a dollar for a house call isn't bad. A poor man might work a day for a dollar. One problem was that a lot of the fees were never collected: the patient wouldn't pay. Doctors were not usually wealthy men, said Worthington Hooker, partly because patients "feel a less urgent obligation to pay than they do to pay others. I know not any other reason for this than the *intangibility* of the favor which is bestowed by the physician."[58] Richard Arnold of Savannah wrote to his wife in 1839, "It runs me almost crazy to think that with hundreds and hundreds due me professionally I find the greatest difficulty in raising a simple fifty dollars." He hoped that as he grew older he would not "be constantly in want of a twenty dollar bill. . . ."[59]

With the fierce competition for patients that existed at that time, with time wasted in house calls, and with uncollected bills, the doctor's fees would not add up to much in the way of wealth. Charles Rosenberg estimates that a doctor beginning practice in New York City in the 1860s could expect to make about four hundred dollars a year, "adequate but not munificent salaries."[60]

We shall shortly see the doctors' fortunes changing dramatically. But although they began to become pillars of the community, able to "make their visits with gloved hands in stylish carriages," few family doctors ever became wealthy men. "Every physician knows that it is almost impossible to get rich by the practice of medicine, unless it is through a money-making specialty," said Daniel Cathell in 1882. "The truth is, when a doctor dies, his family is usually left poor and helpless, unless he has acquired money otherwise than by practice."[61]

Early doctors fell short of gentlemanly status, but I don't want to make them out as rowdies or ruffians. Nevertheless, clearly something of the boor clung to these undereducated American practitioners from the very beginning. Boston's William Douglass, himself an "M.D." and full of airs over it in addressing his British audience, said in 1755, "In our plantations a practitioner, bold, rash, impudent, a liar, basely born and educated, has much the advantage of an honest, cautious, modest gentleman."[62] Nor do I want to suggest that the typical doctor somehow brawled and battled his way about town; however, as doctors got together, the stories they would chuckle at tended to be of exactly this kind of rowdiness. Here is more on Dr. Dictionary, whom we have already met.

> Because of his incessant bragging he was ofttimes referred to as "Bugle."

One day, as he entered the room wherein the "County Medical" was meeting, one of the younger doctors, who was looking through a window as if at something in the street, blared out—
"Blow, bugle, blow:
Set the wild echoes flying;
Blow, bugle; answer echoes,
Dying, dying, dying."
Dr. Dictionary . . . walked up behind the young doctor, pulled him out of the chair by his ears, dragged him to the top of the stairway and kicked him to the bottom.[63]

Just imagine. In the 1950s that kind of behavior would have produced headlines in the local paper; there would have been lawsuits, people expelled from the Medical Society. The profession would have been horrified.

A couple of doctors in Burlington, Vermont, named Knox and Dixon, were noted as big, burly men, not at all averse to a mixup. Once when the two were "playing billiards in the old American Hotel"—this must have been in the 1850s or 1860s—

a fellow came into the room, just drunk enough to be disagreeable, and began shouting and dancing about, getting in the players' way, bumping against them, and making a general nuisance of himself. Knox finally said, "Dixon, what are we going to do with this fellow? I can't put up with him any longer."

Dixon was over on the other side of the table, near the window. "Hand him over here," he said.

Knox tossed the obnoxious gentleman over the table and Dixon caught him on the fly and threw him through the window. The room was on the ground floor.[64]

Daniel Cathell, in his widely read advice manual, would later counsel doctors against permitting themselves even the hint of this kind of behavior. Not only should you not throw people through windows; you shouldn't even hang out in pool parlors: "Do not let your office be a lounging place or a smoking room for horse-jockeys, dog-fanciers, gamesters, swaggerers, politicians, coxcombs, and others whose time hangs heavily on their hands. The public looks upon physicians as being singled out and set apart. . . ." He instructs them, "Do not squirt tobacco-juice around you at your visits, or have your breath reeking with its fumes, or with those of cloves, cardamom, alcohol, dead beer. . . . Appearing in your shirt sleeves, wearing rough creaking boots . . . chewing, smoking, skylarking, etc., will show weakness, diminish your halo. . . ."[65] Apparently, this is the way doctors had been carrying on.

As a result, traditional doctors enjoyed rather little respect. Of course one can find individual exceptions, but the overwhelming public view was that of Marion Sims's father, upon hearing that his son was going to study medicine. Young Sims said, "Father, I know that I have been a great disappointment to you. I knew from the outset that you wanted me to be a lawyer. It is impossible for me to be a lawyer. I have neither the talent nor the gifts necessary for the profession." Then he told his father what he was going to do.

The father responded, "My son, I confess that I am disappointed in you, and if I had known this I certainly should not have sent you to college."

Sims replied, "I did not want to go. . . . But if I must study a profession, there is nothing left for me to do but medicine."

The father: "Well, I suppose that I cannot control you; but it is a profession for which I have the utmost contempt. There is no science in it. There is no honor to be achieved in it; no reputation to be made, and to think that *my* son should be going around from house to house . . . with a box of pills in one hand and a squirt in the other . . . is a thought that I never supposed I should have to contemplate."[66]

That is the point of departure for the doctors.

CHAPTER THREE
The Traditional Patient

NOW LET'S turn to the patient. Much of what follows—attachment to magic, terrible drugs, shrugging off of symptoms that would send us bolting for the emergency room—will not be comprehensible unless we remember how often death once appeared in the midst of life. If you were born a male in Massachusetts in 1850, you would have had a life expectancy at birth of thirty-eight years. The figure is so low because it includes infant mortality, in an era when one child in eight would not survive to the age of one. But even if you made it to age twenty, you'd still live only to about sixty.[1]

Sixty is not bad. What is distinctive about death before the end of the nineteenth century is the randomness with which one could be carried away at any age, just as one was founding a family, let us say, or thinking about the prospect of a grandchild. Today the occurrence of death is far less random. At age twenty we know there's an excellent chance we'll see seventy. Almost certainly we'll make it to forty or fifty. Our own times of mortality cluster in old age.

In Adams County, Mississippi, including Natchez, around 1850 there was no clustering in old age: death could strike at any time of life. In November 1849, Clark Raymond, age twenty, was carried away by a "bilious fever." Martha Goodall, twenty-seven, died of "debility." H. Hamerton, who had come to the Mississippi delta from England, died in November, single and "suddenly" at the age of thirty-five. The "fevers," "consumptions" (most of which were probably TB), "intestinal inflammations," and "debilities" of which 117 adults in Adams County died in 1849 and 1850 were typical of the pattern of death all over Atlantic civilization in the pre-1870 period.

Cholera, a common killer at that time around Natchez, had not been known in America or Europe before the nineteenth century. Lung tuberculosis was probably the most common cause of death everywhere, not just in Adams County. That and stomach cancer have been the major wasting diseases historically in most places. Number two, in Adams County and generally, were the acute fevers, whose courses would all be short. Mississippi was full of them. William Smith of New York came to the Delta to die at twenty-five of "fever"; likewise William Rice, dead at twenty-seven of "typhus fever." Then follows a long list of what are basically terminal symptoms: jaundice (including acute sepsis, liver disease, or obstruction of the bile duct), convulsions, apoplexy (stroke), and dysentery (bloody diarrhea). Finally, there are the freak accidents: in Adams County the Irishman Michael Kelly, dead at an unknown age of murder; the black slave Stephen, age nineteen, owned by R. W. Phillips, dead in March 1850 of "inguinal hernia," meaning that a piece of bowel had become caught in an opening in the wall of the abdomen, cutting off the blood supply of that part of the intestine and killing the young man of "peritonitis." One gets a sense that death could strike at any age.[2]

What was true of causes of death in Adams County prevailed generally. Forty percent of the adult male deaths in seventeenth-century London were from tuberculosis of the lung, 27 percent from "fever," 12 percent from "dropsy," and so on.[3] Two quite different patterns of illness thus appear for adults: long sieges in which the patient finally gives up after months of pain and struggle, the gynecological cancers, stomach cancer, and tuberculosis being the classic examples; and brief, acute attacks of infection, by viruses in the liver and bacteria in the belly and central nervous system (thus yellow fever, dysentery, meningitis). The pattern for infants is quite different but does not now concern us, because traditionally so few sick infants were ever taken to a doctor.

THE SYMPTOM PYRAMID

All the symptoms that a person feels can be thought of as adding up to a kind of pyramid. The grave symptoms, few in number, are at the top, the minor symptoms such as colds, coughs, and itches at the bottom. Figure 3-1 suggests the obvious: patients don't run to the doctor for every symptom they have. The percentage of their symptoms that they define as disease and refer to a doctor for treatment can be indicated as a level on the pyramid. The argument of this book will be that traditional patients sought treatment or took time off for relatively few of their symptoms: only the most alarming ones, such as coughing up blood or abdominal edema, or only the most disabling ones, such as broken bones or immobile joints. A major part of the patients' story will be the expansion of the symptom pyramid to include lesser and lesser complaints, as time goes on.

FIGURE 3-1. *The Traditional Symptom Pyramid.*

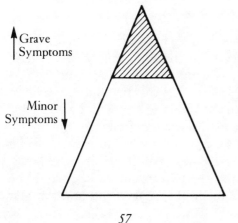

Grave Symptoms

Minor Symptoms

The entire pyramid represents all the symptoms an individual perceives.

The cross-hatched area represents the symptoms an individual defines as "illness" for which he or she seeks help or rests.

What evidence suggests that traditional patients sought help only for major symptoms? The diaries that the doctors themselves leave behind contain few patient complaints of "feeling a bit numb in the foot" or "pain in the stomach." Let's take the patients Dr. Richard Kay, of Baldingstone in Lancashire, saw on 13 August 1746:

- *A young woman sick for five days with a bad fever who, the night before, "went out of door and rambled in the fields insensibly, lying down in a field, and, the night air abating her fever, she became sensible of the dangerous situation and went home." So Kay bled her.*
- *A previous female patient "seized very bad in her belly who has had a dangerous fever and been very much threatened from the violence of her pain at first, with a mortification of her bowels. . . ." She had lost a lot of blood and "matter" in her urine and stool.*
- *"A young man beginning a fever."*
- *"A girl with a strumous disorder under her chin"* (swollen thyroid, TB of the lymph glands?).
- *"An ancient woman with a bad pain in her hip."*
- *"A young wife near her time of delivery and under some discouragement lest she should not do well."*
- *"A brother and sister both consumptive."*
- *"A woman with a sore leg."*
- *"A young woman with a very sore stinking leg."*
- *"A man with a strumous disorder in his arm"* (a *"struma"* was a swelling).

Kay noted, after his fourteen-mile ride had ended on that 13 August, "These particulars have been the occurrences of the day, and to mention which every day would be abundantly too tedious and prolix."[4] Of these eleven patients, a third would today be in the hospital: the woman with the stinking leg, who had a major bacterial infection; the woman disoriented from her high temperature; the woman with a raging systemic infection, losing blood *both* in her urine and her bowel. Another third, the possible case of thyroid disorder and the two consumptives, would be the object of very aggressive medical management; and the rest would certainly be urged by friends and loved ones to seek medical treatment: the old woman with the bad pain in her hip, and so on.

Dr. James Clegg, who practiced in the Peak district of Derbyshire around the same time, had a somewhat less active practice and kept less thorough notes, but he was not being called out for headaches. Ann Gee's case is typical:

24 January 1742. Slept not very well in the night, got up pretty early, but was soon called out to Ann Gee of Lydiat. I ordered her a clyster [enema]. . . .

26 January. I was called to visit Ann Gee, found her better and more easy. I take her disorder to be the gout in the stomach and entrails and am afraid of the iliac passion. . . . (The days pass. He mentions other patients, like Mr. Kirk's son, "who is under the common disorder and is very feverish.")

On 1 February, two days after the death of Clegg's own wife, Ann Gee died as well. Her "gout in the stomach" was thus a terminal symptom, perhaps of stomach cancer. But that January visit had been the *first time* he'd seen her, so clearly Ann Gee had cared otherwise for her symptoms up to then.[5]

Thus far, most of the patients on whom the doctors report have been quite ill. How about patients reporting on themselves? At what point did individuals decide that their own symptoms justified medical attention? That point was quite high. Let's look at the illnesses of Reverend James Woodforde, forty-nine, a country parson in the Norfolk village of Weston, starting in the late winter of 1789, a period chosen from his diary as typical of his middle years. He had actually been quite well in the preceding weeks and months, reporting mainly on what he ate for dinner and the friends he saw. But then on 25 November he was "exceeding ill all the day long" and ate "nothing but some pea soup and a small bit of pheasant." (The Woodforde family dined well.) That night he was "very bad indeed . . . my stomach quite sore by coughing and profuse sweats and when in one of those sweats was obliged to jump out of bed to stand on the stone-hearth, being so violently attacked with the cramp, twice so." Thus the next day he could scarcely try anything save "a small bit of roasted neck of mutton" and vomited that at once. He gave himself an emetic.

Two days later, on Friday, 27 November, Parson Woodforde sought help, not from the doctor but from his brother, who "recommended to me last night to carry a small piece of the roll brimstone [sulfur] sewed up in a piece of very thin linen to bed with me, and if I felt any symptom of the cramp to hold it in my hand or put it near the affected part." That the parson then did and felt that the sulfur forestalled a leg cramp. Parson Woodforde's stomach complaint then turned into a cough, and after ups and downs he thanked God in his diary on 7 December for "a tolerable good night." A week later he was still "rather low the whole day long" and on 13 January 1790 had another bout of stomach pain, "which I apprehended proceeded from gouty wind there likewise from bile." He was ill the whole day with vomiting and took a mixture of rhubarb and ginger as a laxative. This cycle of gastrointestinal complaints wavered on until 6 April 1790, when Parson Woodforde acquired a new problem, gout, his first attack, and one that would plague him steadily over the coming years.

The months passed. There were various other laments: "a pain in my right under jaw owing to a loose tooth," in November 1790; an inflammation of his right eyelid in March 1791, which he treated by rubbing the tail of a black cat on it, and for which, a week later, he consulted one of the local doctors, a Mr. Thorne. This was the first time Parson Woodforde had called a doctor since we began following his story two years previously. Mr. Thorne recommended he wash his eye with cold water.

Consider the succession of Parson Woodforde's complaints: vomiting with spasms that left him weak; weeks passed feeling "low," "indifferent," punctuated by wakeful nights; the quite sharp gouty pains in his big toe, and so forth. For none of these symptoms did he deem medical aid necessary: He treated himself with laxatives and tried magical home remedies such as rubbing himself with the parts of dead animals.[6] We have dwelled at

length upon Parson Woodforde because he was a perfect proto-
type of the traditional patient. Only for the most exasperating
discomfort did he call a doctor.

Were traditional patients less sensitive to pain and discomfort
than we are, or just more stoical about them? This is a difficult
question, because the degree of pain one feels is subject to all
kinds of mental censorship, including the level of pain the surrounding culture deems bearable. I am astonished at what some
of these people were able to endure. Joseph Mathews told the
story of the young doctor pulling his first tooth, possibly taken
from his own Kentucky practice which started in the 1870s. "Mr.
Planter," a wealthy farmer, appeared at the doctor's late at night
and wanted a tooth pulled. Doctor and patient went off to the office; he put "the victim" into a high-backed chair, standing on a
couple of boxes piled behind it. "You ask the gentleman to open
his mouth and to place his finger upon the aching tooth. This he
does and you find it to be the last 'molar' on the upper jaw."
Doctor Mathews then described how tough it was to pull the
tooth, all the wrenching and tugging and sweating and "inward"
cussing. "Great beads of perspiration stand out on your forehead,
you hold your breath and pull with the power of Hercules. . . ."
The tooth didn't budge. He spit on his hand(!) and renewed the
attack. Finally the tooth came out. The farmer rinsed his mouth,
and the doctor discovered that he'd pulled the wrong tooth. He
said nothing; the farmer paid him fifty cents and walked out into
the night. The point is not how hideously incompetent the young
doctor was, but how stoically throughout Mr. Planter endured
the pain: a healthy tooth yanked out by a young maniac and the
farmer didn't cry out and walked home.[7] My God. Did those
people feel the pain as much as we do?

We won't be able to resolve this issue. Traditional people may
have felt various symptoms as acutely as we do, or perhaps they
did not. The question is, once they felt a symptom, how willing
were they to define it as a disease and call the doctor or take bed
rest for it? Not very willing. As I shall demonstrate, medicine
was held in such low esteem that traditional patients preferred to
dose themselves or to seek out an "alternative" healer. Only after
their own remedies and the drugs of the alternative healer had

failed would they consult a doctor, because it was he who had the "truly powerful" drugs.

PATIENTS TREAT THEMSELVES

Traditional patients loved home remedies, prepared from local plants, in the same way that postmodern patients adore the patent medicines for colds and coughs that fill the drugstores. The home-made teas and the postmodern antihistamines and "orthomolecular vitamin therapies" are equally useless. They acquire a following only because most of the minor diseases that plague us are *self-limiting*, which is to say that they get better on their own without treatment. We understand today why this is so: invading microorganisms excite the body's immune response; antibodies are formed to counter the foreign antigens, and ultimately the body's natural defenses carry the day: the "cold" goes away, whether you take antihistamines or not.

This naturally self-limiting nature of disease has long been recognized. Oliver Wendell Holmes said in 1871, "In the natural course of things some thousands of persons must be getting well or better of slight attacks of colds, of rheumatic pains, every week in this city [Boston] alone. Hundreds of them do something or other in the way of remedy . . . and the last thing they do gets the credit of the recovery. Think what a crop of remedies this must furnish, if it were all harvested!"[8] Holmes, with the physician's contempt for lay remedies, saw people as just stumbling blindly from one product to the next until the *vis medicatrix naturae* (the healing power of nature) finally made them get better spontaneously.

But in fact the traditional patients had their own theories about the way the body works and treated themselves in what they considered rational terms on the basis of these theories. In the popular mind, two kinds of medical problems existed: those requiring drastic, immediate evacuation of the "poisons" and those requiring "tonic" restoration of the body's forces. Each drew upon quite different remedies.

In an era when iron-deficiency anemia and undernutrition

were common, it was not difficult for people to acquire the notion they were somehow "run down," and to seek tonics that would restore them. "Almost everyone is filled with the belief that he is debilitated," wrote Daniel Cathell in 1882 of his Baltimore patients. "Say to the average patient, 'you are weak and need building up,' and you will instantly see by his countenance that you have struck *his* key-note. So much is this the case, that many of the sick, fully impressed with this idea, will want you to treat them with tonics and stimulants...."[9] People reveled particularly in the idea of a "spring tonic," something to drive the accumulated sludge of winter away. Thus in Lancashire, for example, lime flowers, wintercress, and sorrel were once taken as "blood purifiers," as were a mixture of "brimstone" and treacle, or the simple liquid in which vegetables had been cooked.[10] Indeed, doctors were quite sympathetic to this "very common, and very old notion, that what are called *cooling medicines* should be taken at particular periods of the year, especially in the spring." Thus it was, continued Manchester's James Harrison, that "many a poor child has been condemned to a pot of brimstone and treacle merely because it was the spring-time."[11] Note, moreover, how closely parallel to academic medicine these popular theories about "heating" and "cooling" the body ran.

Similarly, folk theories about *acute* diseases ran alongside official medicine: get those poisons out of there. (*Plethora* was the official term.) Whenever anything went seriously wrong with the body, evacuation was the patient's design for self-help, just as it was the doctor's. People believed so implicitly in these strategies of purgation that jokes such as the following, incomprehensible to today's reader, would seem quite humorous:

Some Kentucky farmer, so went the story, was suffering from "obstruction of the bowels, and all efforts to have them move had failed. Even the best known 'yarbs,' etc. had been tried, but to no avail."

So a nearby doctor was sent for. "Waal," he said, "I'm only a hoss doctor; never tended a human in my life. For a hoss in this condition I would give a half pound of salts, but I guess a quarter of a pound would do for a man." So he gave the dose and left.

The next day he rode by and asked a neighbor chopping wood

near the house, "Neighbor, hev you heard from the sick gentleman over the way this morning?"

"Oh yes, Doc," said the man.

"Kin you tell me if the medicine acted that I gave him?"

"Oh yes, Doc, it acted."

"I am glad ter hear that," said the doctor. "Kin you tell me how many times hit acted?"

"Well, Doc, as well as I can remember, it acted well nigh onto twenty times before he died and nine times after he died."[12]

In the people's battle for purgation were enlisted time-honored laxatives: buckthorn syrup or rhubarb that one could prepare oneself; jalap, "Epsom salts" (magnesium sulfate), castor oil, senna, and aloes that one could buy from the apothecary. But if the fever were truly raging, the illness desperate, then people would take out the salts of mercury. Isabella Beeton, author of the widely read text *Household Management*, advised worried parents to give their child twelve grains of calomel and two grains of tartar emetic for croup. Indeed, always keep such metals as antimony and mercury in the family medicine chest, she counseled.[13] "The public insists on being poisoned," said Holmes. "The popular belief is all but universal that sick people should feed on noxious substances." A doctor friend of Holmes had been called "to a man with a terribly sore mouth [a sign of mercury poisoning]. On inquiry he found that the man had picked up a box of unknown pills, in Howard Street, and had proceeded to take them, on general principles, pills being good for people."[14] The nineteenth century did see something of a backlash against mercury; yet a great many people continued to trust it as the one drug that would get "those poisons" out of their digestive tracts after all else had failed.

Popular medicine involved more than purgation, though. Whenever you had a skin eruption, the idea was that something had "burst" down inside, thus expressions like "only a burst," or "he's burst himself." How might you get a burst? Drinking too much water was one way; hence the logic of not giving new mothers anything cold to drink for several days, on the grounds that it would either "burst" or "founder" them.[15] (The reasoning was, I think, that some forms of childbed fever were accompanied by scarlatina rashes. Hence, if you denied a new mother water, you might prevent the postpartum infection that caused the rash.)

These internal poisons could also be evacuated via the skin: thus the logic of making sick people sweat in cases of measles, scarlet fever, or other acute infections. The cure comes with the sweating. Here again, people thought they were making sense of observed facts. In an infection the body's defenses produce substances that make the temperature control center (in the hypothalamus of the brain) raise its "set point," the temperature at which the body should be. So in flu, for example, you might get a new set point of 101 degrees. When, finally, the immune system has overcome the invader and these temperature-raising substances are no longer appearing, the body now "realizes" it's too hot, and sweating begins in an effort to decrease the temperature to the normal set-point. Thus sweating usually follows the "crisis" in an acute infection, the point at which the battle has been won. Hence it was a simple deduction to imagine that sweating might *help* the body get over disease. "It is . . . a common notion that sweating is always necessary in the beginning of a fever," wrote William Buchan. "The common practice is to heap clothes upon the patient, and to give him things of a hot nature, as spirits, spiceries. . . ."[16]

Enlightened eighteenth-century physicians, who believed in "cooling regimens," shuddered at the smelly, sweaty steambath that was the traditional sickroom. "If, in consequence of great heat or delirium [patients] attempt to get out of bed, they are confined to it by force; nor are they suffered to change their bed- or body-linen, till the fever is quite removed; by which means the air becoming more putrid, aggravates the symptoms. . . ."[17] By extension, the association of sweating with cure, and chill with disease, which prevailed in so many traditional minds, led to popular fear of the night air and insistence on closing the windows: the Illinois farmers of the nineteenth century would sleep with their windows shut tight to keep out the "night air."[18]

Bleeding, the great ally of purgation, was similarly in demand. "Amongst common people," said William Buchan, "the very name of a fever generally suggests the necessity of bleeding."[19] Mrs. Beeton gave patients exact instruction on how to do it:

> Place a handkerchief or piece of tape rather but not too tightly
> round the arm, about three or four inches above the elbow. This
> will cause the veins below to swell and become very evident. . . .
> The operator should take the lancet in his right hand, between the
> thumb and first finger, place the thumb of his left hand on the vein
> below the part where he is going to bleed from, and then gently
> thrust the tip of the lancet into the vein. . . .[20]

Samuel Gross recalled, from the early days of his practice in Easton and Cincinnati, patients coming in requesting to be bled as a spring and fall tonic, "a means, as was believed, of purifying the blood and relieving congestion. Sometimes a person would come with a request to be bled in the foot, on the assumption that it was a great remedy for headache!"[21] Plenty of additional evidence suggests that bleeding was an object of profound faith among traditional patients, rather than a detested imposition of the doctor. People didn't like being bled until they fainted ("bleeding until syncope," it was called), but overall they thought it salutary.

Thus far, popular theories have run fairly close to traditional medical theories. Where the two parted company was over "magic" in treatment. Since the seventeenth century the medical profession had rejected any invocation of magic in the cure of disease, be it astrology, the imputed powers of the moon, or mystical powders left behind by leprechauns. The populace, by contrast, remained root-and-branch credulous until late in the nineteenth century. In my previous work on the history of obstetrics I encountered numerous examples of women who feared that witches would put the "evil eye" on them in childbed and make them sick, that malefic forces would remove their own newborn and substitute a "changeling," that birth deformities were caused by looking at a full moon out of doors during pregnancy, or that a woman would fall sick if, when she was having her period, she walked across the grave of a new mother. We shall better grasp the dramatic change represented by the popular embrace of scientific medicine, late in the nineteenth century, if we bear in mind that in an earlier time people said things like, "Poor Mr. So-and-So is a little off the book just now—a little wrong in the upper story; but then it is the full of the moon next month."[22]

A key magical concept was that of ridding oneself of disease by transferring it onto someone or something else. A doctor in Cardenden, Scotland, thought that "the commonest cause of criminal assaults on little children is the wish to get rid of venereal disease," that is, by "transferring" it to the little girl the infected man can end his own malady. "I saw lately," he added, "a case where a nurse-girl deliberately 'smit' a younger girl with impetigo contagiosa [a bacterial skin infection] to relieve herself of the complaint."[23] The Fifeshire practice of making a "puppy poultice" similarly incorporated this principle: a local wisewoman advised a man with a "poisoned arm" to chop up and apply "hot to the diseased surface three puppy dogs." So a neighbor "with a cross-bred litter doomed to the tub readily handed them over . . . and on went the slaughtered innocents. . . . The arm got better."[24]

These magical remedies persisted in the folklore of southern Illinois toward the turn of the century:

- *To cure "sore eyes," "pour hot milk over the place where the patient's afterbirth is buried."*
- *A red string wound tightly around the left little finger will stop a nose-bleed.*
- *Drinking one's mother's urine will prevent the drinker from ever having the mumps.*[25]

An Illinois wisewoman named Aunt Glory explained to Dr. Thomas Shastid how to treat poliomyelitis: "Why, I'd take and I'd bile me a big yeller yam, then strain off the bilin's an' mix it with corn meal. I'd then sprinkle it with sheep drippin's an' let it stand out one night . . . in the dark of the moon. Then I'd say certain words over it, which I ain't a-gwine to tell ye. An' then I'd give the patient a whole tablespoonful o' that there liquid every single hour, an' in a day he'd be plumb well."[26]

Within decades of the advent of modern medicine, the Aunt Glorys of this world, whose lore had endured since the birth of humankind, would fall silent.

Whether magic was added in or not, the practice of self-dosing was enormously widespread. By a people who lived near the land, the medicinal qualities of the local plants were as readily mastered as the names of the city streets are by us. What do you take for diarrhea? Some raw sweet potato, they said in Lafayette County, Florida, to "stop the stomach running off." Problems with manliness? Try the sting nettle. Tea made from its roots will "give a man courage."[27] In Appalachia every one knew that the roots of the wild indigo, if harvested in the fall, would serve well as a "febrifuge [drug to reduce fever], tonic, purgative, and antiseptic." The coralroot made a good diaphoretic (drug to cause sweating) and a sedative.[28] Every region of the United States, United Kingdom, continent of Europe—and as far as I know every other settled place on the globe—once had its own medical folklore.

That almost all of this lore was hokum is unimportant. What interests us here is that traditional patients turned to these plants as an alternative to the doctor. And often when desperation drove them to a medical consultation, it was not the doctor's curing hand they sought, not his rich medical knowledge nor his skilled procedures. They sought out the doctor because he was a conduit to drugs that they could not compound for themselves, drugs they thought "really worked," drugs that would agitate and shake the body and thus, they hoped, provide relief. "I remember when apomorphine [an emetic] first came into use," wrote Shastid, probably referring to the 1890s:

> You shot a tiny bit of the substance under the patient's skin. And then the patient in a perfectly gentlemanly or ladylike manner . . . gave a soft-like heave—a so-so sigh such as anyone could use in Sunday School and not attract attention from the teacher—and up would come—well, whatever . . . had formerly been below. But patients would have none of that gentility sort of medicine. "Peared like nothin' ain't been a-doing," they would say. They wanted emetics that "would jest nacherly knock the socks offin your stomach."
>
> So it was with all the other remedies, Shastid continued. "Anything to cure a chill must make you mighty hot. Anything to cure a fever must make you mighty cold. A sleeping medicine must make you saw wood. A tonic must tone you 'so's you could jest feel 'er all thoo yer anatomy,' " said the patients.

Added Shastid, "Otherwise, why bother about sending for a doctor?"[29]

ALTERNATIVE HEALERS

Indeed. If you could get some "alternative healer," "empiric," "irregular," "medicine man," or "quack" to prescribe something truly powerful for you, why bother with a doctor at all? An important indication of traditional patients' lack of respect for the art of medicine was the readiness with which they sought out "nonregular" medical practitioners, meaning anyone with pretensions to heal who did not subscribe to one of the mainline medical systems. Only a minority of those who called themselves "doctor" had ever attended a medical school or received a "regular" education. Of the 10,200 practitioners listed in one British medical directory in 1856, only 2,400 had degrees either as surgeons or apothecaries.[30] The others could be anyone who walked in off the street and decided to call himself "doctor." (This would be true until 1858.) In five New England counties, in the period 1790–1840, two-thirds to three-quarters of the practitioners were not medical school graduates. Of two hundred physicians in Eastern Tennessee in 1850, only 38 percent were medical school graduates or had taken as much as a course of medical school *lectures!*[31] The others could believe or practice anything, and it is predominantly among them that we find the "alternative healers."

The concept of the alternative healer really embraces three types: the outrightly "quackish" medicine men who traveled about selling snake oil; the traditional alternative healers, such as midwives, bonesetters, cataract gougers, or sow gelders (who performed operations on humans, too); and those who subscribed to alternative systems of medicine, such as Christian Science, homeopathy, Thomsonianism, and the like. All were important rivals to the regular physician.

Quacks is short for *quacksalvers*, or people who applied salves of quicksilver (mercury). "Quacking out" in the marketplace, they stood in contrast to regular physicians who weren't supposed to advertise themselves. The essence of quackery was retailing "secret remedies," often called "patent medicines," which meant not that the formula itself was patented but that the name was trademarked. These early medicine men sold their own formulations, mainly purgatives and salves for "skin diseases," among which principally was syphilis, an absolute specter because people had little idea of how it was acquired or whether they might have it and were terrified that their noses might fall off.

Thus there was fertile ground for the "Elixirated Spirit of Scurvy Grass," the "Pectoral Lozenges," and the "Worm Powders" of a Restoration quack named John Russell; for the "Bilious Pills" of the American Dr. Lee; the "Venise Treacles," "Scots Pills," and "Daffy's Elixir Salutis's" that flooded Britain and the New World in the seventeenth century and after.[32] "People still shut their eyes and take every thing upon trust that is administered by any Pretender to Medicine," wrote William Buchan in 1769. " Implicit faith, everywhere else the object of ridicule, is still sacred here." It was therefore especially vexing to Buchan that the "ignorant peasants" were suspicious in particular of the medicines of the doctor.[33]

The quacks sounded so confident that one can see why the desperate might have been drawn. Here is one, an herbalist named Bigwood, testifying at an autopsy at Marshfield, England, in 1875. He claimed the doctor of the deceased had abandoned the case as hopeless:

> I told [the patient] that his liver did not throw any blood, and that it was very dry. I thought by his countenance that his liver did not throw any blood, as he looked as sallow as death. I sent him a bottle of medicine next day which contained seven different sorts of herbs. They were herbs governed by the sun. . . . I use a hundred different sort of herbs. I give medicine for every part of the body where it is afflicted.

The herbalist explained that he had been practicing for twelve years. "I have raised men very near the grave with that medicine and pills. . . . I judge all complaints by astronomy. If I have the date of a man's birth, if he lived in London and sent to Gorsham to tell me he was bad, I could tell what his complaint was, and what to prescribe for him."[34]

This was to be close to the last gasp of the medicine man. Modern medicine would shortly transform the nature of quackery.

A second variety of alternative healer was the local wisewoman, bonesetter, midwife, and numerous other sorts of "paramedical" who for centuries had provided basic medical care to small towns and villages not served by regular surgeon-apothecaries (few degreed physicians were found outside the cities). Many of them were women, tied into a larger network of "women's culture" that had as its special mission the handing down of medical folklore from generation to generation. This women's culture of medicine once embraced millions of women patients. One such was Mrs. King of Northfleet, whom Dr. John Woodward saw for the first time around 1710, by which time she had many complaints. She had started out in the 1690s with an ulcerated leg and had been "in the care of women for above two years before any surgeon was called in."[35]

Pig castrators were also traditional healers of humans. In the second half of the nineteenth century the English village of Aysgarth had a celebrated sow gelder who was also known for his recipe for "infectious jaundice" (probably group A hepatitis). His jaundice remedy, which he passed on to his daughter, contained barberry bark, which he got from "the herb garden of Bolton Castle." He handed it out free.[36] These jaundice doctors would also shortly go the way of all flesh.

A third alternative was the medical "sects." Unlike the wisewomen and sow gelders, the sectarians, or "irregulars," had integrated medical theories of their own, theories opposed to those of mainstream medicine. One group of sectarians, for example, was the *Thomsonians*, followers of the New England farmer Samuel Thomson, who had acquired a fanatical devotion to the supposed healing powers of the lobelia plant. Lobelia in mild doses stimulates the central nervous system as nicotine does and in powerful doses acts as an emetic. After Thomson's *New Guide to Health* was published in 1822, a craze for self-induced vomiting by using lobelia swept the land.[37]

A later group of sectarians were the *homeopaths,* followers of the German Samuel Hahnemann. They subscribed to a doctrine of "minute doses" of any drug: the smaller the dose, the greater the effectiveness of the drug. In reality, their cures were effected either by suggestion or as a result of keeping "nature's healing ways" undisturbed by the harmful intervention of the physician. Because the homeopaths offered such a clear alternative to the customary bleeding and purging, they attracted quite a following in the second half of the nineteenth century, including many physicians. Around 1871 perhaps one of every eight doctors was a sectarian, and millions of patients believed implicitly in the homeopathic "dilutions" of drugs to thousandths and hundredthousandths of their normal strength.[38]

Evidently, traditional medicine inspired so little faith that everywhere ludicrous rivals ballooned up, hawking puppy poultices, magical cures, plants to make you vomit from really deep down, and "dilutions" of medicines, whose very philosophy flew in the face of science and reason. We shall see the phenomenon's recurring in our own time, as patients once again turn from mainstream medicine to "alternative healers."

TRADITIONAL DOCTORS HAD LITTLE AUTHORITY OVER PATIENTS

If traditional doctors ultimately were able to keep most of their patients away from the bonesetters and homeopaths, it was because only the doctors were thought capable of providing access to "truly strong drugs," via the elaborate prescriptions they wrote for druggists to compound. But once this role as drug conduit is set aside, traditional doctors had precious little authority over their patients. Today, too, patient "compliance" with complicated drug regimens is considered a problem, but it pales in comparison with the refusal of the traditional patient to believe that the doctor had any specialized knowledge at all.

For one thing, the laity were reluctant to cede to medical opinion in licensing and in the operation of hospitals. In the early licensing legislation of the colonies, it was up to politicians and judges to decide who was competent.[39] The lay governors of the large London charity hospitals would hold hearings on the competence of surgeons with only lay people present and would make appointments to medical and surgical staff without even the pretense of consulting the hospital's doctors. If the board of governors of Guy's Hospital early in the nineteenth century wished to hear from the medical staff, the doctors would be "summoned" to their presence.[40]

In the 1830s in Mount Meigs, Alabama, when a Mr. Adams fell sick with a swelling and fluctuation in his upper right side, he called in two doctors, J. Marion Sims and Dr. Baker. The doctors disagreed. Baker believed the illness was liver cancer, Sims, an abscess filled with pus. So Sims "proposed a council" to break the deadlock. "Mr. Billy Dick, who was the great authority in that neighborhood, to whom everyone appealed and looked for advice, and three or four of his neighbors, were called in."

"Gentlemen," Sims said, "our consultation results in a difference of opinion between us." So he asked Billy Dick and his pals to decide whether medical therapy or a surgical operation was appropriate to the case. The council of neighbors decided for surgery, as Sims hoped they would (the patient indeed had an abscess).[41] The assumption everybody shared here was that medical knowledge was nothing very arcane and that an Alabama cracker's opinion was just about as good as a trained surgeon's.

Patients had just as little hesitation about *challenging* the doctor's diagnosis or plan of management. Connecticut's Worthington Hooker supposed such a case. "A lady is sick under the care of her physician." Her loved ones are anxious and full of concern and ask the doctor many questions about medicine and her prognosis. So far, so good. But then they go on to engage him in medical debate. "They ask him, perhaps, if he is not afraid that such a remedy will produce such an effect . . . and they may even go so far as to attribute some unfavorable symptom to some medicine that has been administered."[42] Thus, no hint of awe at the doctor's all-knowing wisdom.

If in postmodern medicine the "noncompliant patient" is one who doesn't take hypertension pills, in traditional medicine it was one who *completely disregarded everything the doctor said.* In the 1870s, Henry Sutler, of Pittsfield, Illinois, was such a disobedient. Although he was a kind man and successful in business, his weak point was that "he never liked anybody to tell him what to do." But when he came down with typhoid fever he had to obey his wife and his doctor, Thomas Shastid's father, up to a certain point.

"Then Henry Sutler's condition began to improve. Henry did not understand typhoid fever [an infection of the bowels], but he thought that he did. After the fourth week, when he had no more fever and scarcely any pain, *he* informed *my father* that he was all right now, that he was going to get up shortly, dress himself and set about his work."

Dr. Shastid demurred and said Henry risked the danger of hemorrhaging from the bowels if he were to get up.

"Henry persisted. My father resisted. Henry begged his wife to bring him his shoes, his shirt, his trousers. Father told her not to bring them." Unless Henry promised not to get up, Dr. Shastid threatened to "gather up every particle of clothing that you have in the house, take it away home with me and burn it." Henry promised.

"Father and I then went away happy.

"Scarcely, however, had we driven half a quarter when we heard behind us a woman's shrill screaming. Turning, we saw Mrs. Sutler standing on her front porch, crying and frantically gesturing to us to come back.

"At the house again we arrived just in time to see Henry Sutler faint and fall to the floor. Yes, he was dead, and his trousers were full of blood."[43]

We shall shortly learn what true "medical authority" means. Why didn't the traditional patient respect it? Consider the sign on the front of Dr. Popjay's house in mid-nineteenth-century England: "I Popjay Surgeon Apotecary[sic] and Midwife etc; draws teeth and bleeds on lowest terms. Confectionary Tobacco Snuff Tea Coffee Sugar and all sorts of perfumery sold here. NB New laid eggs every morning by Mrs. Popjay."[44]

Would you have stood in awe of such a doctor?

CHAPTER FOUR
The Rise of the
Modern Doctor

O F THE two central characters in our story, the modern
doctor and the modern patient, the doctor comes on
stage in the period between 1880 and 1950. We will
consider as "modern" the men who graduated from medical
school in these years, because it was at school that all these new
ideas were learned. The essence of their "modernity" was the
doctors' ability correctly to diagnose disease: not to *cure* it, but to
recognize what it was the patient had.

NEW IDEAS IN MEDICINE

The doctor's ability to make an accurate diag-
nosis stemmed from a revolution in medical thought that had two
basic components. The first was knowing what was going on in
the body by linking up changes observed in the tissues after death
to the patient's signs and symptoms during life. The second was

75

the new science of microbiology that made it possible, for the first time ever, to say how threats in the world around us—in this case, germs—produced disease.

Remember, a patient's symptoms can be baffling, if they are all one knows about the case. A man is sitting in front of you wheezing and hacking, spitting up a bit of blood, reporting night sweats, and feeling exhausted. What's going on? "How do you put all this together clinically?" as doctors say. Around the time of the Napoleonic Wars, a Frenchman named René Laennec started paying careful attention to exactly what he heard and felt in the chest, then comparing it to what he found in the same patient at autopsy. Can you hear through his chest wall the words the patient whispers? A sort of gurgling, cavernous sound comes from within? Each word is followed by a puff, as though "blowing out a candle"? It's tuberculosis. Shortness of breath? A big, round chest? "The absence of the noise of respiration in the chest"? It's emphysema, a condition in which the lung tissue is destroyed, and gas exchange comes to a halt.[1] Sure enough, when Laennec opened up these gravely ill individuals at autopsy (for all of them died), he would find the tubercules in the chest that are distinctive of miliary tuberculosis, or the big gaping patches in lung tissue that indicate emphysema. Thus Laennec and the whole school of Parisian "pathologists" who followed his lead in the 1820s and 1830s, were able to isolate a host of distinctive diseases that previously had all been placed into the category of "peripneumonia" and treated alike.

But one can learn only so much from examining organs after death. True, lung diseases bring about some pretty distinctive changes; but often, gravely diseased organs may not look very different at death from healthy organs, or, at least, many different diseases produce roughly the same postmortem appearance. What does change in disease is the cellular structure of the tissues, and to see this one needs a microscope, because you can't see cells with the naked eye.

Back in the days when I was first beginning research into the practice of medicine, I knew nothing about tissues or microscopes. At an autopsy I was observing, the pathologist was throwing bits of tissue from each organ into two jars, one for the right side of the body, one for the left.

"How can you tell later what organ's what?" I asked, since the little bits all looked more or less the same to me.

"We look at them under the microscope," he said.

"You mean they all look different under the microscope?" I cannot now believe I asked such a dumb question. He nodded patiently.

Let's take, for example, two diseases that look quite different under the microscope, peptic ulcer of the stomach and stomach cancer, totally different maladies with different courses and treatments. To the naked eye the diseased stomachs in both cases appear pretty much the same, and it took the next big leap forward in pathology to enable them to be sorted out: the invention of a new kind of microscope with compound lenses, in the 1820s, and the introduction of chemical stains for tissues. Stains are important because you can't just put a piece of tissue under a microscope and start observing it: it looks like a big mess. First, incredibly thin sections of the tissue must be sliced off with a microtome. Then the slice of tissue has to be "fixed" to prevent its decomposition, and then it is stained so the nuclei of individual cells will stand out, making it possible to observe details. The development of fixatives and stains awaited the expansion of modern chemistry. So it was only in 1865 that the effective stain haematoxylin (from the logwood tree) was introduced, and eosin (from the organic chemical aniline dye) appeared in 1876.[2] (In hospital laboratories today you can hear mentions of "H-and-E" stains, which refer to these stains.)

Thus, one main arm of the advance in medicine was in *pathology*, the study of diseased tissues. This new intellectual operation of reasoning back and forth, from symptoms to physical changes in tissues, was quite straightforward but of enormous consequence. For example, by distinguishing peptic ulcer from stomach cancer by means of microscope examination, one was able to clarify the way that the symptoms of the two diseases differed. By the time of World War I, doctors would be able to ask whether the pain in the stomach was relieved by eating and to guess from the answer that the ulcer was probably benign; or to find a "rolled edge" in the X-ray after the patient had swallowed a solution of bismuth and to suspect that it was malignant.

The second great arm of the advance was the germ theory of

disease. Infections were once blamed on the "malignant north wind" or on " miasmas" (noxious emanations from the ground), rather than on microorganisms. Indeed, the Manchester doctor James Harrison mocked his patients for their foolish belief in the contagiousness of TB. "That consumption is catching is a popular opinion, which, in this country at least, is not recognized by the profession."[3] Therefore, it caused a stir when in 1876 a country doctor in the Prussian town of Wollstein demonstrated that *anthrax*, an obscure disease of woolsorters, could be transmitted artificially from animal to animal and that the anthrax bacteria in the blood of the previously healthy animal could be cultivated in a dish and seen under the microscope. Then, on 24 March 1882, the same doctor, Robert Koch, announced that similar bacteria caused tuberculosis.[4] The discovery stunned everyone. If "germs" caused major diseases, it would be possible to figure out where the germs lived and how to avoid catching them—and thus to avoid getting TB, scarlet fever, gonorrhea, typhoid, or any of the other bacterial infections that up to that time had been ascribed to "bad heredity" or "a sudden chill."

These two advances, pathological anatomy and the germ theory of disease, were to transform medicine. They would also upgrade the public image of the doctor and, therefore, also the doctor's power to heal diseases that arose in the mind. But let us take our story one step at a time. These new ideas entered the world of the family doctor slowly. They did not come by way of the medical press: although widely reported there, they were frequently disbelieved by an older generation of men. The new ideas entered medical practice by way of medical school.

Harvard's was the first American medical school to impart these ideas. In 1869 Samuel Eliot Morison became president of the university, and two years later he presided over a complete reorganization of the program in medicine, emphasizing laboratory sciences such as microscopic anatomy (called *histology*), pathological anatomy, chemistry, and physiology. The program was made three years long; later a fourth "clerkship" year was added, to be spent entirely at patients' bedsides. Three big new laboratories for microscope use and physiology research were created, and the number of chemistry desks for the three hundred undergraduates in medicine rose, in 1871, from sixteen to one hundred. "Learning by doing" was to be the new philosophy: looking at germs and diseased tissues under the microscope and understanding how they added up to the symptoms and signs real patients would have.[5]

One Harvard graduate later remembered the course in which Oliver Wendell Holmes had taught the class to use the microscope, toward the mid-1870s. One day one of the microscopes was missing when the students handed them back. Said Holmes to the class: "Such men as are engaged in the study or practice of medicine are supposed to be gentlemen. Therefore I do not suppose that any member of this class could have had anything to do with the disappearance of that microscope. I prefer to suppose that some inmate of the neighboring institution [pointing with his thumb] has escaped from it" and purloined the instrument. The "neighboring institution" was the nearby Charles Street Jail, and we do not know whether the microscope was returned.[6] But the story illustrates a problem that has plagued faculties of medicine ever since: students are so keen to see germs and diseased cells that they try to take the "mikes" back to their rooms.

The revolution spread, in fits and starts, to other American medical schools. Students at the Chicago Medical College started learning to use the microscope in the late 1870s because "German pathology was the fashion."[7] That is, the center of learning had spread from Paris, where it had resided in the first half of the century, to Berlin, Leipzig, and Vienna.

William Macartney remembered learning, as a medical student at the City University of New York in the 1880s, how to prepare slides and stain tissues. The director of the lab would come down the aisle: "Holy Smoke! You're getting your light with your reflector from that fly on the ceiling instead of from the window as I told you." "For heaven's sake, don't try to crush the slide with your coarse adjustment. Do you think you are handling a stone-crusher?"

He went to one young student's desk. "What's that on your slide?"

"I don't know, sir. I've had no time yet to examine it."

"Well, what do you see?"

79

"So far, just a series of more or less parallel pink and white stripes."[8]

As this med student and hundreds and thousands of others after him would learn, those parallel stripes were the tubules of the kidney, and one could diagnose kidney disease by finding in them the little black dots that indicated infection (stained white cells rushing to meet the bacterial invaders), or the light pink, featureless indications that the very core of the kidney itself was being destroyed and that the patient would soon die.

The most "scientific" of the new medical schools was Johns Hopkins in Baltimore, opened in 1893, twenty years after the death of a merchant by the same name who left in his will funds for a university, a hospital, and a medical school. You had to have an undergraduate degree and a knowledge of French and German even to be admitted to the medical school. And with such giants of the time as William Osler and William H. Welch on the faculty, Hopkins soon became a synonym for all that was advanced and distinguished about medicine.

Contrast the following typical week in the life of a Hopkins student, in 1906, with the know-nothing apprenticeships and useless lecture going of the traditional medical student:

October 15. Recitation and lecture by Dr. Welch. He called on me. [Picking out students and calling on them is a basic torture test in medical schools.]

October 16. Stewart and I work on optics. Higgins has some excitement over the appearance of the clerk [presumably female] in the registry department.

October 17. Work on astigmatism.

Ocotber 18. Drizzly day. Color demonstrations by Dr. [William Henry] Howell.

October 19. Surgical clinic this morning by Dr. [John M. T.] Finney: inguinal hernia and inner canalicular myxoma of mammary gland [a breast tumor].

October 20. Barker's clinic. Three cases of typhoid complications, one tuberculous pneumonia, six arthritides [cases of arthritis], and a boy with heart, spleen and liver on wrong side.

October 21. A rainy day. Seventy at Sunday School today. Wrote letters all afternoon.

October 22. A blue Monday. Rabbit autopsy; death caused by inoculation with staphylococcus aureus. Savoy Quartet made a little music tonight.[9]

The diary fairly breathes science—pathology, bacteriology, experimental (on animals) medicine, clinical medicine—the new spirit on every page.

From such commanding heights as Harvard and Hopkins, and later the University of Chicago and the University of Rochester, the new medicine radiated outward. Traditional knowledge began to seem so inadequate that it insulted the very sensibilities of a population fascinated generally with science and technology. In 1878 the Illinois State Board of Health upgraded requirements for medical graduates who wanted the board's certification, and other states followed along, forcing medical schools everywhere to begin improving their offerings. In 1891 a national association of state boards was founded; in 1904 the American Medical Association founded its Council on Medical Education, whose purpose was to prod along the squalid little proprietary medical schools. And so when in 1910 Abraham Flexner issued his famous report on medical education, it merely set the capstone on thirty years of improvement in the training of young doctors.[10]

THE MODERN DOCTOR AT WORK: DIAGNOSIS

The point of all this scientific training was not to produce young scientists. It was to produce doctors who would have some sense of what was going on when a patient came in with a pain in the chest or blood in the urine. The basic technique doctors have of matching symptoms to an underlying lesion (an abnormal change in structure or function of an organ) is called the *differential diagnosis*. In traditional medicine a "differential" was not possible, because doctrines of "laxity of the fibers" and the like were so unspecific: you'd have only one analysis for whatever presented itself. With modern medicine, however, the differential took on considerable practical importance, because the therapy, and the prognosis (chances for recovery), would depend on the particular diagnosis. When John Wheeler was a medical student at Harvard in the 1870s, Dr. Calvin Ellis taught him diagnosis:

"He took a long, thorough, systematic history of each case, catalogued every symptom, made a list of all the diseases which the aggregation of symptoms could possibly suggest and then, by comparing the patient's symptoms with those of each disease, would decide whether, in this case, that disease could be present."[11] This list of possibilities, then, is the differential diagnosis, and one selects the final, correct diagnosis from the list by going on to do a physical examination and lab tests. These examinations and tests make the real difference between modern and traditional medicine. They gave the modern doctor his power and influence, and for that reason I shall describe in detail the examinations that a post-1870s doctor could perform in order to establish the diagnosis.

After taking the history, the doctor looked the patient over quite carefully, not just examining the color of the skin and the eyeballs—steps the traditional doctor had prided himself on—but poking and prying. Silas Weir Mitchell, a Philadelphia neurologist, told the story of a "young physician," possibly himself, confounding his seniors by poking around a bit.

> The case was one of a young man who several times had been found at morning in a stupor. The attacks were rare, and what caused them was unknown. The young physician, much embarrassed, was civilly asked to examine the case, and did so with a thoroughness which rather wearied the two older men. When they retired to an adjoining room, he was asked, as our custom is, to give, as the youngest, the first opinion. He said, "It is a case of epilepsy. He has bitten his cheek in the fit." Dr. P. rose without a word and went out. Returning in a few moments, he said, "You are

right. I did not look far enough back. You will reach, sir, a high
rank in our profession."[12]

Throughout the nineteenth century, techniques were elaborated to extend the "inspection" of the patient beyond merely
looking at him. They are known medically as auscultation, palpation, and percussion, and although they are losing ground today,
they were once extremely important.

Auscultation means simply listening, and one does it with a
stethoscope. René Laennec, the pathologist whose comparison of
chest sounds with autopsy findings was discussed earlier, was
hearing the various chest noises with a primitive stethoscope, a
device he invented in 1816 by rolling up a paper tube and applying it to the chest wall.[13] Only much later did the device make
any impact on the practice of medicine. It was not introduced to
the United States until after the publication of Henry Bowditch's
1846 book *The Young Stethoscopist*, and even then the stethoscope remained confined to the commanding heights of medicine,
until in the 1870s the schools began to teach its use. Although
Robert Pusey, a Kentucky doctor who had graduated in 1860
from a good medical school, owned a stethoscope, "he did not,"
his son explains, "have confidence in himself with it. I have seen
him many times examine the chest with the stethoscope at my
suggestion, but soon he would have his ear down on a towel on
the chest wall; then he knew what he heard."[14] When Thomas
Shastid, an Illinois doctor who'd graduated in the 1880s from Columbia, wanted to listen to the chest, he used a stethoscope, but
when he wanted to hear the *bowels* of a patient named Sam Creek
(to see whether they were passing food through normally), he
"laid across the man's naked abdomen a handtowel, and then,
down on the towel, I laid my sleepy head."[15] Norman Moore, a
London physician prominent around the turn of the century,
"used to tell his students of a physician of the old school who
carried a stethoscope, not from any personal conviction of its efficacy as an aid to diagnosis, but in deference to the prejudices of
his younger colleagues."[16]

But younger doctors did use their stethoscopes, and the device,
which was improved steadily throughout the century, greatly ex-

panded their ability to tell what was going on. Noises in the lung? A whole "differential" of possibilities. Noises in the heart? A host of "murmurs" (damaged valves) come to mind, some of which are innocuous, some life-threatening. Noises in the arteries? A result of turbulence caused by the rushing of the blood around obstructions. The obstructions, like atherosclerosis, would be of great interest.

The British doctor Arthur Conan Doyle, who also created Sherlock Holmes, described in a thinly fictionalized account his own beginning days of medical practice in the 1880s. He arrived in town with an absolute minimum of equipment: "In my box were a stethoscope, several medical books, a second pair of boots, two suits of clothes, my linen and my toilet things." But he had a stethoscope! Thus he was able to perform a proper work-up of the ancient, alcoholic naval officer who was among his first patients. The young doctor found "mitral regurgitation, cirrhosis of the liver, Bright's disease, an enlarged spleen, and incipient dropsy. I gave him a lecture about the necessity of temperance. . . ."[17] Of those conditions, the damaged heart valve ("mitral regurgitation") was the only one he found with his stethoscope, but a traditional doctor would not have spotted it.

The rest of the officer's problems Doyle's young doctor identified by using two other techniques of physical examination: palpation and percussion.. Laennec had popularized them as well. *Percussion*, actually begun by a Viennese doctor in the 1760s, is simply tapping one's finger against the patient's body to hear the resonance it produces. Or rather, you put one finger on the patient's chest and then tap *it* several times with the other finger. Highly resonant noises mean the cavity beneath is hollow, which is a good thing: no tumor, no pus. Dullness, on the other hand, means trouble: a lung lobe is filling up with pus, meaning pneumonia, or a tumor is obstructing a bronchus.

Palpation, from the Latin *palpo*, "I handle gently," developed in fits and starts with the nineteenth-century progress of pathology. Doctors learned to figure out, from autopsies, what it was on the inside that they were feeling from the outside. And so the medical students memorized the differential diagnosis for swollen kidneys, for swollen this, for swollen that. Is it painful for the patient when you press down on the abdomen and then take your fingers away? "Rebound tenderness," a sign of peritoneal irritation, such as infection. Is the thyroid gland enlarged? Five things on the differential and a separate technique for pinning down each one. Every first-year med student would learn exactly where the normal liver and spleen were, knowing that if those could be felt sticking down below the ribs they were enlarged and something was wrong.

Finally, in this first burst of aids to diagnosis, the family physician would acquire a microscope, not to look at bacteria or biopsy sections taken from the liver, but to examine the urine. The microscope was essential, of course, for anything having to do with microorganisms or for telling whether tumors were benign or malignant. But the GP didn't do that. He sent out such work to labs. He was also interested, however, in knowing whether that abdominal pain was appendicitis (the term was invented in 1886) or a bladder infection. If you put a drop of urine onto a slide and look at it under the microscope, you can tell whether pus, blood, bacteria, or sloughed-off tissue is present; if so, the problem is coming from the urinary tract. And if the urine is normal, you know that the problem is elsewhere.

The microscope had already reached the commanding heights of medicine by the 1860s and 1870s, but not until the first generation of scientifically trained young physicians had installed themselves in practice did its use spread to family medicine. In 1882, Daniel Cathell advised doctors who wanted to rise socially to display for their patients their "diplomas, certificates of society membership, pictures of eminent professional friends and teachers, anatomical plates," and also their microscopes.[18] By the turn of the century it was bon ton in medicine to have the makings of one's own "private laboratory." The GP "attempts it now . . . with his few beginning test-tubes, his bottle of nitric acid and his Fehling's solution [to test for sugar in the urine] and the binocular microscope under that large glass globe on the marble-topped table in the front window in the parlor."[19] Thus the microscope was both a practical tool and a badge of "scientific medicine."

What we have thus far described is really the first stage of the revolution in diagnosis; it is the revolution of the "brilliant clinician," the doctor who observes keenly, taps a bit here, listens a bit there, reflects long about the differential of what he has seen, and then formulates a stunning diagnosis. That is the practice of bedside observation depicted in Luke Fildes's 1891 painting of *The Doctor*, who is sitting beside the little sick girl. No instruments are in sight, although perhaps he has a stethoscope in his pocket. The Fildes image of the wise old doctor was exploited to great effect in the 1940s by the American Medical Association (AMA), in its campaign against health insurance.[20] It is an image that has gripped the imagination of the public: the bedside doctor whose diagnosis depends on the quickness of his own hands and eyes, and on years of experience in separating the blur of bewildering signs, atypical cases, and confusing symptoms that are the real world of disease.

The very distillation of brilliance, in this first stage, was represented by the "spot" diagnosis: the diagnosis born of such familiarity with pathophysiology that the doctor need scarcely look at the external signs of illness to know what was happening inside. For a "spot" or a "flash," you could dispense with stethoscope and percussion because you had spent a lifetime using them and already knew what they would reveal. The spot diagnosis was not publicized outside the medical world—it might have suggested irresponsibility or superficiality—but heroic "spot" tales were widely circulated inside, fortifying the profession's own pride in its flair, its "clinical instinct."

In 1934 one distinguished doctor recalled Christian Fenger's swiftness in diagnosing a particular case. "Ignoring my carefully written history, he pulled down the bed clothes, gave two or three prods in the right iliac region [right lower part of abdomen] and curtly announced 'osteosarcoma of the ilium; inoperable' and walked away."[21]

The Mayo Clinic's Dr. Walter Alvarez recalled his own residency in San Francisco, before World War I, with Dr. Emile Schmoll:

> Dr. Schmoll was the most brilliant "snap diagnostician" I have ever known. I remember the day a man came in and Schmoll, noting a glass eye, asked, "Was that eye removed for a little black tumor?"

"Yes," said the man.
"Now you have pains all over?"
"Yes."
Turning to me, Schmoll whispered, "Black cancer all over him."
And he was right. The man was soon dead.[22]

We see in these anecdotes two things: the profession's reverence for years of bedside experience, as opposed to biochemical lore, and the enormous value for the clinician of a solid knowledge of pathology, derived from the microscope and the autopsy table. James Mackenzie, a British cardiologist, illustrates this in his description of one of his mentors at the Royal Infirmary in Edinburgh in the 1870s:

A "powerful young man was brought in evidently ill." He'd had shaking chills and a high fever, but aside from that nothing was obviously wrong. "While we were puzzling as to the nature of the trouble, our teacher came into the hospital and I brought him to this patient. He merely looked at his face, felt his pulse and turned away and said, 'Going to have pneumonia,' and then, in a low voice, 'He will do no good.' The diagnosis was correct. The patient developed a pneumonia and died in a few days." It was the "undefinable impressions," explained Mackenzie, that permitted such snap diagnoses. Only a lifetime of bedside medicine would permit one to recognize that in pneumonia cases there is a "slightly dusky tinge of the countenance, with a faint blueness of the lips, and the pulse is large, with no sustained force, and rapid—a pulse difficult to describe. . . ."[23] These undefinable impressions enhanced greatly the doctors' regard for their own art.

In a second wave of diagnostic advances, the clinician's instinct would be supplemented by some very hard and reliable data on what was going on, and then the confidence of the public would be won as well. In roughly the years 1900 to 1940 the average family doctor was to acquire a new technology for diagnosing that was both effective in its own terms and inspiring to the patient.

As we saw above, a good clinician is alert for signs (information that *he* detects in the patient, such as heart murmurs) and "symptoms" (information the patient reports). With these signs and symptoms one can diagnose many of the ailments of mankind. The problem is that these distinctive clinical landmarks often show up only late in a disease, when the patient is about to die, the lung entirely destroyed, the heart faltering. *Early* in disease these signs and symptoms are often lacking or highly ambiguous, a phenomenon that exasperated William Mackenzie in his early days in general practice: "I found that most of the patients had no physical signs, and often such physical signs as I detected had no seeming relation to their complaints."[24]

Into this breach strode the X-ray machine, first used medically in 1895, when Wilhelm Roentgen made an X-ray of his wife's hand. Take the example of aneurysms of the thoracic aorta—pouches in the wall of that great artery that fill with blood, balloon out, and may burst, with fatal results. Before the X-ray, their evidence could sometimes be divined after an elaborate song and dance with palpation, percussion, and the eliciting of a number of obscure signs that might or might not reveal something (does the patient's chest sound different with his mouth open than closed?). But an aneurysm shows up nicely on an X-ray film because of all the fluid in it and can easily be spotted in a film of the chest, appearing as a big gray shadow above and beside the heart. All this was appreciated within a couple of years of Roentgen's discovery, and by 1906 medical textbooks, such as the famous one by William Osler, were counseling doctors to send their patients for X-ray if they suspected an aneurysm.[25] (Not that the doctor could do much about an aneurysm after he diagnosed one.)

GPs don't spend a lot of time diagnosing aneurysms, but they did, in those days, agonize endlessly about lung TB. There the X-ray had its greatest impact, freeing the family doctor from the cult of obscure signs and enabling him to see whether there was "cloudiness" in the film of the lungs. "I recently admitted to hospital a girl aged 10 years suffering from asthma," wrote one doctor in 1930. "A skiagram [X-ray film] showed a large calcified gland" in a certain part of the lung, evidence of healed TB. OK, no problem. But three weeks later "her sister aged 3 years was brought to see me. The only abnormal sign was a slight impairment of the percussion note at the base of the right lung. The breath sounds over this area were normal, and the child's appearance was healthy." An X-ray of the lung, however, showed extensive pleurisy (a discharge into the lining of the lung). "The condition was almost certainly tuberculosis. Here, then, were two children in the same family suffering from a mild tuberculous infection, in one case healed and in the other still active. The mother denied symptoms, but consented to be examined."

The mother did have a few signs, but appeared healthy. Her X-ray, however, showed extensive tuberculous changes in both lungs: "definite evidence of a tuberculous fibrosis of both lung apices."[26] There wasn't much the doctor could *do* for this family, aside from advising them to rest, maybe sending the daughters to the countryside, and trying to keep them from infecting others. But he had made the *diagnosis*.

Most physicians did not acquire their own X-ray machines. Even in the 1950s fewer than half of all American GPs had one in their office.[27] GPs sent their patients out for the X-ray, but even so, the machine's existence enormously fortified patients' confidence in the doctor. Patients would come in asking for an "X-ray all over" to see whether they were all right. Even a lot of doctors misunderstood the device's limitations. One sent a female patient who was short of breath to the radiologist, "saying he knew she had valvular heart disease but wanted me to use the X-ray to see just how badly the valves were affected."[28] The machine was useless for that purpose, but in viewing fractures, finding ulcers, and differentiating tuberculosis from flu it was amazingly useful.

Another technological form of diagnosis is measuring the pressure of the blood as it goes through the arteries. This is important because high blood pressure (*hypertension*) can cause strokes and kidney failure, to say nothing of heart failure, as the heart slowly weakens from pumping against the body's contracted blood vessels. Before the invention of measurement devices, doctors had virtually no knowledge of the existence of high blood pressure. Osler's textbook did not refer to "increased tension" of the blood until its fourth edition in 1906.[29]

The principle of determining blood pressure is quite straightforward. The doctor puts a rubber cuff around the patient's arm and pumps it full of air until the expanded cuff cuts off the circulation of the blood. He then puts his stethoscope against an artery in the pit of the elbow and listens, while slowly releasing the air in the cuff. The point at which he can hear blood starting to circulate through the artery again is the maximum, or *systolic*, blood pressure, in other words, the pressure just as the heart is contracting. The point at which the blood ceases to make noise in the artery—because it is now flowing so smoothly—is the minimum, or *diastolic*, blood pressure, the pressure when the heart is at rest. (We shall require a bit of this elementary physiology when we look at the dying of Franklin D. Roosevelt.) Thus blood pressure might be expressed in such terms as "120 over 70."

The technology for these measurements was worked out in the last quarter of the nineteenth century. In 1912, doctors at the Massachusetts General Hospital started routinely taking the blood pressure of every patient they admitted.[30] By the 1920s most family doctors had blood pressure cuffs and measuring devices (*sphygmomanometers*).[31]

Yet far more important in assessing what's happening to the heart is the direct measurement of its electrical activity. This is done with the *ECG*, or *electrocardiograph*, which is the last technological device we shall discuss. By attaching electrodes to a person's chest, arms, and legs, the physician can measure spread of electric current through the heart muscle. Accordingly, the ECG tracing is useful in keeping track of damage to the heart muscle suffered in a heart attack (because the current no longer passes through the fibrosed scar tissue) or in watching the left side of the heart enlarge as the heart, beginning to fail, pumps harder and harder. Since over half of all deaths in America today result from heart problems, the significance of this kind of measurement is obvious.

Although the ECG was invented by Willem Einthoven in the Netherlands in 1901, it wasn't until 1910, in Thomas Lewis's appendix to Mackenzie's *Diseases of the Heart*, that the device was introduced to medicine[32]—and even then, slowly. The first ECG tracing in Osler's textbook does not appear until the ninth edition in 1923.[33] Only in the 1930s are the various leads that show activity in the heart from several dimensions worked out. The Sandorn Cardiette, which became available in the mid-1930s, then made the use of ECG accessible to the general practitioner, "provided he was trained to interpret its tracings."[34] One study in the late 1930s estimated that GPs would become sufficiently capable of using the ECG, fluoroscopy, and other measurement devices that only 3 of every 100 heart disease cases would have to be referred.[35] That figure may have been optimistic, but it is true that by the early 1950s almost half of all GPs had ECG machines in their offices.[36]

For our purpose what is important about the ECGs is not their technical ins and outs, but the climate of scientific precision they created in the doctor's office. In 1953 the British journal *The Practitioner* published typical floor plans of American doctors' offices. Illustrated were ECG rooms; rooms for fluoroscopy, X-ray, and basal metabolism tests; recovery rooms for patients having minor operations, offices for secretaries and record storage, and dressing rooms for two or three patients at a time. "Obviously, this plan is extravagant by any British standards," noted the authors, consumed by envy, who then went on to describe the American doctor and his secretary. "On being shown into the consulting room by an attractive secretary in a light grey dress with a yellow scarf, we were surprised to find the doctor in black patent shoes, light grey suit, white shirt, and primrose yellow tie."[37] These poor Brits, just pulling themselves out of their war-torn ruins: welcome to scientific medicine.

These aids to diagnosis mattered for three reasons: (1) they permitted the doctor actually to make the right diagnosis in the majority of cases; (2) they would, as Daniel Cathell put it, "aid you greatly in curing people by heightening their confidence in you and enlisting their co-operation"[38]; and (3) they permitted the doctor to give the patient a prognosis.

Patients didn't really care all that much about the complexities of aortic aneurysm. They wanted to know whether they were going to get better. "Let it be understood," said a San Francisco doctor in 1923, "that patients are not so keen to know the minutiae of the diagnosis as they are to learn how long they are to be sick. They will insist on knowing when they will be well and 'how much it will cost.' "[39] This the doctor was able to tell them, in ballpark terms, once he knew exactly what ailed them, and all kinds of prognostications were worked out: "Now if we could say, as I hope before long we can: 'Pneumonia when due to the micrococcus lanceolatus ends by crisis, when due to the strepto-coccus by lysis'—what a godsend it would be!" wrote Harvard's Richard Cabot in 1906. *Crisis* was sweating, then a quick recovery; *lysis* was a slow recovery. A patient would want to know which lay ahead, instead of hearing such predictions as "Sometimes pneumonia ends by crisis, sometimes not."[40]

All this scientific medicine, in other words, would impress the laity by persuading them that the doctor had the power to see the future. As James Mackenzie put it, "The patient has not only a confidence in the doctor's power of diagnosis, but also believes he possesses the knowledge which will enable him to foretell the progress of the disease. . . ."[41]

THE DOCTOR AT WORK: TREATMENT

It was good that the modern doctor had the power to foretell the patient's future, because he could do relatively little else to help him. The fact is that, despite the advances we have just seen, the modern doctor's power to cure was only a little better than the traditional doctor's. But for our discussion, that fact is relatively unimportant. What did matter around 1900 was the patient's confidence in the doctor as a man of science. The few new drugs that burst upon the scene increased this confidence.

I'd like to leap ahead briefly to the argument of coming chapters. The problem today is not that patients don't believe in their doctors' scientific qualities. They do: but that scientific status centers almost exclusively on drugs. The torrent of effective drugs perfected since the 1940s has given medicine a gleaming high-tech allure.

Patients of today go to the doctor because they must go through him to get the drugs they know are truly powerful. This infuriates many of them, for like traditional patients they know very well what they want. The doctor is there merely to write it out for them. By contrast, the modern doctor of 1900 possessed inspirational qualities that enabled him to heal patients by suggestion: meaning, with an arsenal of drugs that were by and large worthless.

We must distinguish between the diseases the modern doctor could actually cure, those he thought he could cure, and those the patient thought he could cure. What drugs did the doctor have that actually worked? First of all he could relieve pain, not just the physical pain that goes with burns and bruises, but the pains of depression, anxiety and mental upset that arise in the mind. To patients, these pains can be every bit as real as the physical pains of cancer. Even though doctors have generally thought of lifesaving as their main function, "It is the relief of the pain that chiefly interests the patient," said a country doctor, "and skill along this line is the big factor . . . in general practice."[42]

Since the days of Theophrastus in the third century B.C., doctors have known about opium for pain. And opium, or the juice of the poppy (the milky exudate of the unripe seed capsules of *Papaver somniferum*), taken orally, does provide some relief. But the potent painkillers in opium are the twenty-odd "alkaloids" it contains, and these started to be isolated and reproduced synthetically only in the nineteenth century. Morphine (discovered in 1806) was the first, followed by codeine in 1832, and heroin in 1898.[43] Raw opium can't be injected because of its impurities, but these alkaloids *can* be, and they give a terrific rush as they travel through the blood to hit the brain. The injecting of morphine began in 1844. Of course there's always a lag between the first time something is done and the time it achieves popularity.[44] John Black, an obstetrician in small-town Delaware, bought his first hypodermic syringe in Paris in 1866, four years after finishing medical school. It had gold needles, "and to this day it has served me well."[45]

Before the narcotic control legislation of 1914, doctors administered morphine with astonishing liberality. "Above all else, have with you a supply of morphia granules," Daniel Cathell exhorted his colleagues, "and show your power over pain." The doctor might "administer a nightcap of morphine to the Rev. Mr. Cantsleep at 8 o'clock, to Mrs. Allnerves at 9, to Colonel Bigdrinks at 10, and to Miss Naryawink at 11 o'clock," and thus—in addition to addicting his patients—be adored by them as a "healer."[46] We have, for example, "Jimmy," a patient in late-nineteenth-century small-town Illinois, who "began complaining about outrageous pains in his legs. His general practitioner, thereupon, once each week or ten days, would administer a hypodermic of morphine. Then the man would sleep deeply. . . ."[47] Under such therapeutic regimens, the United States in 1891–1892 consumed 587,000 pounds of opium.[48]

The organic chemical industry of the nineteenth century created a number of synthetic drugs for patients who were in psychological distress but whom the family doctor did not want to risk addicting to morphine. Because they figured prominently in medical practice until quite recently, I mention them briefly:

- Chloral hydrate *was first made by the German chemist Justus Liebig in 1832 and first used as a sedative and sleeping potion in 1869. "Chloral," a standard prop in any melodrama before World War II, circulated in the world of lonely divorcees and tense businessmen. It relieved anxiety and insomnia but tasted awful and upset the stomach.*

- *The* barbiturates *were derivatives of Adolph von Bayer's barbituric acid. The first of them,* barbital, *was introduced into medicine in 1903 under the trade name* Veronal. Phenobarbital, *sold as* Luminal, *followed in 1912, and over the following years came fifty or so other derivatives. They were basically sedatives and were enormously popular among family doctors because of their ability to calm patients with high blood pressure, relieve epileptic fits, and assuage anxiety. A small-town doctor in Ontario called Luminal "indispensable." "I bought Luminal tablets in five-thousand lots every few months. . . . One patient who comes to mind took five grains three times a day for months. . . . He was a tense and highly excitable person, but the use of Luminal quieted him and helped keep his blood pressure within reasonable limits, contributing to his longevity of 94 years."[49]*

From the cornucopia of the German organic chemical industry poured forth a series of highly useful minor painkillers. Sold under names like *Tylenol* and *Anacin* today, they were once drugs that doctors prescribed for patients, although they (like all other drugs in those days) could be purchased over the counter as well:

- Acetaminophen, *first used in medicine in 1893, was an off-spring of a drug called* antifebrin *that had hit the market six years earlier. Acetaminophen had marvelous results against fever and pain.*[50] *It's the main ingredient today in a number of antipyretics and analgesics.*

- Aspirin *is the current generic name for a drug that in the United States now sells between ten and twenty thousand tons annually. It goes back to an ingredient in the bark of the willow tree. In 1838 a chemist made salicylic acid from this ingredient, and twenty years later somebody else figured out how to make this acid artificially from phenol. Thus the* salicylates, *derivatives of salicylic acid that turned out to be effective against the pain of maladies like gout, were born. Then in 1899 a chemist made a further change to salicylic acid and sold the patent to the Bayer Company, which proceeded to call it* aspirin. *Aspirin, like acetaminophen, relieves pain and fever and also works against* inflammation. *Thus the doctor acquired for his bag a drug that would partially relieve arthritis, rheumatism, and other inflammatory conditions of muscle and bone. In the early years it was advertised only to physicians in medical journals (an "ethical" drug) and not to the public.*

The other effective drugs in the doctor's bag were somewhat limited in scope:

- *Not many people got malaria, but doctors had for it a drug derived from the bark of the cinchona tree:* quinine. *The Jesuits brought the bark back from South America in the seventeenth century, and early in the nineteenth century the active principle, quinine, was isolated. Quinine is not particularly effective against fever in general but does work specifically against the parasite causing malaria.*

- Ether and chloroform, *first used medically in the 1840s, were terribly important in childbirth and surgical operations; they were reassuring to have in one's bag, in the event that one ended up removing gallstones or an appendix on a patient's kitchen table, a not uncommon event before World War I, referred to at the time as "minor surgery."*

- *An* antitoxin *against diphtheria developed early in the 1890s; inoculating children with it in advance could counter the ef-*

fects of the toxin *that the disease produces. The sensation that the drug caused among the public was important in fostering the image of the doctor as a miracle worker.*

- *Drugs to help the failing heart. We have already seen* digitalis *tried in the eighteenth century for heart disease, and then falling into oblivion after people became disillusioned with its failure as a panacea. It was revived early in the twentieth century by James Mackenzie[51] and would help succor the dying President Roosevelt. For short-term relief in* angina (*pain from the heart's shortage of oxygen*) *doctors in the later nineteenth century gave the* organic nitrates: amyl nitrite, *first used for angina in 1857, and* nitroglycerin, *first taken under the tongue for angina twenty years later. Both drugs open up the arteries of the heart for brief spells and permit an increased flow of blood to reach the heart muscle.*

- *Syphilis was not very common, but there was a widespread sigh of relief when in 1910 Paul Ehrlich announced the discovery of a specific drug against it: another German organic chemical product with arsenic attached. The Germans marketed the drug as* Salvarsan, *and so essential was it thought to be in the practice of medicine that after World War I broke out, Congress suspended the German patent and permitted several American laboratories to continue making the drug under the trade name* Arsphenamine. *It did not actually cure syphilis, but it checked the progress of the disease and ensured that the patient wouldn't transmit it.[52]*

- *Finally, to conclude this chronicle of what the doctor could do, the discoveries of insulin in 1922 and of liver extract as a cure for pernicious anemia in 1926 caused an enormous sensation. But they come already toward the end of the period I have designated as modern, and the prestige of the modern doctor had by that time become established.*

That was it. Those were the diseases medicine could cure or palliate. The doctors' prestige clearly rested on qualities other than their talents as "healers." Yet they thought of themselves as healers and believed, falsely, that they could cure a much wider range of afflictions. I want to illustrate this point briefly, because it helps account for their own self-esteem, an important factor in our story.

It is not that physicians continued to be attached to the *traditional* drugs that didn't work. The therapeutic nihilism of the 1880s and 1890s had discredited most of the elaborate compounds of yesteryear. But doctors were attached to a number of "modern" drugs, especially patent medicines, that had little value: to germicides, antiseptics, the bromides and iodides, aconite, strychnine, camphor taken internally, and collargal to stimulate a "colloidal reaction" in infections; there is a long list. "Is there a medical man on earth who would stand with folded arms," asked Daniel Cathell in the 1920s, "and let intermittent and remittent fevers take their course without drugs?" Sepsis, gout, peritonitis, hysteria: Cathell claimed that the physician could treat them all. If there were such a "medico anywhere who does not sincerely believe in his power to help Nature to help herself in many of the twenty-four hundred diseases . . . to which mankind is subject, he is a medical infidel, and should at once take down his sign and burn his diploma."[53] However, drug treatment in the 1920s was quite ineffective for most of the diseases he listed.

The patients' expectations of what the doctor could prescribe, however, exceeded what even the doctors themselves thought possible. The traditional patients' implicit confidence in the doctor's drugs had not weakened by the early twentieth century, even though the modern doctors themselves retained far less confidence in pharmacy. The few *effective* drugs of the early twentieth century merely confirmed patients' belief that medicine could offer true cures. Therefore, they expected every consultation to end with a prescription.

Consider the pediatrician called to treat "little Jimmy with the measles." There was no drug for people who had contracted measles (nor is there today, although we have a vaccine). So the scientific doctor would simply "leave detailed instructions for nursing care and [go] without having given a prescription for drugs; the tidings of this remarkable procedure may safely be expected to have spread through all the neighbourhood by nightfall." When little Jimmy's cough and fever hung on after two months, "and the child was kept in bed . . . and still no drugs, suggestions came pouring in from lay advisers. Some wagged their heads, and some said, 'Why send for such a doctor?' " William Houston, a distiguished Georgia physician who gives us this anecdote, urged the doctor to resist these entreaties for a prescription. "The young practitioner does well to remember that his client sent for him, very likely because he thought him freshly supplied with the latest utterances from the oracles of modern science, and that 'modern' is now a word to conjure with."[54]

The inrush of science into medicine had thus created an incipient tug-of-war between doctor and patient: the patient, terribly impressed at the doctor's new skills of diagnosis and prognosis, all the more readily believed that new drugs would cure. The doctor, although inclined by training to therapeutic nihilism, would easily give in and fill out a "script," partly from fear of losing his practice and partly from a very human desire to ease anxiety. After all, the drugs were innocuous, so why not oblige the patient? Later we shall turn to the much fiercer tug-of-war taking place today, over drugs that are not innocuous.

The Modern Doctor and the Death of Franklin Delano Roosevelt

Can you think of any patient better doctored than the president of the United States? He has, night and day, a personal physician at his side. At his call are the best consultants in the country. In the early 1940s the country is in the midst of a terrible war, its forces under the president's command. Nothing could be more urgent than preserving his health. Franklin Roosevelt's ordeal with high blood pressure, heart failure, and stroke lets us see therefore, exactly what the modern doctor could, and could not, do.[55]

FDR had been crippled in both legs by a severe attack of polio in 1921. He suffered a bout of flu late in 1943, and after that had a series of what seemed like colds. He felt tired, and his stomach had started to swell out. When Dr. Howard Bruenn, a distinguished cardiologist who was at that time serving in the Naval Reserve, saw the president on 27 March 1944, "he appeared to be

very tired, and his face was very gray. Moving caused considerable breathlessness."

Dr. Bruenn performed fluoroscopy and X-rays of the chest the
following day and gave the president an ECG. (Why his earlier
doctors hadn't done this is a mystery.) The president's heart was
enlarged, his blood pressure was 186 over 108, and the ECG
tracing (see Plate 17) was alarming. Dr. Bruenn diagnosed "hypertension, hypertensive heart disease, cardiac failure (left ven-
tricular), and acute bronchitis."

"These findings and their interpretation were conveyed to
Surgeon General McIntire. They had been completely unsus-
pected up to this time."(!) The president's regular doctors had no
idea what was going on until Dr. Bruenn applied this new diagnostic technique.

But now the question was, what to do? How did you treat a
president who refused to take to his bed and who could not, for
obvious reasons, be heavily sedated? They gave the president
aminophylline (a mild heart stimulant similar to caffeine) and
phenobarbital, and when he didn't respond to that, administered
digitalis three days later. One of the things you do with congestive heart failure is try to get the blood volume down. Therefore,
Dr. Bruenn suggested giving the president another new drug to
make him urinate, a mercurial diuretic, which was different from
the old calomel compounds in being soluble and therefore inject-
able. But the committee of doctors looking after the president
voted this down, deciding that "in view of the complexity of the
situation as little medication as possible be used at this time."

The president responded to the digitalis. Two weeks later
X-rays showed that his heart had grown smaller and that his
lungs were clearing up from the congestion caused by his episode
of heart failure. But his blood pressure remained 210 over 120.
Indeed, his hypertension would ultimately kill him.

Bruenn became, essentially, the president's shadow. They traveled for a rest to Bernard Baruch's estate, Hobcaw, in South
Carolina. They traveled by private train across the country to
San Diego, where on 20 July 1944 Roosevelt accepted the Demo-
crats' nomination for a fourth term. Dr. Bruenn would see the
president every morning around nine, ask him how he felt, exam-

ine his heart and lungs, and take his blood pressure. "At no time did the President ever comment on the frequency of these visits or question the reasons for the electrocardiograms . . . nor did he ever have any questions as to the type and variety of medications that were used." He was a perfect "modern" patient, in contrast to the postmodern variety that we shall see later.

Bruenn sailed with the president on the heavy cruiser USS *Baltimore* into the Pacific, then back to Washington. FDR was on and off "phenobarb" and "dig" over this time, and as the election campaign swept him up in October, his blood pressure was lower. The therapy was working.

In January 1945, Bruenn and the president sailed for Yalta. At this point the picture started to darken. The Big Three—FDR, Churchill, and Stalin—would usually start conferring at four in the afternoon, talk for three or four hours, and then have dinner. "On February 8, after an especially arduous day and an emotionally disturbing conference" [they were settling the future of Poland], the president "was obviously greatly fatigued. His color was very poor (gray)." And his blood pressure showed, for the first time, *pulsus alternans*, alternating strong and weak beats that are a sign that the heart is in trouble. Back at sea FDR bcame further upset over the shipboard death, from a stroke, of his military aide and close friend General Edwin Watson. Now wide swings began to appear in his blood pressure, even though he otherwise seemed well.

FDR returned to Washington for a bit. But "by the end of March he began to look bad. His color was poor, and he appeared to be very tired." On 29 March he and Dr. Bruenn left for Warm Springs, Georgia, where the end came. FDR's blood pressure had been as high as 240 over 130. (Normal is around 130 over 70.) His arteries were under extreme pressure.

"On April 12 I saw the President at 9:20 A.M., a few minutes after he had awakened. He had slept well but complained of a slight headache and some stiffness of the neck."

After a morning spent going over state papers, and during which "his guests commented on how well he looked," Roosevelt "suddenly complained of a terrific occipital [back of head] headache. He became unconscious a minute or two later."

FDR's blood pressure was now 300 over 190. "It was apparent

that the President had suffered a massive cerebral hemorrhage."
Dr. Bruenn gave FDR a number of drugs to strengthen the heart.
But the president never regained consciousness, dying at 3:35 that
afternoon.

The following features are interesting for us:

1. *If FDR had had his first episode of congestive heart failure
fifty years earlier, he would have been a goner. James Mackenzie revived digitalis only in 1908, and phenobarbital didn't
come along until 1912. Thus in all likelihood "modern medicine" procured FDR another year of life.*

2. *Despite modern medicine, there was nothing FDR's doctors
could do for his high blood pressure. They had only a tranquilizer at their disposal, nothing with any specific action on the
blood vessels, whose puzzling narrowing causes the blood
pressure to rise.*

3. *In contrast to traditional doctors, FDR's attendants definitely
did know "what was going on." With X-rays they could see
how big the heart had become, and by interpreting ECGs (see
Plate 17) they learned that the heart wasn't getting enough oxygen: deep inversion of "T waves" in leads I and CF. The diagnosis was clear. (The "T wave," corresponding to the recovery
of the ventricles, normally appears as a little blip above the center line. In lead I especially, we see it dipping down.)*

   *But remember that Dr. Bruenn represented the commanding
heights of medicine. In ordinary practice things were sometimes a little less clear. FDR's personal doctor had had no inkling at all that the president was experiencing heart failure. A
man like Arthur Hertzler, the country doctor who went on to
become a distinguished Kansas physician, confessed in his 1938
autobiography, "I have never learned to determine heart murmurs; but, after all, if one can estimate what the heart is doing
. . . he gets along very well in ordinary clinical work. At least,
that is the ointment I used for salving my ignorance."[56] And a
1953 survey of GPs in North Carolina discovered that a third
of them did not understand what they were doing when they
treated patients for congestive heart failure; they failed to explain to patients the need to restrict salt in their diet, and so
forth.[57] So even though modern medicine had acquired some
ability to "make the diagnosis," we must remember that this
skill had real limits.*

4. *Finally, the main reason FDR was followed so carefully was*

101

that he was president. In those days elderly patients in particular were not treated aggressively for congestive heart failure and would mainly be given morphine and prescriptions for bed rest until the end came.[58]

We will shortly see how different postmodern medicine is on most of these points.

THE MODERN DOCTOR RISES IN HIS OWN SELF-ESTEEM

Flushed with very real diagnostic and partly imaginary therapeutic successes, the modern doctor began to think increasingly well of himself. I am not trying to prick anybody's balloon; any group can retrospectively be made to sound ludicrous in its self-congratulation—historians, too. But the doctors' improving self-image enters our story in a curious way: once medical men began imagining themselves to be socially a notch or two above everybody else, their ability to cure psychological disease increased correspondingly. One precondition for healing by suggestion was the patient's implicit belief in the doctor's healing power. This belief was much easier to inspire when the doctor stood several rungs higher socially than the patient.

To understand how medicine came to be identified with upper-middle-class life we must remember that after around 1910 it began to be difficult to get into medical school. For example, in 1914 Harvard began limiting the size of its incoming class to 125.[59] The number of doctors in American society began declining as proprietary medical schools folded because of new regulations. Doctors started to be a scarce commodity, able to charge more for their services.

A "better sort" of medical student, in social terms, appears. Harvard's President Charles Eliot wrote of the Medical School in his 1879–1880 report,

An American physician or surgeon may be, and often is, a coarse and uneducated person ... unable to either write or speak his mother tongue with accuracy. . . . In this University, until the reformation of the School in 1870–71, the medical students were noticeably inferior in bearing, manners, and discipline to the students of other departments; they are now indistinguishable from the other students.[60]

And as these bright, upscale young men poured onto the wards they would beam forth a new image of crisp, socially smart science. A visiting European physician wrote in 1912 of his medical impressions of America, "Whenever I met of a group of those smartly-groomed internes, with their clean-shaven, energetic faces, I could not help saying to myself as they sized me up: 'They are evidently speculating whether I have not got chronic appendicitis.' "[61]

Once out in practice, a young doctor had to make his way in society. We are no longer talking about barely eking out a living by lancing boils. We are talking about community *leaders.* The doctor "will be made a more important man in the community," said Charles Dunn in 1913. "He will be called into public as well as private affairs. And as one who can manage the health of a nation, or of a community, he has a greater function than . . . prescribing for an individual. Medicine will become a part of statecraft; doctors will direct affairs more, and lawyers less."[62]

How do you become a community leader? Young Doctor Franklin Martin, fresh out of medical school in Chicago in the 1880s, first had to be taken on at a "desirable" boarding house. He went to a tony one with a "long waiting list," run by two maiden ladies, down on Wabash Avenue.

"Proudly, but rather doubtfully, thinking of the long waiting list, I [said], 'My name is Dr. Martin. . . . I was wanting to inquire about board.' "

When Miss Ellen heard that he'd been living in his office, she frowned and said no. But then "Miss Nellie, a comely niece and the third of the triumvirate," saw that he was an eligible male and implored her aunt to take Dr. Martin on, thus launching his social career in Chicago.

Next step for Dr. Martin was getting a desirable pew at Plymouth Church, then enrolling in "Bourniques' Dancing Academy" on Twenty-fourth Street, then being included at the performance of a drama club, "a select group of young people residing in the vicinity."

The better to distinguish themselves from the medical rabble of the day, Dr. Martin and some friends founded "The Chicago South-Side Medico-Social Society," and for twenty years they met at the Southern Hotel: "Dinner at seven o'clock sharp; formal dress and white tie," followed by a paper. "Parliamentary rules were insisted on."[63] This is the behavior of the parvenu, the arriviste, but these young men were on their way up.

GPs in smaller towns as well were becoming "local squires." "Remember that a doctor's family should move in good society 'and wear good clothes,' " wrote a Kentucky doctor. "You should consider that the wife is to be the 'first lady' at the same time that you are playing the role of first citizen of the county. . . . Yes, you will find that your profession will be remunerative enough for you to live like a gentleman."[64]

How did one live like a gentleman? There were new rules, unfamiliar to many rough-hewn frontier practitioners but part of that grand tradition of the Royal Colleges in England to which American medicine now aspired:

- *As a gentleman, you joined clubs and community organizations, where you would meet "all the active people of your locality. You can learn to know those of the better class," and especially meet "more men each week at the luncheon table."[65]*

- *A gentleman did not dun clients for payment, as though he were some kind of grocer. Michael Lepore reflected upon the pre–World War II years: "Physicians of that era were trained and bred to feel that financial matters were below the dignity of a true physician. This was the era when almost no one spoke of fees and bills were seldom sent to patients. . . . Collection agencies were anathema, and advertising of fees was only for quacks." As Cathell warned, a gentleman should not come across as "Dr. Grabber," "Dr. Badegg," or "Dr. Hogg."[66]*

- *A gentleman did not get into fist fights. Contrast the brawling frontier physicians we saw previously with the horror of young*

Dr. *"Stark Munro"* (*Conan Doyle's fictitious alter-ego*) *at be-coming involved in fisticuffs when he arrived in town to set up practice. On a stroll he noticed that "a crowd of people had gathered, with a swirl in the centre. I was, of course, absolutely determined not to get mixed up in any row." But nonetheless he couldn't help seeing that "a woman, pinched and bedraggled, with a baby on her arm, was being knocked about by a burly brute of a fellow whom I judged to be her husband. . . . He was one of those red-faced, dark-eyed men who can look peculiarly malignant when they choose" and was drunk to boot. "Dr. Munro" then stepped up to the brute and said, "Come, come, my lad! Pull yourself together."*

Instead the brute hit the young doctor, and Dr. Munro re-sponded in kind. "So there, my dear Bertie, was I, within a few hours of my entrance into this town, with my top-hat down to my ears, my highly professional frock-coat, and my kid gloves, fighting some low bruiser on a pedestal in one of the most public places, in the heart of a yelling and hostile mob."[67] Just what a tony young doctor needed, in other words.

- *The gentleman-physician would be at pains to locate his office in a "genteel neighborhood." Don't suggest to the public "de-fective ambition or distrust of your own acquirements," coun-seled Dr. Cathell. "Clean hands, polished boots, neat cuffs, gloves, fashionable clothing, cane, sun umbrella [!], all indicate gentility." How does a gentleman get around? "You should get a respectable-looking horse and carriage, as soon as circum-stances will possibly justify."[68]*

- *The gentleman, finally, would take care to treat patients and laity appropriately. "Freeze off all attempts to 'Hallo Doc!'" advised Cathell. Don't make a practice of giving your photo-graph to everyone, he went on.[69]*

This last makes the doctors sound like snobs. But there were advantages for patients in the doctor's presumed gentility. The "first-name" issue much vexes doctor-patient relations today, and many women in particular dislike their physicians' referring to them by their given names. But bon ton in the 1930s called for politeness. Clinicians such as Columbia-Presbyterian's Dr. Rob-ert Loeb insisted that, in Michael Lepore's words, "the poorest and most undesirable patient was accorded the respect owed to his being ill. No patient, whether he was on the ward or in the most expensive private room, was addressed by his first name . . . unless he was a personal friend."[70]

It is bad form for gentlemen to appear to be technicians or un-cultivated, narrow specialists. When we later ask, Why were these "modern" doctors so interested in the patient as a whole, the answer will partly be that it was good manners: a gentleman expresses noblesse oblige, rather than limiting himself to the technical aspects of disease. Michael Lepore looks back, with some nostalgia, upon those years:

> By their own example, in the eyes of their students, caring for the patient became just as important as curing the disease. Who will ever forget having witnessed the aristocratic and fastidious Hugh Auchincloss, Sr., Professor of Surgery at Columbia Presbyterian, clearing a patient's "intestinal obstruction" on rounds by rolling up his gold cuff-linked shirtsleeves and digging out by hand, a large fecal impaction!"[71]

Note that he didn't ask a nurse to do it; he didn't ask the intern to do it; he did it himself because he wanted to show respect for the patient. The stage is now set for the awe-inspiring doctor, who socially towers miles above his patient, to become a healer of psychological disease. But first the patient must be made responsive to the healing touch.

CHAPTER FIVE
The Making of the Modern Patient

*T*HE MODERN patient had two defining characteristics: a greater sensitivity to the body's internal state and an implicit confidence in the doctor, not just as a conduit of drugs but as a healer. This first characteristic, the patient's new alertness to his body, arose early in the nineteenth century, perhaps even sooner among the upper classes, and was quite independent of any changes in medicine. The second characteristic, the modern patient's confidence that "science" could cure, was a direct consequence of the changes in medical practice we saw in the previous chapter. Both these new attributes resulted in a very different kind of doctor-patient relationship, one marked by the patient's willingness to accept "medical authority." It was a relationship that would start to unravel in the 1960s.

What was a "modern" patient? "Dr. Knock" created plenty of them when, in Jules Romains's 1923 play *Knock*, he purchased a rather feeble medical practice in a small French town. The first thing the penniless Knock tried to do was improve business by making people aware of their symptoms. "Les gens bien portant sont des malades qui s'ignorent," he said: "Well-appearing people are just patients who aren't aware of their true state."

So Dr. Knock began giving free consultations, the only way to alert the sturdy peasants of the district to the gravity of their internal states. He received a forty-eight-year-old peasant woman in black, "who breathed of avarice and constipation," and who had never previously been in care.

DR. KNOCK: If you and your husband run that farm yourselves, you must have a lot of work?

THE PEASANT WOMAN: Pensez, monsieur! Eighteen cows, two oxen, two bulls, the mare, the colt, a good dozen pigs, not to count the poultry.

DR. KNOCK: My sympathies. You must have very little time to take care of yourself?

THE PEASANT WOMAN: Very little.

DR. KNOCK: And so you feel sick?

THE PEASANT WOMAN: That's not really the word. It's more like tiredness.

DR. KNOCK: Yes, that's what you call tiredness. (He goes up to her.) Stick out your tongue. You probably don't have much appetite.

THE PEASANT WOMAN: No.

DR. KNOCK: You're constipated.

THE PEASANT WOMAN: Yes, quite.

Dr. Knock then pokes at her kidneys, asks her whether it hurts, and convinces her that she must have fallen from a ladder as a girl and thus acquired an illness that has now been gathering steam for forty years. He also informs her that a cure will cost a lot of money.

DR. KNOCK: But of course, if you'd like to try a pilgrimage, I won't stop you.

THE PEASANT WOMAN: No thanks. That costs a lot too and often doesn't work. (A silence.) But what could I possibly have that's so awful?

DR. KNOCK (draws a cross section of a spinal column on the board and explains to the woman that in the fall her "Türck's fasciculus" and her "column of Clarke" must have migrated a few millimeters in opposite directions): I agree that it's not a lot. But it's very badly situated. So you must have a constant twinging here on the multi-polars.

THE PEASANT WOMAN: Mon Dieu! Mon Dieu!

DR. KNOCK (tells her that to recover she must give herself constant care, lying down with the blinds closed, no solid food for two weeks except a bit of Vichy water): And if you should feel a sort of general weakness, a heaviness of the head, a certain sluggishness as you try to get up, we'll have to act. OK?

THE PEASANT WOMAN: Do as you see fit.

As the play ends, she and hundreds of other inhabitants of the small town have learned to "care for their symptoms," as the "pharmaco-medical spirit" spreads its wings. All now regularly seek prescriptions. Knock and his predecessor, who has returned for a visit, stand in the top floor of Knock's new hospital, looking out over the dusking scene.

DR. KNOCK: Just think that in a few minutes it will strike ten o'clock. For all my patients ten means the second daily taking of the rectal temperature, and in a few minutes two hundred and fifty thermometers will simultaneously slide in. . . .[1]

This was the sort of humor that made French audiences in the 1920s howl with laughter. But they appreciated Romains's point: medical "science" was uncovering a whole new world of patients and symptoms that cried out for treatment.

CONVERTING PEOPLE INTO PATIENTS

We may understand the avalanche of symptoms that began to shower upon modern medicine as having three different sources: new groups in the population that started demanding treatment, new organ systems that patients began singling out as needing care, and a general increase in patients' sensitivity to symptoms of any kind.

In the nineteenth century, what kinds of people would be

starting to see doctors for the first time? Par excellence, younger women and children. The dying elderly of either sex had always been treated. Country doctors in eighteenth-century England saw about equal numbers of gravely ill men and women, but most of them were middle-aged and elderly. Lots of lesser but still annoying conditions affect the human flesh. When these happened to younger women they were usually treated within the women's culture and not medically. Men, on the other hand, did tend to call doctors for the fractures, the hernias, the dislocated shoulders, that have plagued them since time out of mind.[2]

Thus, a major change in the profile of the "modern" patient was the arrival of younger women in the doctor's office, seeking care for themselves and their children. These new patients were so numerous, in fact, that they became the keystone of modern medical practice. (By the 1920s the average woman would go to the doctor 2.4 times a year, the average man 1.8. And although in the traditional period even gravely ill children rarely saw a doctor, by the 1920s the average child visited the doctor twice yearly.[3])

The women, as mothers of families, were taking their children to the doctor. So we must first see how women became installed in the doctor's office. The process began before any great change occurred in the practice of medicine itself, so one cannot argue that "modern science" led women to seek medical attention. Rather, a new pattern of sentiment in family life, an "emotionalizing" of human relationships, made people less stoical about suffering. For example, women's tolerance of "feminine ailments," once considered the curse of Eve, diminishes as pain and debility start to be regarded as major obstacles to personal romantic and sentimental fulfillment. Similarly, parents' tolerance of the pain and suffering of their children grows less as infant mortality is reduced and parents become more firmly attached to the children. This injection of sentiment into all kinds of connections that previously had been governed largely by the calculus of self-interest or by tradition is an enormous subject that I have treated at length in another book, and I shall not elaborate upon it here.[4] Suffice it to say that the sentimentalizing of family relations helped bring physicians into intimate contact with female patients.

In the early nineteenth century both doctors and women were aware of the physician's new access to the intimate side of women's lives. Worthington Hooker explained in 1849 that in enlisting the trust of the patient, the doctor is acting not merely as man of science but as a "confidential friend." "If he has been the physician of the family for any length of time ... this feeling of affectionate reliance is deep and ardent; so much so, that it is a severe trial to the sensitive mind to be obliged to consult a stranger. . . . Especially this is so when the patient is a female." The doctor is received in the "very bosom of those families," entrusted with all the secrets and burdens of the heart of the mothers and daughters. "I refer to the sympathy which he has felt with them in their seasons of suffering, anxiety, and affliction."[5] So a physician capable of listening, of empathy, was required to treat the complaints of a newly sentimentalized population.

Why so many women in the doctor's office? "There are several accidental reasons which increase the number of female applicants," wrote a doctor in small-town England in the early 1840s. "Men are less inclined to resort to physic for every passing ailment; they have less time and opportunity for doing so; from greater vigour of constitution and a more nourishing diet they are less seriously affected; their nervous system is less excitable and their moral sensibility less acute."[6] The man's analysis reflected all the male prejudices of his time against women, but he nonetheless was picking up a tremendous historical change: women were now seeking treatment for all kinds of genital, rectal, and internal complaints that previous doctors—whose knowledge of women was limited to "furor uterinus," the complications of childbirth and breast cancer—would not have seen.

This transformation occurred before the scientific revolution in medicine of the 1870s. After that revolution, doctors and women were drawn even more tightly into mutual dependence: the women on doctors for relief from a range of "nervous complaints" that will be an important subject in the next chapter, the doctor on women for his very livelihood. Looking back in the 1890s on forty years of medical practice, John Black, a small-town physician in Delaware, said, "Most of the practice of medicine has now to do with women and children."[7] These women went to the doctor not just because they were ill, but because they had started to acquire an implicit confidence in their doctors as healers. Few physicians understood this better than the Philadelphian S. Weir Mitchell, who, in addition to making important contributions to the development of neurology, played much the role of the "society nerve doctor." "No group of men," he wrote in 1887 (typifying the patronizing attitude toward women of his age), "so truly interprets, comprehends, and sympathizes with woman as do physicians, who know how near to disorder and how close to misfortune she is brought by the very peculiarities of her nature." He found women "far easier to deal with, far more amenable to reason, far more sure to be comfortable as a patient, than men in the same social bracket."[8]

That doctors appreciated the financial importance of their new therapeutic alliance with women is evident from the advice manuals written for the profession. Why is it useful to get an M.D. degree? asked the London surgeon Charles Keetley in 1878 (in Great Britain the degree *bachelor of medicine*, or *M.B.*, conferred permission to practice). "The chief value of the letters M.D. is that they produce an undoubted impression on the general public, especially upon the ladies; that they are necessary to the holders of some medical appointments, and that they are almost essential to consulting physicians."[9] And Daniel Cathell, whom we have already encountered many times as a streaming font of cynical advice, was categorical on the subject: "No one can succeed fully without the favorable opinion of the maids and matrons he meets in the sick room. The females of every family have a potent voice in selecting the family physician. I have often thought the secret why so many truly scientific aspirants fail to get practice, is that their manner and acquirements do not appeal to the female mind."[10]

Even in locating his office, the successful physician would keep the women in mind: "Endeavor to secure rooms on a shopping street," said a San Francisco doctor in 1923, "since this is the place where the women will come. . . . If you can get the women coming to your office, the men will follow." And once you had the women there, he added, furnish the office so they would feel comfortable. "One thing every treatment room should contain is a corner shut off by a small screen where the women may arrange their things and adjust their apparel. On a stand should be some of the toilet articles that women commonly use—a large mirror and a hand-mirror, comb and brush, powder jar and puffs."[11] All this was not merely a ploy to enlarge one's clientele. It represented a genuine belief, however misguided we may find it by today's standards, that women patients required treatment that would reach to the heart.

The women took their children with them. A major new group of patients were the pediatric ones. We find it hard today to comprehend how the illnesses of children were once medically neglected. In the diaries of eighteenth-century physicians, the only mentions of children occur in the context of disasters like smallpox epidemics, or the terminal diphtheria of an especially beloved child. Society generally displayed a casualness about infant death, of which the eighteenth-century villagers in Yorkshire's Chapel en le Frith were typical. James Clegg, who was both minister and doctor, tells us in his diary that on 14 March 1749, "I was called to baptize a child of William Carrington's of Whitehough Head called Peter. . . ." A week later, with no intervening references, we learn that "I was at home all the forenoon, in the afternoon I assisted in burying the child of Will Carrington (which I had lately baptized) at our chapel."[12] What happened? Why hadn't the Carrington family called him sooner? Called him at all for a failing infant? (This apparent parental indifference is something of a chicken-egg problem. Parents doubtlessly withdrew emotionally because they feared their children might die young. Yet precisely this emotional withdrawal, whether caused by fear of loss or other factors, *contributed* to the high infant mortality. On this see Shorter, *The Making of the Modern Family*, Chapter 5.)

During the nineteenth century children were discovered as patients. To be sure, medical writers had turned their attention to children from the mid-eighteenth century onward, urging mothers to employ breastfeeding and in other ways improve their care. But medical calls on child patients, physical examination in the office, and the general conversion of the child into a patient did not figure in the lives of most families until the second half of the nineteenth century. The new situation was a sign of parents' confidence in medicine as well as of their devotion.

How easily, however, could this devotion be manipulated! "I will suppose a case," said Hooker.

> A child is taken sick, and the parents are full of anxiety. The physician sees at once that the case is not at present a grave one, and that remedies will probably in a short time give relief. If he be honest he will say so, and remove the undue anxiety of the parents. But if he be disposed, as many are, to make capital out of the anxieties of his employers, he will say that the child *is* very sick, and perhaps that "it is well you have called me so soon," or "I wish that you had called me before, but I think on the whole that the little one *can* be relieved." Every physician knows how readily the imagination of a parent may be excited in relation to the symptoms of disease in a ailing child.[13]

Hooker was warning against monsters. In general, I do not accept the interpretation that the doctors were cunning fiends, drumming up business. I think that physicians, just as parents, saw in the child a precious little being who required a sentimental approach entirely unlike that for the adult. This special sentimentality was the justification for the emergence of pediatrics as a separate field late in the nineteenth century, for in terms of knowledge, pediatrics is little different from general internal medicine. Pediatricians had to learn the special sadness of illness in children. If they did not, they could not bear the burden (just as many doctors today cannot bear the burden of terminal illness in children, with the result that such fields as "pediatric hematology" are spoken of in hushed tones by the rest of the profession). A doctor who does not adjust his own sentimental reflexes for children "goes to extremes, loses judgment, and does too little. I once saw a very young physician," Mitchell said, "burst into tears at the sight of a burnt child, a charming little girl. He was practically useless for the time."[14] Thus the sentimentality of the nineteenth century created new kinds of patients, and new kinds of doctors to deal with them.

Another way the modern patient differed from the traditional one was in the discovery of new kinds of symptoms. The late nineteenth century saw an attentiveness to areas of the body that the old-style patient had seldom considered. After 1900 the cardiovascular system came to preoccupy millions of people, especially when there were problems with pressure of the blood. Before 1900 patients had been quite absorbed in what happened to the blood once it was *outside* the body: whether it crusted properly in the barber-surgeon's cup. But patients after 1900, aided by the doctor's pressure cuff, became obsessed with the course of blood inside the body: hence occurred a massive rise in awareness of hypertension and hypotension around the turn of the century, a direct consequence of the physical examination.

Many feared their blood pressure was insufficient, generally a baseless fear unless one is actually dying. "Owing to a misconception of the true facts of the case," wrote a London physician in 1938,

> I venture to assert that a large proportion of the population are at present firmly convinced that their blood pressures are too low, and suffer accordingly. I assure you that for some time past whenever I begin to apply the armlet to my patients they almost invariably remark, "I'm afraid you will find it too low, doctor!"[15]

In the cossetted little world of the continental health spa, ceaseless agonizing about supposed hypotension was the order of the day, echoes of which are heard even now. A London doctor asked in 1967, "How comes it that so many patients from other European countries seek treatment for liver disease or low blood pressure? Surely these are people who once went to a doctor when they were anxious or unhappy and came away believing in a mythical illness. . . ."[16]

High blood pressure, unfortunately, is not a mythical illness, and people who have it do well to seek treatment. Again, it was discovered only at the beginning of our century, and then was ascribed to every cause imaginable: infected teeth, constipation, "a disease of American life," "fast-paced city existence," and so on. None of these holds up. But what is important is that suggestion inspires worry, which can bring on high blood pressure. "Doctor, I've got high blood pressure," a patient might have said to Philadelphia's David Riesman, as one might say, "Doctor, I've got malaria."[17] Thus patients wait anxiously for the doctor to strip off the armlet, remove the ear pieces of the stethoscope, and announce the verdict. To some extent, therefore, it is true that "the instrument creates the condition," as William Houston of Augusta, Georgia, wrote in 1936. "Not only is hypertension developed through fear of the verdicts of the instrument, but it is kept alive by meddlesome interference with the patient's eating habits. Each time the patient sits down to eat he has to remember not to put any salt on his eggs, not to eat any pork. The list of *Verboten* follows him throughout the day."[18]

Thus a whole folklore of hypertension weaved itself through the life of the modern patient: the fetishizing of taboos on salt, eggs, fat, and "stress." To what extent any of the items on the endless list actually *causes* the disease is still unclear, but the folklore would convert great numbers of people into patients. "If the doctor is in need of attentive clients," wrote Kansas doctor Arthur Hertzler, "he can increase his revenue by telling the patient that she has high blood pressure. He need not be more specific. The patient knows no more than we doctors about high blood pressure, but it is something that one can fix on."[19] And indeed to prevent patients' fixing on it, many physicians decided, rightly or wrongly, not to tell them they had high blood pressure. (They told the relatives instead!)[20]

For converting people into patients nothing matches the stomach and bowels, organs that produce a great many symptoms. This is a risky generalization, but I have the impression that despite their massive purging, traditional patients were not especially preoccupied with their digestive organs as such. When peasants purged themselves it was not because they had abdominal pain or were constipated, but because they thought getting rid of those foul liquids was the key to health in general. By contrast, modern patients tended to be quite attuned to whether their stomachs hurt, how much gas they had, how hard the colon felt as they pressed upon it from without, and whether they had a daily bowel movement. We shall return to these matters again in a different context, but here I want to establish that they are rather new historically.

A wonderful account of the new fashionableness of bowel complaints is Doctor Axel Munthe's description of ministering to middle-class Parisians' "colitis" around 1890. *Colitis* meant then a change in bowel habits, in the direction of either constipation or diarrhea, accompanied by pain (but not bleeding). Today it would be called *irritable bowel* syndrome. Whether that's what these bourgeois Parisians actually had is unclear, but they *thought* they had it: "A new disease was dumped on the market, a new word was coined, a gold coin indeed, COLITIS! It was a neat complaint, safe from the surgeon's knife, always at hand when wanted, suitable to everybody's taste."

Word got around that Munthe understood its pangs. "Colitis spread like wildfire all over Paris. My waiting-room was soon so full of people that I had to arrange my dining-room as a sort of extra waiting-room. It was always a mystery to me how all these people could have time and patience to sit and wait there so long, often for hours."[21] Munthe was playing with these "fashionable ladies"; but whatever their real problems were, it's clear that they were highly attuned to their abdomens.

In the first half of the twentieth century diagnoses like "chronic appendicitis," "enterospasm," and "chronic abdomen" blossomed. All basically mean abdominal distress that doesn't seem to correspond to any physical lesion, and all were diagnosed far more often in women than men: part of this great drawing in of females to the net of "patients." "As a rule [the young doctor] learns in years of private practice that there is much abdominal pain which has no name and which does not kill," said Herbert Hawkins, a London physician, in 1906.[22] "The subject of the chronic abdomen," said another London physician, "is usually a woman, generally a spinster, or, if married, childless and belonging to what are commonly termed—rather ironically nowadays—the 'comfortable' classes. . . . An abdominal man, on the other hand, is by comparison a rare bird, and when caught has a way of turning out to be a Jew—or a doctor."[23]

This sensitivity to the stomach was to be found in little burghs like Halstead, Kansas, as well as Knightsbridge. According to Arthur Hertzler, "the stomach is the organ most commonly mentioned in office practice. . . . Many women patients tell of some distress in the stomach, just to make the history complete." By "stomach," some of these patients meant "the front of the body." Upscale individuals would mean the upper abdomen. Still others, "when they say 'stomach,' mean stomach."[24] Another doctor felt this to be a familiar office figure: "a woman who has had periodic attacks of intense pain in the abdomen ... for more than thirty years."[25]

A final aspect of the making of the modern patient was a generally increased sensitivity among men and women to all body symptoms, whatever their origin. Whether the peasant was aware of his ankle's itching or his nose's twitching is a question we can't answer, since he didn't seek out a doctor or take medicine for it. My argument is that the modern patient was more likely to define the constant itches and twitches that our bodies send us as "illness," and that, thus defined, this illness would more readily entail some kind of careseeking. Thus the "symptom pyramid," the symptoms that patients considered to be disease and for which they sought help, was very much larger for the modern patient than for the traditional (Figure 5-1).

Thomas Mann's novel *The Magic Mountain*, published in 1924, draws the archetype of the modern patient, a man sensitive to his own internal workings. The novel is set in the Swiss spa of Davos, in those days a peasant village with a number of rest homes (sanatoriums) for the cure of tuberculosis. And Hans Castorp, the young "antihero" of the novel, is quite attuned to his own internal condition from the moment of arrival. That is the logic of the health spa: to make one start interpreting various in-

FIGURE 5-1. *The Modern Symptom Pyramid.*

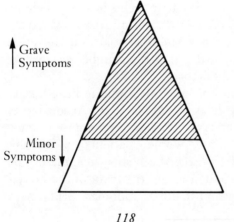

Grave Symptoms

Minor Symptoms

The entire pyramid represents all the symptoms an individual perceives.

The cross-hatched area represents the symptoms an individual defines as "illness."

The modern patient defines as "illness" a much higher percentage of his or her symptoms than does the traditional patient.

ternal physical sensations as disease. But Hans Castorp actually does have tuberculosis. The really quintessential modern patient is his perfectly healthy Uncle James, who has come to visit Hans and then flees upon discovering himself turning into a patient. Uncle James "had become inwardly aware," thought Hans Castorp later. "After only a week up here, he would find everything down below [back home in Hamburg] wrong and out of place. . . . It would seem to him unnatural to go to his office, instead of taking a prescribed walk after breakfast, and thereafter lying ritually wrapped, horizontal on a balcony."[26] Thus, as they became patients, the Uncle Jameses of this world were seeking care for a higher percentage of their symptoms than ever before.

What symptoms did the modern patient perceive, and how many reached a doctor? One preliminary point: many of the traditional patient's diseases—smallpox, yellow fever, to some extent malaria, hookworm, diphtheria, cholera, typhus, plague—were no longer around by 1920. The terrible infectious killers of the past had largely been banned by the beginning of our own century, thanks not to medical therapy at all, but rather to the public health movement.[27] So if we ask what did the modern patient have, the answer will not be cholera.

The distinctive new symptoms were the runny nose, the cough, the sore throat, the sneezing and sniffing and hacking and blowing that constitute the "upper airway infection," or upper respiratory infection (URI), as it is known today. In a nationwide survey of thirty-nine thousand white Americans in 1928–1931, almost 30 percent had suffered a "minor respiratory illness" in the past year. Only 7 percent, by contrast, had had the next most common affliction: accidents and injuries, followed then by stomach upsets, skin diseases, and measles.[28] These are the illnesses that people felt worth reporting to the investigators. Thus, colds dominated the list.

I am struck by the relative absence of references to colds in the memoirs of patients and physicians who lived before 1850. Was it that traditional people had fewer colds? That they were less sensitive to them and deemed them unworthy of mention? That the acute infectious killers dominated the pre-1850 picture? Impossible to say. But it is interesting that the wealthier people become, the more likely they are to report colds. This same nationwide U.S. survey found that the higher your social class, the more you have certain diseases, notably colds ("minor respiratory"), cuts and bruises ("accidents"), and skin problems[29]—or *report* these afflictions. Another piece of evidence: In 1947 doctors in the Sheffield area treated 41 percent of their patients for respiratory complaints, whereas a century earlier in Sheffield, "diseases of the air passages" amounted to only 30 percent of the case load.[30] As the population as a whole became better off, their sensitivity to colds and coughs presumably increased.

One would expect that rising prosperity made the average American of the 1920s healthier than he was in the 1820s. But he considered himself to be sicker. The nationwide U.S. survey found, for example, that in 1928 to 1931, eight out of ten Americans had some illness in a twelve-month period: that is to say, your chances of getting sick were a bit less than once a year. And the *higher* the class, the more frequent the illness,[31] which suggests to me that people in a middle-class society were more attuned to their internal states than those in a frontier society.

This increased sensitivity produced the bewildering mix of symptoms that is the hallmark of illness in the rich. Here is Cathell on the subject: "You will probably find . . . the poor much easier to attend than the higher classes; their ailments are more definite and uncomplicated. . . . With the wealthy and pampered, on the other hand, there is often such a concatenation of unrelated or chronic symptoms, or they are described in such a diluted or exaggerated tone, that it is difficult to judge which symptom is most important."[32] In sum, the onrush of modernity was producing in patients a greater sensitivity to internal well-being.

This sensitivity made the modern patient more dependent upon doctors. Far more often than in traditional times, patients would consult a physician for an illness. In a London suburb in the 1930s, 30 percent of the people who had chronic symptoms had seen a doctor. Of seven hundred items of illness reported by a sample of Londoners in 1953–1954, 27 percent had reached a doctor. Americans were even more likely than the English to seek care for their symptoms: in a small town in upper New York State in the late 1940s, 68 percent of the twenty-two hundred reported illnesses that had been treated medically. The nationwide U.S. health survey asked people whether they had seen a doctor when they were sick in the last year. Seventy-eight percent said yes. In fact, the average American then saw a doctor 2.9 times a year, which is about half as high as it is today.[33]

We may sum up:

1. *Beginning in the nineteenth century, people probably became more willing than those living earlier to define vague collections of internal sensory impressions as "illness" and thus to become "patients."*
2. *This modern sensitivity focused upon the airways and the digestive system.*
3. *Modern patients were much more likely to "seek help" than traditional patients had been.*

DRUGS AND QUACKS

But what kind of help? As we saw in the traditional era, self-dosing and "quacks" provided alternatives to established medicine. Indeed, whenever people lose confidence in official medicine they turn to unsanctioned patent remedies and unofficial healers. How do we reconcile Listerine and Christian Science, both of which flourished in the 1920s, with the new confidence in medicine that I have ascribed to the modern patient?

The sales of patent medicines were immense, and represented as much as 16 percent of the average family's medical bill. In Shelby County, Indiana, for example, the average family might fork out eleven dollars a year for these potions, in an era when eleven dollars was a lot of money.[34]

Of the drugs sold by an average urban drugstore in the 1920s:

- *Forty-two percent were patent medicines, meaning that the trademark was patented and the ingredients secret.*
- *Thirty-two percent were medicines prescribed by doctors: some of those compounded by the pharmacist, some "ethical" drugs advertised only in the medical press.*
- *Sixteen percent were various "home remedies," like chamomile*

121

*or cherry cough syrup, that the druggist would sell out of big
jars (a further 10 percent were "miscellaneous").*[35]

Thus prepackaged medicines, manufactured by nationwide
companies, had become big business in the Roaring Twenties.
Sales of drugs in general had climbed from $51 million in 1905 to
$120 million in 1929, and half of all those were patent medi-
cines.[36]

The big sellers were products like Listerine, which Lambert
Pharmaceuticals spent $3 million to advertise in 1926; Konjola, a
tonic, of whose $3.5 million sales, $2 million was plowed back
again into advertising; Castoria, a laxative selling 20 million bottles in 1929; Bromo-Seltzer, Vicks VapoRub, and so forth.[37] The
fact that many of these remain household names today is evidence
of the gripping power upon the public of huge advertising cam-
paigns for products that have basically no medical uses.

The fact of the matter is that people in every epoch of history
have loved self-dosing, and the novelty for the modern patient
was doing it with commercial preparations rather than homemade
teas and poultices. "It is not the scarcity of sources of drugs and
medicines that constitutes a problem in Shelby County," wrote
Allon Peebles in 1930 after an intensive study of that little farm
district.

> It is rather their very abundance.... The people of Shelby
> County, as is probably true of many other communities, are still in
> the drug-taking age as far as the treatment of illnesses is concerned.
> Their faith in the efficacy of bottles of brightly-colored medicine is
> strong.... It was a common occurrence for the writer to see a row
> of bottles on a table in the doctor's office waiting for little Mary or
> Mrs. Brown to come to get them.[38]

In England the same story held true: "Many patients have a
deep-rooted objection to washing, to fresh air and to anything
else that will do good," wrote one doctor in 1927. They were suspicious "in fact of everything except medicine out of a bottle,
which they will swallow by the bucketful."[39]

While middle-class families tended to keep aspirin and "antiseptics" like Listerine on hand, the working classes placed
great faith in "kidney pills," "liver pills," and "stomach medi-

cines." One working-class woman whom Earl Koos interviewed in "Regionville," New York, in the late 1940s, said, "My husband and I take C——— Liver Pills regularly. We get to feeling stuffy if we don't, and keeping your liver flushed out gets rid of the stuffiness. . . . Once in a while I take S——— Kidney Pills, too. It's good to flush out your kidneys once in a while. . . . If I do this, I don't get sick."[40]

When a team led by Gladys Swackhamer interviewed a number of working-class households in Manhattan in 1938, they discovered how extensively many families relied upon patent medicines. Take "Mr. and Mrs. Wright," for example, a middle-aged couple with three children, who had recently lost their home in the Depression. "Mr. W. is very nervous as a result of his financial difficulties. He has always suffered in the winters from bronchitis and was an invalid because of it for a year before his marriage." Mrs. W., on the other hand, suffered from "bleeding piles" (hemorrhoids). She also had a hernia and wore a hernia belt "passed on to her by her sister." These people had various problems, none of them curable with drugs.

Yet Mr. Wright "gets so desperate that he tries various remedies. He used a liquid put up by a druggist he knew but it did not help much. The insurance collector recommended a patent medicine and now he is taking that." Mr. Wright had recently "developed a rash on his hands and arms," for which he used an ointment. Mrs. Wright took a laxative daily (not only useless but harmful). How much of the thirty-five dollars that Mr. Wright earned weekly as a hardware jobber was thrown away![41]

Swackhamer discovered that the 365 families interviewed used drugs extensively, "selected on the basis of advertised merits and drug clerk's advice. Laxatives were purchased in the greatest quantity of all; remedies for colds, coughs and sore throats were a close second. . . . Three out of four households reported frequent use of proprietary medicines." In fact, the people in one out of every eight households used a laxative, headache pill, or sleeping pill daily.[42]

Doesn't this fondness for self-dosing contradict my hypothesis about the modern patient's trust in the doctor? Two points in response.

First, I think the increase in people's sensitivity to their symptoms, or the greater readiness to define symptoms as illness, was probably so considerable as to saturate the ability of official medicine to treat them all. People simply had more symptoms than they had time, money, or inclination to spend on the doctor, and so when they thought it appropriate they treated themselves. Here I part company with such scholars as Paul Starr, who feel the medical profession made people dependent upon medicines prescribed by the doctor. Remember that people could buy without a prescription any drug the doctor might prescribe, once they became familiar with the name (alcohol and narcotics excepted). Limiting over-the-counter sales began only with the Food, Drug and Cosmetic Act of 1938.[43]

Second, many popular drugs started out being advertised *to doctors only* and spread to the general public only as people became familiar with them from prescriptions. In other words, many patent medicines flourished precisely *because* the trusted medical establishment had recommended them. Of course, since time out of mind nostrum makers had hyped their wares with "testimonials" from "Doctor X" or "Doctor Y," but that was in the days when anyone could call himself "Doctor."[44] A licensed M.D. prescribing a product was more impressive, and in the 1920s perhaps a third of all prescriptions were for *proprietary products*, meaning either patent medicines (a term the doctors hated) or other drugs sold already packaged by commercial firms.[45] Thus Sal Hepatica, Listerine, and BiSoDol all started out as ethical specialties (advertised to doctors only), and wound up being advertised directly to the public only after their names had gotten around by word of mouth.[46] One illustration: in 1929, *Hygeia*, the mass-circulation health magazine published by the AMA, recommended that people not use aspirin except on their doctor's advice. Aspirin was then halfway in its drift from ethical specialty to mass marketing.[47]

In 1908 the editor of one prominent medical journal wondered whether accepting drug advertisements at all was wise, because drug therapy as a whole was "upon such an uncertain basis," meaning that many medicines were valueless or harmful. But, he said, by the time "its claims ... seem absurd" to doctors, the public had gotten wind of it.

> As soon as [an ethical drug] becomes much used by the pro-
> fession, the public will become familiar with it and it will become
> purchasable over many counters. That is not only the fate of every
> good preparation but it is what the manufacturers are striving for
> in advertising it. They hope ultimately to vend it directly to the
> public when the physicians have created a great enough demand
> for it and made it sufficiently popular.[48]

In his 1906 play *The Doctor's Dilemma,* George Bernard Shaw
puts into the mouth of "Sir Ralph Bloomfield Bonington," the
distinguished London physician, the words,

> Ah, believe me, Paddy, the world would be healthier if every
> chemist's shop in England were demolished. Look at the papers!
> full of scandalous advertisements of patent medicines! a huge com-
> mercial system of quackery and poison. Well, whose fault is it?
> Ours, I say, ours. We set the example. We spread the superstition.
> We taught the people to believe in bottles of doctor's stuff; and
> now they buy it at the stores instead of consulting a medical man.[49]

Because drugs diffused so rapidly from ethical specialty to
mass market, pharmacists often asked doctors to prescribe items
the pharmacists themselves could compound from scratch, rather
than prepackaged commercial "proprietaries."

"Dear Doctor," began a form letter put out by a pharmacists'
association. "On the drug market today, as you know, are thousands of 'specialty preparations' offered for the use of physicians. . . .

"Such 'specialty' items lend themselves to ready sales to a laity
learning the 'catch name.' Self-medication is closely related to
these attractive and easily learned titles." The letter observed that
once people had learned the titles they could repeat them "to the
druggist or to an ailing friend" without the doctor's knowledge.[50]
But although it is true that thousands of patent medicines *not*
sanctioned by doctors flourished on the market, the big-money
items usually had passed from doctor to patient.[51]

How had doctors become caught up in this snare of prescribing
valueless drugs? Partly it was from a lack of knowledge. Many of
the patent medicines and proprietaries were, in effect, laxatives,
though they might contain aromatics, bitters, alcohol, bromine, or

whatever. And far into the twentieth century doctors continued to prescribe laxatives on the grounds that constipation might cause "autointoxication," i.e., poisoning your system from the contents of your colon. This view, though still widely held today by quacks and cranks ("colonic irrigation" therapies abound), is baseless. The fecal material in one's colon does not infiltrate the wall to "poison" the rest of the body, and constipation, unless it lasts for weeks, can at worst make one uncomfortable. But early in this century many doctors believed implicitly in the horrors of "intestinal toxemia." A discussion at an annual meeting of the American Association of Obstetricians and Gynecologists in 1911 makes harrowing reading. Doctors stressed the need for *several* bowel movements daily to rid the system of "poison." "The vast majority of humans are chronic rectal constipates," said one. "Foul breath, dulled minds, sluggish muscles prevail. . . ."[52] So of course these physicians would prescribe laxatives, thus reinforcing the age-old pattern of purgative abuse we have already encountered in traditional patients.

Yet even when a doctor realized the uselessness of most drugs, patient pressure would force him to write prescriptions for them anyway. Shaw knew that the average physician could refuse to prescribe patent medicines only at the cost of losing his practice. In the preface to *The Doctor's Dilemma* he said that doctors "must believe, on the whole, what their patients believe, just as they must wear the sort of hat their patients wear. . . . When the patient has a prejudice the doctor must either keep it in countenance or lose his patient." Thus in essence, "private medical practice is governed not by science but by supply and demand; and however scientific a treatment may be, it cannot hold its place in the market if there is no demand for it."[53] I find this a delicious irony: patients were flocking to doctors in the first place for "science," yet a doctor who behaved truly "scientifically—prescribing nothing, because almost none of these substances had any impact on infections—would lose a patient.

In the modern patient's mind was engraved the rule (chiseled no less indelibly today): "Every consultation should end with a prescription." The patient had to bear away a bottle or a "script," or he wouldn't be happy. An English country doctor described his patients' attachment to "a bottle" as so great that even during the epidemics of influenza that swept back and forth in the inter-war years, epidemics that the doctors' training told them no drug could touch, physicians nonetheless would have the pharmacists pack "into our cars a large basket of appropriate remedies, which were doled out to our grateful patients. . . ."[54]

American patients were not one whit more scientific about the uselessness of drugs. Doctors might learn therapeutic nihilism in medical schools, but on the firing line other rules prevailed. S. Weir Mitchell wrote in 1901, "I once expressed surprise in a consultation that an aged physician, who had called me in, should be so desirous of doing something, when I as earnestly wished to wait. At last he said, 'Doctor, it is not the child I want to dose; it is the mother's mind.' "[55] Despite the folksy country doctor mantle he pulled about himself, Arthur Hertzler, who later became a professor of surgery at the University of Kansas, was quite a sci-entific man. Yet even he remembered of house calls, "One left some medicine in case of a recurrence of the trouble; this was largely the bunk, but someone had to pay for the axle grease and just plain advice never was productive of revenue unless fortified by a few pills. It was about as important as the deacon's 'Amen' during the preacher's sermon—it did no harm and it was an evi-dence of good faith."[56] I dwell on this, because when we encoun-ter patients in the postmodern period, the drugs they demand will no longer be innocuous "bunk" but very powerful and often mood-altering chemicals.

The best evidence of the modern patient's attachment to scien-tific medicine is the decline in quackery that had occurred by the 1930s. The reader will remember how abundant was the supply of traditional rivals to the physician: the plenitude of medicine men and bonesetters and wisewomen. And rightly so, because the traditional physician's head was as filled with therapeutic mumbo-jumbo as were the heads of his rivals. But the scientific medicine of the 1880s and after had the power to convince and to detach the patient from the "irregulars" of yesteryear.

Of course, quackish cults were still to be found. In the 1920s Morris Fishbein catalogued many of these, which included Lim-pio Comerology, the work of one Caroline M. Olse and her husband Emil Olse of St. Louis, who dispensed preparations Q-33 and Q-34 to make "clean eating physically successful." In those years could be found Naprapathy, an offshoot of chiropractic; "orificial therapy," devoted to enlarging the various openings of the body; and "practotherapy," a school of enema therapy of the now familiar "get-those-poisons-out-of-there" variety.[57]

But though such cults existed, they did not have a wide following. The nationwide survey of American patterns of illness in 1928–1931 found that of all calls to healers among 8,800 families, only 10 percent involved the attendance of a "nonmedical practitioner," i.e., a quack. The 26,000 people of Shelby County, Indiana, for example, could call upon 31 physicians for assistance, 6 Christian Science practitioners, 5 chiropractors, 1 osteopath, and 1 chiropodist. In the United Sates as a whole, in the 1920s, one could weigh against the 143,000 regular physicians some 8,500 practitioners of Christian Science, 7,600 osteopaths, 15,000 chiropractors, 500 naturopaths, 300 electrotherapists, and so forth.[58] Thus, the relative number of irregulars was nowhere near as great as it had been early in the nineteenth century, when the rival sects and self-styled doctors outnumbered the graduates of regular medical schools.

Nor were Americans in the 1920s seeing the irregulars for diseases like cancer. Of the 121 calls performed by Christian Scientists, naturopaths, midwives, and others included in the survey, 18 percent were for births (midwives), 15 percent for skin complaints, and 13 percent for rheumatism.[59] I am loathe to continue using the term *quackery* to describe all these activities, since some of the paramedicals doubtless possessed wisdom that scientific medicine had not yet made its own. The point is, rather, that by the 1920s most American patients had come to trust their doctors implicitly, for the rivals had fallen away.

TRUST IN THE DOCTOR

Before I establish the point that the modern doctor had enormous power over the patient, I want to discuss the twin sources of this great influence.

One source was the modern doctor's new-found social status. By World War I he had become a local notable, a person of standing in the eyes of the community. We touched on this phenomenon earlier, when describing how doctors saw themselves. Physicians' fellow citizens also looked up to them in the 1920s and 1930s, more than ever before.

Mrs. X, "an obese American widow of 51," entered the Massachusetts General Hospital on 9 November 1924. She had a history of abdominal pain, a "cold in the chest," and a "complete paralysis of both legs following an injury to her spine eleven years before." She recounted her personal history. It included a background of poverty and work as a dressmaker. After her first husband had died, she lived with another man and "had to bear taunts and insults in public about her poverty...." She felt friendless and much depressed. She was treated with electrical therapy and massage, and her "paralysis" began to disappear.

Of interest is her attitude toward her doctors. "As soon as motion had begun to return to her limbs, and she became thoroughly convinced that she would soon be able to walk, she concluded that the physician who was effecting this 'cure' must be Christ returned to earth." And even after her doctors had dispelled this idea, her main impetus to recovery seemed to be her desire to please them. "On one occasion only, when she had repeatedly refused to try to walk without his presence as a mental support, her physician was obliged to fall back on her desire to please him, and to request her to do it 'for his sake.' On the other hand, she frequently stated, when told to do something by anyone else, that she 'would do it because her doctor would be pleased and for no other reason.' "[60]

After conducting a survey of general practice in England, Joseph Collings was able to write in 1950, "The general practitioner enjoys more prestige and wields more power than any other citizen, uless it be the judge on his bench. . . . The powers of even the senior managers are petty compared with the powers of the doctor to influence the physical, psychological, and economic destiny of other people."[61] As I quote these lines in the 1980s they already have a quaint, archaic ring: Collings's survey had caught the profession at the very apogee of its prestige.

The "Regionvillers" whom Earl Koos interviewed in the late 1940s had similarly respectful views of the local practitioners. "Who, in your opinion," he asked, "are the five persons you believe to be the most important in Regionville?" All who answered except three named at least one doctor. It was not just because of the physicians' personal influence over them that they felt this way. It was the men's income, the houses they lived in, the cars they drove. Said one man, "I put Doc X on that list not because he takes care of a lot of our families when they're sick—that's important—but because he's who he is. He's one of the best-educated men in town, and makes good money—drives a good car, belongs to Rotary, and so forth. . . . But people look up to him, not just because he's their doctor, but because he's *the doctor*."[62] The point is clear, then, that doctors enjoyed great status in modern patients' eyes not just because of what they did but what they *were*.

A second reason, however, for their great personal influence upon patients was the halo of science that clung to the profession. Tire company executives, accountants, clothing-store owners all had high incomes and drove big cars, but they lacked a similar ability to influence others' personal lives. Modern patients were willing to submit to the doctor because they saw him bathed in the particular glow of science. It was science that so distinctively separated the modern doctor from the traditional in the patients' eyes. To return to "Regionville": when residents who had changed physicians were asked why they had done so, the most frequent response by far was the belief that the first doctor had not "kept up with medical progress." Despite the fact that Doctors V and Z, both of whom had been around many years, were "slow to collect their fees" and "easy to get along with," people shunned them because they hadn't kept up. "We had Doctor V for a long time, but gave up on him last year. It just wasn't any use—he was still giving the same old 'bitters' and pills. I don't think he even knows about some of the new things the other doctors use today."[63] These men fell out of favor because they were insufficiently scientific.

The public's respect for science was interwoven with the revolution in scientific achievement that swept across all fields of endeavor, not just medicine, in the second half of the nineteenth century. Just think of the number of former "arts" that acquired a "scientific" basis for their authority: from meteorology to metallurgy to the study of handwriting to the study of the mind. Sherlock Holmes, after all, was such an impressive late-Victorian figure because he seemed to have mastered all of these. Medicine was merely one of many arts that acquired a scientific underpinning. Therefore, we cannot date exactly the public's initial *prise de conscience* of the doctor as scientist. It was certainly palpable when Daniel Cathell in 1922 wrote the final edition of his marvelous guide. "Never omit to call for a glass of water and a napkin with which to cleanse your thermometer," he counseled. "Wash it thoroughly several times and dry it carefully before the eyes of everybody present.... Everybody will like to see the sanitary precaution."[64] It was, of course, the budding sciences of microbiology, physiology, and public health that had made these rituals necessary in the eyes of both doctors and laity.

But to the extent that we can give any precise date to the crystallizing of the public's infatuation with medical science, I think it would be the arrival in 1894 of the first diphtheria "antitoxine," which subsequently broke the back of several diphtheria epidemics. This was the first genuinely therapeutic "specific." Diphtheria, a disease of childhood, acts by causing the lining of the throat to swell, threatening suffocation, and by disseminating a highly potent toxin in the blood that affects all the organs. The "antitoxine," as it was known, specifically countered this toxin, giving the person's natural immune system time to overcome the bacteria.

In a series of earth-shaking discoveries between 1890 and 1894, French and German bacteriologists had figured out how to grow a pure culture of the diphtheria bacteria: inject the germ into research animals such as cab horses, and then, once the horse's own immune system had produced sufficient antibody in its blood, take blood from the horse and use the serum portion of that blood as antitoxine to be injected into humans. Of the deeply scientific basis of all this there could be no doubt. On 7 October 1895, the *New York Times* quoted the Johns Hopkins pathologist William H. Welch: "The discovery of the healing serum is entirely the result of laboratory work. It is an outcome of the studies of immunity. In no sense was the discovery an accidental one. Every step leading to it can be traced, and every step was taken with a definite purpose and to solve a definite problem."

From the beginning, the antitoxin's discovery and diffusion in the United States had excited an enormous amount of public interest. It was a media sensation, followed in its minutest details by millions of people. The story began on 9 November 1894 with the *New York Times* headline, "Diphtheria's New Treatment," followed by an account from the London *Times* of "Dr. Roux's remarkable communication to the Buda-Pesth Congress some six weeks ago. . . ." The article urged haste: "Hundreds of children are at the present moment lying under the shadow of painful death, and the annual period of the greatest incidence is still before us. If only a fraction of these lives can be saved. . . ." What drama already!

Then American reports of the antitoxin's success started to stream in. The *New York Times* missed nothing, giving quite prominent play to highly technical reports from medical journals as soon as they appeared. Thus of one: "This is the first important and conclusive contribution from America to the growing mass of evidence. . . . We are glad that it has been furnished by New-York" (21 November 1894).

By 24 November there were about fifty cases of diphtheria in New York City. Seven had been discovered the previous evening. Four schools were ordered closed. The existing supply of antitoxin in the city was exhausted. Since the first of November, twenty children had died.

Two days later a supply of the desperately needed antitoxin arrived from Europe by steamer. "Mr. Fink," of the pharmaceutical firm of Lehn and Fink at 128 William Street, decided to make it available to doctors with urgent cases at a nominal cost.

I shall not detail all the developing drama, but the reader will realize that what we have here is a media spectacular. All the components are present: gravely ill children (today read: "Child needs liver transplant"); overworked doctors struggling against all odds; and selfless philanthropy by community leaders. By June 1895, the *Times* was able to conclude that the antitoxin was not only a "specific" against disease but a "preventive": if you inoculated children in advance, they wouldn't get diphtheria. Later stories went on to talk about "revolutionizing certain lines of medical science" and applying the principles of the antitoxin to other diseases.[65] It would be hard to underestimate the public awe for medical science that all this caused. By the early 1920s mass-market periodicals such as the *Ladies' Home Journal* were running medical columns explaining to the public quite complicated points of immunology.[66] The doctor had passed from an unsavory boil lancer to a folk hero.

Physicians didn't acquire all this new prestige entirely unaided: they rode on the coattails of the surgeons. Because surgeons get so many of their patients as referrals and rarely see them after surgery, they don't belong in the narrative of doctor-patient relations I'm relating here. Yet public awe at the triumphs of surgery lent a reflected luster to the physician's image, and so the stunning accomplishments that began to be performed in the operating room in the 1880s demand our attention for a minute.

Before the 1850s, the only major operations possible in surgery were cutting for bladder stone, amputating limbs, setting fractures, and a host of grisly procedures in obstetrics. The risk of infection made the body's major cavities—cranium, thorax, and abdomen—virtually inaccessible, to say nothing of the terrible pain involved in something like a hip amputation, which by itself could send the victim into fatal shock. Then, in 1844, Horace Wells had his famous tooth extracted while under the influence of nitrous oxide, and the whole modern chapter of pain relief in surgery began. Access to the body's cavitie· became possible with the discovery of antisepsis and asepsis (killing germs, or keeping them away) in the late 1860s, and therewith infection-free operations on the stomach, colon, gallbladder, uterus, lung, and brain—hitherto unimaginable—could be contemplated. If, for example, the stomach were cancerous, the malignant portion could be cut away and an artificial opening made into the remaining part to connect with the intestine. If the gallbladder were filled with stones and inflamed, the stones could simply be removed. If a person's life were slowly being extinguished by a growing tumor within the cranium, the skull could be entered, the tumor excised, and health once again restored.

133

When on 19 July 1911 young Doctor Pat Nixon, a freshly minted Johns Hopkins medical degree in hand, checked into the Rochester Hotel in Rochester, Minnesota, the first thing that struck him was that "the hotel—and in fact the whole town—is full of patients, pre- or postoperative. And my how they do talk, especially the women. Each of them has had or is to have a very serious operation." So the next day Nixon went to see some operations. Here's what William Mayo, one of the two brothers whose father founded Rochester's Mayo Clinic, had lined up that morning:

- *Hysterectomies for fibroids;*
- *Exploratory laparotomy [opening the abdomen];*
- *Resection [removing part of] of cecum, or colon, and part of transverse colon for carcinoma ... Time, one hour;*
- *Nephrectomy for hypernephroma [removing a cancerous kidney];*
- *Resection of rectum for carcinoma.*[67]

Each day Nixon catalogued what he saw: operations on the appendix, uterus, tubes and ovaries, thyroid, breast, jaw: the list was endless. The two Mayo brothers and their chief of surgery, Edward S. Judd, were extremely energetic and skilled and made the Mayo Clinic a magical name for hill people in little hamlets in Missouri whose doctors were unable to find out "what the trouble was."

Ten years later Edward W. Morris, superintendent of the London Hospital, sat at his desk: "I see in today's list of operations— just arrived as I write—that there are twenty-seven major operations this afternoon, of which eight are extensive abdominal operations. If such a list had been attempted fifty years ago what would have been the mortality? Fifty percent at least. Yet such a list is a matter of daily routine."[68]

This onmarch of surgery, more than any other single factor, elevated the doctor in the public's eye to demigod status. Daniel Cathell noted somewhat bitterly in the last edition of his book,

The laity invariably admire and appreciate the quick and keen man who can see and take the responsibility of anything, anywhere at the critical time. . . . Capital operations in surgery illustrate this: the manual parts—expertness with the knife, etc.—are highly spectacular, and deeply impressive, and receive vastly more praise from the public than knowing when to operate, and how to conduct the after-treatment.[69]

"Demigod status," the reader might wonder, is that not a bit strong? Yet how else may one describe the heroes of the silver screen who strutted back and forth in the 1930s and 1940s? To moviegoers in small towns, the actors had a godlike appeal, and many of them played surgeons. Perhaps the most famous of the "doctor" movies of the 1930s (which included the *Doctor Kildare* series begun in 1938), was David O. Selznick's *Dark Victory*, released in 1939 and starring Bette Davis as the rich, doomed young heiress "Judith Traherne," with Ronald Reagan and Humphrey Bogart in minor parts. Bette Davis, first looking at the script, had asked, "Who is going to want to see a picture about a girl who dies?" But the film was a major critical and box-office success. Judith Traherne, dying of a brain tumor, falls in love with her doctor and marries him. But the doctor, "Steele," is not just any doctor. He's a neurosurgeon; one who, moreover, after years of high-pressure surgery for a Park Avenue clientele, is getting out and going off to do "medical research." At the film's start a bit player, Carter, joshes him about his decision:

CARTER: Well shine my golden halo—you and Pasteur!
STEELE: Probably you're right. But somebody's got to find a serum that will be to these growths [brain tumors] what insulin is to diabetes—what antitoxin is to diphtheria—and really earn his title Doctor of Medicine.[70]

Surgeon, physician, it all ran together in the public mind. They were all heroes.

The doctors in Sidney Kingsley's 1933 play *Men in White*, which Lee Strasberg directed, go on endlessly about their research. Each vies with the other in monkish dedication to spending a life operating on humanity. The stage directions that bring in "Dr. Hochberg," a German scientist who's immigrated to New

York, played in 1933 by J. Edward Bromberg, read: "He carries himself with quiet, simple dignity. There is strength in the set of his jaw; but the predominating quality expressed in his face is a sweet and simple goodness." Can you imagine the reactions of a cast today on hearing those directions?

The entire play pictures the surgical staff of "St. George's hospital" as selfless giants on the earth, whose magnificence dwarfs both nurses and patients. One intern says to the female lead: "Don't worry, sweetheart! The chances are none of us will live to grow that old. Most doctors die pretty young, you know."

Another intern adds: "That's right. The strain gets them around forty-five. Heart goes bad."

Well, in fact, these titans do have a human side. One of them sleeps with a nurse, whom he impregnates, providing the play's denouement. At the end he decides to swear off women and dedicate his life to research.[71] The play won a Pulitzer Prize in 1934.

The point is that the modern doctor had a great deal of personal influence over the modern patient. It was influence derived from his social position, his scientific aura, his portrayal in the mass media—and it could be *therapeutically extremely useful*. In the late twentieth century we can only with difficulty imagine what these men permitted themselves. In *Men in White*, for example, Dr. Hochberg goes up to the big businessman who is his patient in hospital, takes the cigar out of his mouth, and throws it away. Then he orders him away from the phone and into bed. The big businessman complies.[72] Today there would be talk of "assault." The hospital ombudsman would be called. The "Dr. Hochbergs" of this world, as we will learn, now find themselves very much on the defensive.

We can see to what extent this authority was the product of the doctor's bedside manner (as well as of his social position) in observing how obedient other doctors were once they became patients. Sometime in the 1940s Dr. Frederic Wertham, a distinguished psychiatrist, fell ill with a clot in a leg vein and required an operation. He was on the table:

> The surgeon's voice was deep, calm and authoritative. It was not raised at any time. . . . I developed a very disagreeable pain in the

right calf during the operative procedure . . . I remember that several times I moved the leg, seeking to ease its position—not exactly an appropriate behavior in the situation. I recall very distinctly the surgeon's voice saying quietly but definitely: "Don't move your leg, Dr. Wertham." My emotional response to this remark is difficult to describe. From that moment on, it was unthinkable that I should move my leg, however it felt. The remark had such an authoritative effect on me that—pain or no pain, impulse or no impulse—the idea of moving my leg did not come up again.[73]

Indeed one of the complaints doctors have when they become patients is that their physicians fail, as Dr. Max Pinner, himself a physician, put it, to "take them in charge." Instead, doctors continue to treat other sick colleagues as doctors, failing to "give definite orders or advice" and saying "explicitly or implicitly, 'You know what to do.' " But Pinner, a respirologist, didn't know what to do. "Even if I did know, such an attitude fails to give the psychic relief that every patient expects from his physician."[74] Precisely: this authoritative bedside manner is a source of "psychic relief."

It is a crucial fact that the modern patient was taken much in charge by the physicians of the post-1880 period. From one of these small towns in Illinois Thomas Shastid remembers the "hard-boiled" doctor:

The first time I ever saw this medico he was standing in his own waiting-room arguing vigorously with a small, dark, much frightened man patient. "You talka de Italiano?" inquired the patient, who seemed to be getting the worst of the argument. "No, I don't talka de Italiano," roared the doctor. "But I *do* talk turkey. And I'm telling you now in that language that you got to do as I say—*as I* say, do you understand me—or else. . . ."

The little dark patient, deeply impressed, slipped out of that office silently and with only deep respect, even worship, in his eyes.[75]

By extension, this great medical authority over patients could transform itself into *moral* authority as well, and modern doctors often found themselves consulting with patients about personal problems or issuing moral decrees. James Nicoll, a GP in Surrey, England, remembered,

> I can claim that in these years I had become what I set out to be long ago—namely, the father of my people. Once upon a time they or their parents would have gone to ask advice from a clergyman. Nowadays [the 1940s] they go to their doctor.... During the years that I have been in practice no less than three maidens have consulted me as to whether they ought to accept proposals of marriage which had been made to them.[76]

It sounds rather benign, if quaint—advising "maidens" whether to get married. But to show how extreme could be the leverage that the bedside manner conferred we have the old doc (the "Y. of P. man") in Marion, Illinois, who was telling Shastid

> a story of a big buck negro whose wife had left him and gone to live with another big buck negro, of which the first buck was very greatly afraid. The first buck asked this Y. of P. man if he knew of any means or medicine, "conjure or somepin'," which would have the effect of bringing his wife back home to him.
>
> The doctor gave me a cunning look and a laugh, then said, "The nigger had money, so I knew the thing he wanted."

"Did you actually get her back home?" Shastid asked.

> Sure thing. I gave the fool feller a vial, containing exactly seven drops of the spirits of lavender, diluted with seven teaspoonfuls of water. Then I told him that, beginning on the first of next month, he was, at exactly midnight, for the first seven nights, to take a certain teaspoon, which also I supplied him, and with it to deposit on the very center of his back-door just one teaspoonful of my conjure medicine....
>
> "Another thing that helped to make the 'medicine' effective was that I charged him seventy dollars for it—ten dollars a teaspoonful precisely," said the Y. of P.

Shastid asked, "But wasn't the darky pretty mad when he found out she did not return?"

"Oh ho! But she *did* return. I *saw* to that. Had I been unable to see to it I would not have sold the man the medicine. It would not have been ethical."(!)

"How did you see to it?" Shastid asked.

The Y. of P. man rose, and bending down to Shastid's ear whispered softly, "You see, before this woman had ever married *any*body, she came to my office, saying she was just about to die. In fact, getting down on her knees, she prayed to me to save her." It turned out that she was suffering the effects of a septic abortion, given to her by "an old woman from back in the country." The Y. of P. man tried to fix her up.

"But always afterwards," he said, "she was terribly frightened when she saw me, for fear I was going to have her arrested for getting an abortion started. In fact the woman was now and then so terrified that she was almost insane."

So the Y. of P. man now told her, "You know what you done six or seven years ago." She threw up her hands and screamed. "Quiet," he told her. "And you ain't paid your penalty to the legal authorities even yet."

In brief, he told her that if she didn't return to her first husband, he'd turn her in.

"That's exactly what she done, too. And, since then, they've lived together happily—leastwise he himself has done so for he comes up here to my office once or twice a year to tell me how very much he thinks of me."[77]

In the next chapter we will see that this kind of authority could serve good ends as well as bad.

CHAPTER SIX

Disease of Psychological Origin

THE REASON I have been emphasizing the patient's will to believe, and the doctor's ability to inspire, is that from one-third to one-quarter of all diseases a family doctor sees are probably of psychological origin: that is, they arise in the mind and can be cured with the therapeutic power of the consultation. Here we strike a new note. Until now this book has been concerned with organic diseases, diseases of physical origin—infections, tumors, heart failure. These all arise from some external invasion of the body or from some physical deterioration, such as hardening of the arteries. But the symptoms that most people experience on a week-to-week basis have little to do with tumors and scarlet fever, which are catastrophic, exceptional events. They are more likely to be diarrhea, skin rashes, and loss of appetite. And many of these kinds of symptoms arise not from some physical pathology in the intestines, the skin, or the stomach, but from signals being sent to these organs by the mind. Thus, much of what a family doctor sees in daily practice is "psychogenic."

A Few Explanations

Diseases of psychological origin are not new. People have always known that if you get into an argument, your stomach hurts afterward, or if you're about to take an exam you get diarrhea. Paul Dubois, the Swiss psychiatrist whom we shall encounter shortly, was able to treat uneducated patients as well as sophisticated ones because they all grasped intuitively that the mind affected the body. "The workman and the peasant understand with great acuteness the influence of the moral [mental] on the physical, provided that one takes the trouble to explain it to them in terms which are familiar to them."[1]

Today the code word meaning that the vicissitudes of life produce physical symptoms is *stress*, a concept made popular by Hans Selye in 1950. But doctors have always understood the relationship. The seventeenth-century physician Thomas Sydenham thought that external emotional events could affect the "animal spirits" of the body, causing "hysteria." Robert Whytt, the Edinburgh doctor who helped found neurophysiology, noted in the preface to his 1765 book on hypochondria and hysteria, "Of late these have also got the name of nervous," the causes being not a physical inflammation of the nerves but "passions of the mind."[2]

Yet it was only when doctors acquired the ability to distinguish between symptoms of psychological and physical origin that this notion of psychic causation—which had always existed—could be applied to bedside medicine. There's no point telling someone who has stomach pain to go for "stress counseling" if a carcinoma is the source of the pain. You've got to be able to ascertain that none of the relevant organic diseases is causing the symptoms before you pronounce them to be of psychological origin. This ability was not acquired by modern medicine until the 1860s and beyond.

Thus, in 1869 when John Russell Reynolds encountered a "young lady" admitted as a paraplegic to University College Hospital in London, the first thing he did was try to rule out disease of the spine. After that, by giving her leg muscles small electric shocks he was able to determine they were contracting properly (so the muscles themselves weren't diseased). Her story then pointed him in a different direction. She had been nursing her father, who had himself suddenly become paralyzed a year and a half previously, apparently due to the psychic shock of a bankruptcy. As she went back and forth from her father to her job as a governess, she found

> paralysis constantly upon her mind, her brain overdone with thought and feeling . . . and her heart tired out with the effort to look bright, and be so. Her limbs often ached, and a horror took hold of her, as the idea again and again crossed her mind, that she might become paralyzed like her father; she tried to banish it, but it haunted her still, and, gradually, she had to give up walking, then to stop in the house, then in the room, and then in her bed. Her legs "became heavier day by day"; and she at last reached the state in which I found her when she was carried to the hospital.[3]

We know that she didn't have some kind of organic paralysis, because all they did was rub her legs a bit, walk back and forth with her, and "at the end of a fortnight, she was as strong and capable of exertion as she had ever been in her life." Reynolds described all this as "paralysis . . . dependent on idea," i.e., *psychogenic*.

This kind of psychogenic paralysis affects skeletal muscle. But disturbances of internal organs can also be psychogenic. Digestive problems, for example, can arise either from physical disease (stomach cancer) or for psychological reasons, and separating the one from the other was the work of a number of German internists in the 1880s and 1890s. Until then it was felt that stomach pain or vomiting resulted from a physical irritation or inflammation of the nerves of the stomach. However, these internists insisted that many digestive symptoms were "nervous" or "neurasthenic." "I know ladies," wrote Ernst von Leyden of Berlin in 1881, who have quite normal digestion but are suddenly subject to powerful diarrheas at every agitation." In 1882 a doctor who owned a spa referred to the "nervous dyspepsia and nervous enteropathy" of his clients. Two years later a Berlin internist invented the term *neurasthenic dyspepsia*. Before then *nervous* had meant a physical affliction of the nerves in the brain and spinal cord. Later the term would also mean "of emotional origin"; for example, in 1897 another Berliner, Ottomar Rosenbach, called digestive problems produced by the mind *"emotional dyspep-*

sia." This rich German tradition of "psychosomatic" medicine was picked up in the United States around the turn of the century, notably by the Harvard physiologist Walter Cannon, who believed that a large percentage of gastric cases are "functional in character and of nervous origin."[4] (*Functional* in those days meant that no anatomical damage had occurred; today it tends to mean "caused by the mind.") I have gone through this literature in some detail, not really to revive these largely forgotten men, but to establish that appreciating the "psychological" factors in bedside medicine is neither part of some "age-old" wisdom nor the invention of Sigmund Freud.

Let me tie this together a little more systematically. Figure 6-1 diagrams three different kinds of diseases that arise in the mind: they are psychogenic.

THE "PSYCHONEUROSES"

I put quotation marks about the term because it is used less and less today, as it is discovered that virtually everybody exhibits "neurotic" behavior of some kind, whether they are men who find themselves unable to urinate in a public washroom, sufferers

FIGURE 6-1. *Diseases of Psychological Origin.*

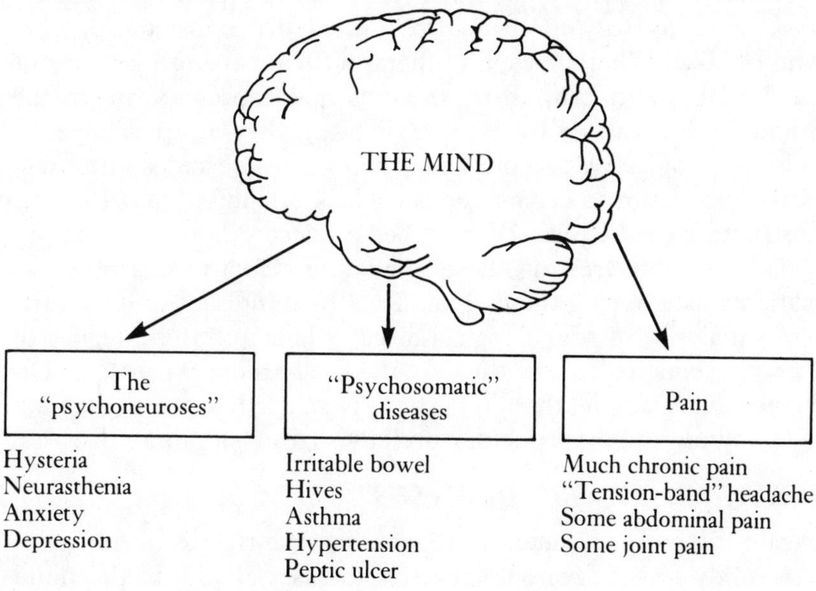

The "psychoneuroses"	"Psychosomatic" diseases	Pain
Hysteria	Irritable bowel	Much chronic pain
Neurasthenia	Hives	"Tension-band" headache
Anxiety	Asthma	Some abdominal pain
Depression	Hypertension	Some joint pain
	Peptic ulcer	

143

from insomnia, or the people who go back to the house ritualisti-
cally to make sure the door is locked or the gas turned off. These
are all "neurotic" traits, and the whole term has become so gener-
alized as to lose its meaning.[5]

When the term *psychoneurosis* came into existence late in the
nineteenth century, it referred to people who exhibited some psychological disorder but who were not grossly *psychotic*, that is,
out of touch with reality. Initially, hysteria and neurasthenia
were the chief psychoneuroses, *hysteria* indicating patients who
were highly emotional and exhibited signs of organic diseases that
they didn't actually have; *neurasthenia*, an old term revived in
1869, referring basically to "nervous exhaustion."[6] For a GP
around the turn of the century, the psychoneuroses were thus
fairly straightforward: "Finding the patient lachrymose and emotional, he calls the disorder hysteria; if depressed and inert, he
calls it neurasthenia," wrote one neurologist rather contemp-
tuously.[7]

After the 1950s, "psychoneurosis" came increasingly to mean
anxiety and depression, because *hysteria* and *neurasthenia* had
become unfashionable terms. The physical symptoms accompanying a depressed mood, let us say, are just the same as the
physical symptoms of neurasthenia and its relatives: sleeplessness, inability to stop crying, loss of sex drive, loss of appetite,
and the like. Whether we find them in the nineteenth century or
in the late twentieth, all these kinds of symptoms arise in the
mind (unless caused by organic disease): they are psychogenic.
The mind of its own accord and without any conscious act of will
drives its victim to crying jags, or a lack of energy, or whatever,
instructing the helpless body to behave accordingly.

Doctors hate treating these intangible symptoms as much as
patients hate having them. Therefore the mind sees to it that the
great majority of psychological diseases falls into the category of
"psychosomatic," where they are medically more acceptable. Diarrhea, for example, though perhaps psychically caused, is an *organic* symptom, and doctors prefer to treat "organic" diseases.

"PSYCHOSOMATIC DISEASES"

Again we require quotation marks, because this term too is increasingly losing favor. It indicates diseases arising in the mind

(*psyche-*) that manifest themselves as disturbances of body function (thus -*somatic*). The mind issues a directive, unconsciously and for whatever perverse reason, to alter the action of the bowels, thus producing constipation or diarrhea; the mind decides to raise a skin rash, or to make a person feel desperate about not being able to get enough air. Where in the mind these impulses arise is not known, but their mode of transmission is the involuntary nervous system, also known as the autonomic nervous system. A lot of body ailments doubtless have some kind of psychological connection, even if they aren't clear cases of psychogenesis. High blood pressure, peptic ulcer disease, and asthma are thought to be psychosomatic in part because episodes often coincide with emotional crises or appear in people with certain personality types.

In the 1930s, when the word *psychosomatic* itself was coined, hypertension, peptic ulcer, asthma, rheumatism, various bowel problems, and skin rashes were all deemed to be of psychological origin.[8] But nowadays we know that things are more complicated. The unconscious doesn't just decide to make the blood vessels narrower, thus causing hypertension. The kidneys, the adrenal glands, and other systems also come into the picture. So doctors now talk about "psychological factors affecting physical conditions," meaning any disease imaginable, from cancer to colds. The interplay between cerebral cortex and body is so intimate that the mind is probably involved in a much wider range of physical events than doctors in the 1930s ever dreamed . Hence the rise of whole new specialties, like "psychoneuroendocrinology."[9] For our purposes it doesn't really matter exactly which diseases are called psychogenic so long as they may be relieved by the power of suggestion, by the catharsis of simply telling one's story to the doctor, or by psychotherapy. More on this in a minute.

PAIN

With the psychosomatic diseases there is, at least, some disorder of function, something you can shake a stick at: the colon works too well or not at all, the skin clearly has little welts on it, the stomach displays a quarter-sized ulcer in its mucosal lining. With psychogenic pain, on the other hand, the problem is entirely in the mind. The sensation of pain arises in the brain and not in the periphery, but it feels as though something out there on the periphery is hurting terribly: the "stomach" or some ill-defined place in the belly, the knee joints, or the head. In contrast to pain of organic origin that is *acute* (meaning that it comes on suddenly and then goes away again), psychogenic pain tends to be chronic. For the sufferer it is very real, although the body parts that feel painful are perfectly healthy.

Medicine has long understood that pain can arise in the mind. John Gregory, the enlightened physician of eighteenth-century Edinburgh to whom we were introduced several chapters earlier, wrote about the pain of nervous patients in 1770. "Although the fears of these patients are generally groundless, their sufferings are real. . . . To treat their complaints with ridicule or neglect, from supposing them the effect of a crazy imagination, is equally cruel and absurd."[10] It has also been long understood that people are *suggestible* about pain. One English doctor recalled, "Some years ago when the local anaesthetic injections began to be used in dentistry, I had occasion to have a tooth extracted. The anaesthetic worked beautifully and I spoke well of it to my patients. . . . Suddenly I began to hear of patients who had severe pain on the day following the operation. On investigation it was discovered that the dentist was telling everyone that it was quite likely this would happen. . . ." Apparently this dentist had had a complaint from one patient who continued to have pain the second day, and from then on had routinely warned all his patients about the second day. The author concluded, "I confess that I was astonished that there were so many suggestible people in the world."[11]

I have treated these "psychological diseases" as discrete entities in their own little boxes. But in real life they all overlap, so that a patient who is suffering from one stands a good chance of being afflicted with others as well. Take depression, for example, a psychoneurosis. One study found that 82 percent of patients hospitalized with depression also had such somatic symptoms as awakening during the night, dry mouth, and feelings of fatigue. In 1982 a special issue of the *Journal of Nervous and Mental Disease* was devoted to "chronic pain as a depressive disorder," with scads of statistics on the way depression causes the sensation of physical pain.

A twenty-one-year-old patient of New York neurologist Joseph Collins wrote to him in 1908 about a problem with eating: he was unable to eat in the presence of other people and would make his mother leave the house at mealtime, to the bewilderment of the neighbors. There were deeper problems as well. "I have never had any inclination or desire to have certain relations with women; on the contrary, I have a feeling of profound dislike for even the thought of it or for anything that suggests it." The young man had, however, become attracted to a certain young woman but responded to her with profuse sweating: "When we returned [from a walk] I went home, changed all my underclothes, which were so wet that they dripped when wrung." The explanation for all this was clear in the lad's mind: "I attribute all my troubles to masturbation, which I began when about 12 years old."[12] Interesting for us is the way all these psychological troubles around sex and eating intertwine with physical symptoms such as perspiration. In psychological disease, "voluntary" and "involuntary" symptoms are usually found together.

The body's major battleground for psychic conflict in bygone times was the colon. Struggles waged in the unconscious would find expression more surely in abdominal pain, constipation, and diarrhea than in any other physical manner. In the 1930s women would say to doctors, "If you would only do something to make my colon more comfortable my nerves would get well." Of 200 patients who attended the Mayo Clinic in the early 1930s for "chronic nervous exhaustion," 69 had bloating, belching, constipation, and soreness of the belly as their main organic symptoms. Or, looking at it the other way around, lots of colon patients had psychological symptoms as well. Of one thousand cases of "unstable colon" on whom Dr. Sara Jordan reported in 1932, 62 percent had such nervous symptoms as dizziness, easy fatigability, and depression. Paul Dubois ascribed to nervous patients "the characteristic trio of functional disturbances, that is to say, dyspepsia, constipation, and insomnia." (Dyspepsia is discomfort around the stomach following meals).[13]

How often would the typical family doctor see these diseases of psychological origin? Very often, by their estimates. "They are legion, these dyspeptic patients, who visit the watering-places every year, and who are never able to eat anything, but who are always in pain," wrote Dubois in 1904 about the spas of bourgeois Europe. And in Halstead, Kansas, it was no different: "The worried businessman often presents himself as a stomach complainer," said Arthur Hertzler, the horse-and-buggy doctor. "The apprehensive look, the epigastric pulsation . . . [are] sufficient to characterize these cases." He emphasized how urgent it was to protect them from the surgeon.[14]

I don't want to submerge the reader in figures, but a few of them are necessary to convey how frequently disease of psychological origin afflicted the modern patient. Take pain, for example. No fewer than four out of ten adults in a working-class housing project in England had taken "aspirin or other pain relieving powders" within the previous four weeks, according to a survey made in the mid-1950s. Indeed, 53 percent of the younger women had done so.[15] Presumably they found themselves in pain.

In the world of the GP, "neurosis" was confronted virtually every hour. The nineteen patients seen by "Dr. E." (who was attending a seminar for GPs at the Tavistock Clinic in London) in a typical day included the following:

- *Mr. I., saturnine Welshman, aged 34. Brought boy to be immunized against diphtheria and whooping cough. . . . Then in his son's presence he said, "By the way, after intercourse I have a strong burning feeling in the stomach and sometimes I do'not want intercourse just to avoid this."*
- *Mr. Z., aged 60, hypertension and Parkinsonism [a neurological disease]. Came for repeat of tablets. Has very real illnesses, but is also an extremely anxious man, and would like to stay and talk. He only refers to somatic symptoms, but he is very anxious.*
- *Mr. F., marital problem; both wife and mother severe hysterics, frequent visitors to the surgery. He complained of impotence last year and after he had been investigated his wife became pregnant. He insisted baby was not his. He is a man with a great deal of violence in him.[16]*

The seminar participants felt that, of Dr. E's nineteen patients that day, "seven suffer from obvious neurosis and a further nine show enough symptoms to suggest that neurosis is very likely present."[17]

Of one thousand patients seen for a medical exam at the Lahey Clinic in Boston in the 1940s, four hundred were deemed to have "neuropsychiatric" problems, of which the great majority were a mixture of "chronic nervous exhaustion," "nervous fatigue," and the like, coupled with digestive problems and tension headaches.[18]

A number of doctors, then, believed the percentage of "psychoneurotics" among their patients to be quite high indeed. Ballpark estimates of psychological disorder by GPs ranged from 25 percent to 75 percent. A small-town Ontario doctor, looking back over a career spanning the 1930s to the 1950s, said, "About 25 percent of my patients had purely emotional disorders or had an emotional overlay of physical ailments." At the other end is Doctor Israel Strauss, speaking in 1947: "I venture to say that in 75 percent of his practice [the GP] will be dealing with patients in whom, in one form or another, the emotional state is the dominating factor."[19]

The physicians who estimated psychological disorder to be present in half their patients were probably unusually sensitive to patients' unhappiness and anxiety. People can be anxious about any somatic condition from cancer to the common cold. Yet even with quite hardheaded hospital-based clinicians, estimates of one-third to one-half recur. Sir Maurice Cassidy, the senior physician at St. Thomas's Hospital in London, said flatly, "Thirty percent of the patients whom I see in consulting practice have no organic lesion." "Every experienced general practitioner will admit that most of his time is spent in dealing with the psychoneuroses." Of 174 predominantly working-class patients admitted to the medical services of the Johns Hopkins Hospital in 1936–1937, the diagnosis in 26 percent was psychoneurosis. (This did not include even the psychosomatic cases.) And Francis Peabody, the distinguished professor of medicine at Harvard, said just before his death in 1927 that he thought perhaps *one-half* of all hospital cases (excluding infections) were psychosomatic in origin. They "may be regarded as patients whose subjective symptoms are due to disturbances of the physiologic activity." "The ultimate causes of the disturbances," he said, "are to be found . . . in nervous influences emanating from the emotional or intellectual life." In response to patient fears that "it's all in my head," Peabody stressed, "There is nothing imaginary about [these symptoms]. Emotional vomiting is just as real as the vomiting due to pyloric obstruction, and so-called 'nervous headaches' may be as painful as if they were due to a brain tumor."[20]

Surveys of the population as a whole in the 1920s and 1930s confirm these high figures. "Nervous" problems in 1917 were *second* in prevalence to coughs and colds; interviewers found that 24 Americans per 10,000 were sick on a given day from "diseases of the nervous system." According to James Halliday, a regional medical officer in Scotland's Department of Health, fully one-third of all "incapacitated persons" in Scotland, 1930–1933, suffered from "psychoneurosis." Among the 335 psychoneurotic individuals in 1,000 consecutive patients surveyed, 26 percent suffered from "neurasthenia or neurosis," 17 percent from rheumatism (in Halliday's opinion a psychosomatic disease), 15 percent from gastritis, and so on. In his view, specific labels had little value. They were "merely evidence that a person is ill and entitled to a sick benefit."[21]

Indeed, specific numbers have little value. I am claiming no scientific precision for this hodgepodge of statistics, impressionistic in origin; biased by the prejudices of the haughty specialist and the tired, cynical GP; and hopelessly inadequate as an indicator of the true level of psychological disorder in the modern patient. One might argue, in fact, that *everyone* is constantly in some state of psychological disorder: everyone is constantly perceiving symptoms of some kind—the twinges and twitches that are our quotidian lot—that may or may not, depending on how much time, money, energy, and self-awareness we have, be defined as illness. I use these statistics merely to estimate the size of the problem. What really interests us is the extent to which modern doctors could *cure* these psychological diseases.

Curing Psychological Disease: Suggestion

When a disease arises in the mind, it's in the *unconscious* mind. An enormous amount of the mental activity in the cerebral cortex occurs without our being conscious of it. We have no rational control over it. We cannot peer into our own unconscious and ask, "What's going on in there?" Yet that unconscious part of the brain is able to peep out. It picks up everything that happens around us. And it can be addressed through therapy. Suggestion is a kind of therapy for tricking the unconscious mind into doing something or not doing it.

People can be afflicted, as we have seen, with paralyses of psychological origin. Try as he might, the patient cannot move his arm. Somehow he has been "suggested" into believing his arm is paralyzed, and no conscious act can unparalyze it. One can also be suggested into feeling pain or into being constipated.

Similarly, the power of suggestion can *overcome* disease that arises in the mind. Although this is no longer done, once the man with the paralyzed arm would have been told that the doctors were going to perform an operation on his spine that would cure him. They would put him out with anesthesia and make a small "sham" incision in his back, and when he awakened he would discover he was "cured." He would have been induced by the suggestion of fake surgery into curing himself.[22]

Suggestion, the reader will see, plays an enormous role in the practice of medicine, even though neither doctors nor patients like to admit it. What interests me is the declining ability of doctors today to cure by suggestion. Therefore, I want to demonstrate how tremendously potent suggestion has been in history. Let us single out two main ways that suggestion is used to cure psychological disease: by surgery, and by medical placebos.

We take an extreme case. Arthur Hertzler has a patient who is a "maiden lady," forty-six. "She had not walked a step for eighteen years. She was lifted from her bed to a wheel chair several times a day by some members of the family." So far we see a pitiable paraplegic, often found in those years, especially among young women. Hertzler did observe, however, that "during the examination she could move her legs any way I directed and that the muscle tone was good." So what did Hertzler do for this sufferer? He removed her uterus. "I explained to the patient that the cause of her inability to walk was due to the pressure on the nerves [of a small fibroid in the uterus] and that its removal would relieve her of difficulty." Three weeks later, after she had

fully recovered from the hysterectomy, he sailed into her bedroom and "abruptly announced that we were going for a walk.
And we did so and she has continued to walk since—lo, these
many years."[23] A pelvic operation had suggested the woman into
a cure of her psychogenic paralysis.

One of the horrifying skeletons in the closet of gynecological
surgery is that during the nineteenth century many doctors removed the pelvic organs of female patients under the quite genuine belief that mental illness arose "reflexly" from "irritation" in
those organs, and that it could be cured by the removal of the
uterus, ovaries, or clitoris. This view that psychic disturbance
was caused by pathological nervous reflexes sent by stomach,
gallbladder, rectum, or uterus had arisen early in the century, and
led to the doctrine that to "cure" hysteria one had merely to remove a woman's uterus or ovaries, some "irritation" always being
present in those organs. These doctors didn't believe that they
were curing "reflex neurosis" (as they called it) by suggestion at
all. They believed their operations provided real, physical relief
for a mind troubled by poisonous nervous signals from the rest of
the body. Of course, their physiological theories were wrong.
Psychic troubles do not arise reflexly from the urethra or rectum
in the way that a knee will jerk if you hit the kneecap's tendon.
But the operations themselves were often successful, as a result of
suggestion. The patients whose organs were removed would discover themselves cured of their paraplegia, or their hysteria, or
whatever.

Henry Marcy, a distinguished Boston surgeon who introduced
the antiseptic treatment of wounds to the United States, believed
implicitly in the theory of "reflex neurosis." When Mrs. D.,
thirty-two, came to him with "a shuffling gait, difficulty in lifting
the feet, and gradually growing worse," he knew just what to do.
He wasn't at all deflected by the news that she was scarcely able
to walk at all *unless wearing her leather jacket.* But when he saw
her in 1898, even "supported by the jacket, she walked alone with
the greatest of difficulty, depending on the aid of a friend to assist
her." So he removed her ovaries and sewed her uterus to the front
of her abdomen. Three weeks later she could "walk better than
for six years. She was discharged from the hospital in four weeks,

walking without the jacket. She improved steadily, resumed her household duties and is at present an active, vigorous woman."[24] Obviously the operation had "suggested" her back into health.

In the following case Dr. Marcy believed himself to be curing a man with reflex neurosis. A thirty-six-year-old merchant was suddenly seized with the delusion that "he has regularly breathed through a hole in his back." He had been from doctor to doctor "without benefit, all having declared the impossibility of his statement, usually laughing at his oddity." Dr. Marcy's eagle eye suspected reflex neurosis, but where could the source of the inflammation be that was sending the pathological signals to the brain? Dr. Marcy "examined him very carefully and found a large, old, suppurating wen [a small cyst in the skin], which caused him pain at every movement." Dr. Marcy removed the wen, and the man was cured of his delusion.[25]

Late in the nineteenth century, thousands and thousands of ovaries and uteruses were sacrificed on the altar of reflex neurosis, to say nothing of the male urethras cauterized, the anuses instrumentally enlarged, the cervixes swabbed with creosote: all to eliminate the source of the irritation that was causing the mind to act up. After appendectomy became common, doctors noted that it was uncommon to find a mature woman who had retained her appendix, a further onslaught against reflex irritation. In 1936 Georgia's William Houston could only "hope" that "the removal of a young woman's ovaries to cure hysterical seizures will no longer be seen." "It has been my misfortune to see a number of patients who had their ovaries removed for hysterical seizure— criminal negligence."[26]

As reflex neurosis finally faded from sight, surgeons abandoned the organs of the pelvis and addressed the kidney and stomach to find out whether they had "dropped" (*ptosis*, as it was called). Dropped organs were thought to cause neurosis and vague, unlocalized abdominal pains. To avoid autointoxication, colons were removed for constipation. Thymus and thyroid were hauled out to reduce "kinetic drive." The autonomic nervous system was sliced and cut for a number of psychosomatic diseases.[27] One bizarre mutilation involved pulling out all the patient's teeth in order to cure fiftyish women of "focal infections," which were thought to cause things like "indigestion, nervousness, loss of appetite, and a marked loss of weight."[28] That this kind of operation flourished until the 1930s is a stunning indictment of the modern surgeon. But the amazing thing is that the patients often got better.

A placebo is a drug given more to please than to benefit the patient. Or at least that is the standard definition. *Placebo* in Latin means "I will please." But placebos often cure the patient, for the act of "pleasing" him, or satisfying him that he is receiving powerful therapy, often turns off the switch in his unconscious mind that was producing the "psychogenic" disease in the first place. Hence placebos, just as surgery, can cure by suggestion.

There were cackles of glee as doctors told one another what they had devised as placebos. Don't prescribe sugar pills, they said, because the pharmacist may mess you up by telling the patient what is in them. Dispensing sugar pills in one's own clinic, however, bypassed the risk of the blabby pharmacist. Because patients thought bitter medicines potent, one doctor advised as placebos "compound tincture of gentian" or "ammoniated valerian" to create "a riot of tastes and smells." Then the pharmacist couldn't spike your wheels, either, because in the *Dispensatory* "he is apt to find a very long list of conditions for which it has been recommended, uses for which not a vestige of scientific evidence exists."[29]

Bottles were mislabeled. One drug company offered for sale to physicians "blank tablets" with *Harvard Experimental Diagnosis Tablets* on the label and sold five thousand of them to a physician in Cambridge, Massachusetts. On the women's ward of the Philadelphia Hospital one staff man "habitually used a solution labelled 'morphine,' which contained none of that alkaloid, but just enough quinine to make it conform in taste to the knowledge of [the inpatients]." He claimed it aided three out of five as well as the genuine morphine.[30]

Patients loved to see injections, believing them superpowerful, and so substances like "calcium gluconate" (calcium and gluconic acid, the chief acid of honey) were widely used. Dr. Charles Wheeler, an internist in the Cornell University Medical College in New York, was horrified to learn that colleagues were injecting calcium and vitamins into *veins* (where the drugs would be carried immediately back to the heart and lungs) and injecting the arsenical syphilis drug arsphenamine as placebos![31]

Note that all drugs exert some kind of suggestion upon the patient, as long as the patient believes in them. As one New York doctor said,

> You cannot write a prescription without the element of the placebo. A prayer to Jupiter starts the prescription. [*Rx* originally meant an invocation to the Roman god Jupiter but later stood for *recipe.*] It carries weight, the weight of two or three thousand years of medicine. The fact that it is signed by a doctor, that it has required a doctor to write out the prescription, that the prescription has to be taken to a drug store to be made up, that the patient has to pay for it, that it has, perhaps, a bad taste, all of these things are placebo elements in a prescription.[32]

Thus, for example, penicillin works by causing bacteria to swell up and rupture and by preventing their reproduction. But it also works by conveying to the patient the doctor's statement "I will take care of you," which is part of the placebo effect. Most drugs today have both the pharmacological and the placebo effects going for them, but before World War II—with exceptions noted in Chapter 4—drugs cured almost solely by suggestion.

It does not matter whether the doctor has confidence in the drug as long as the patient believes in it. The drugs of the 1920s and 1930s were placebos, despite the fact that doctors were bursting with confidence in them. Thus even though the bromides are seen today as medically useless, men like William Macartney, a "country doctor," sang their praises to high heaven. "I am constantly meeting up with cases of 'weak spells' usually attributed to a 'bad heart,' commonly accompanied by a feeling of intense depression . . . a sensation of impending disaster . . . with depression of spirits and, occasionally blank despondency." Dr. Macartney would give potassium bromide. "Many cases of nervous depression of a temporary nature . . . are promptly relieved by one full dose of the bromides," he said.[33] If he had told these patients to stand on their heads—provided he had done so with conviction *and they believed him*—that treatment would have cured depression as well.

Thus, in nervous diseases placebos have a distinguished history. We find the American doctor Augusta Brown in Paris in the 1880s, giving extract of rabbit ovary to "more than a dozen women" who had hysterical fits and palpitations. The result: end of problems, better digestion, more energy.[34] We find Dr. John Banks of Dublin treating a female patient, thirty-eight, who had been bedridden for sixteen years. "Her lower extremities were perfectly powerless. She had not attempted to put her legs under her for years. . . . It was supposed that she laboured under paralysis of the rectum . . . and three times in the week her mother removed the contents of the rectum." Dr. Banks gave her a rhubarb pill and told her it would cure her. "Now she [is] able to walk miles."[35]

In other times and places, these paraplegic women would have been cured at revival meetings or the shrine of Lourdes. But in a society that believes in the science of medicine, medical placebos are able to cure. The secret is to inspire belief in the doctor's healing power. Traditional plant brews had lacked the placebo effect of "medical science," there being none at that time; instead they piggybacked on faith in the medical incantations one was supposed to recite, which were in every peasant's herbal.

I have discussed placebos mainly as treatment for "nervous diseases." But as we have seen, many diseases of "psychological" origin come to the doctor's office as "psychosomatically" caused asthma, peptic ulcer, and the like. What success have placebos with this kind of problem, in which the mental "switch" seems more deeply buried, less susceptible to persuasion than the switch controlling these phantom paraplegias?

The answer is, quite a bit. In the 1950s placebos did just as well as nitroglycerin in some studies of chest pain (angina pectoris). Placebos in those years did as well as aspirin in efforts to treat arthritic pain. And in the treatment of peptic ulcer in that period placebos had an excellent record. For example, a Finnish study carried out in the mid-fifties found that 74 percent of ulcer patients had improved within two weeks of receiving a placebo; only 66 percent of the patients who had received some specific antiulcer drug that was being tested improved. The authors concluded that virtually all of the ulcer medication then in use was placebo treatment, although the doctors prescribing it didn't know that.[36]

Yet for those who prescribed the placebos, there were still certain regrets. There was the "disaster" of being found out by the patient, for that spelled the end of an effective relationship. The questionable ethics of asking patients to pay for drugs that were worthless made many physicians back off. (The whole issue of whether it was ethical to lie to patients at all had not yet arisen.) And there was the social implication of lowering oneself to the level of homeopaths and herbalists by prescribing compounds that, although possessed of therapeutic benefit, had no scientific merit whatsoever. As the Cornell pharmacologist Harry Gold put it, " 'Honest' doctors are not likely to find it easy to give evidence of enthusiasm for coated sugar-pills."[37] Placebos, beguiling though they were, did not represent a full solution to the problem of psychological disease.

CURING PSYCHOLOGICAL DISEASE: THE HEALING POWER OF THE CONSULTATION

What made suggestion potent in the hands of the modern doctor was the whole context of the consultation. The modern consultation, in and of itself, could exert a positive impact upon psychological disease, provided that two things happened:

1. *The doctor showed an active interest in the patient.*
2. *The patient had an opportunity to tell his story in a leisurely, unhurried manner.*

These twin circumstances seemed to have a "cathartic" effect on patients: the conflicts and anxieties that had caused many of their problems somehow were vented in the act of telling. It was this chance to explain oneself, not to the schoolteacher or the minister but to the doctor, that would turn off those hidden psychological switches. For it was upon the doctor that the great veils of scientific medicine and gentlemanly social status were draped.

When Walter Alvarez was practicing in San Francisco around the time of World War I, a "nice-looking, well-dressed married woman of 50" came in to see him. She was furious that Alvarez's chief had dismissed her chronic abdominal pain as neurotic. "Soon, I was asking her why she looked so unhappy, and after sizing me up for a minute, she said, 'I think I can talk to you.' "

It turned out that she had been a madam in a house of prostitution. Alvarez was fascinated and started asking her "how she handled the graft, how much she had to pay the police captain," and so forth. "The next day we had another interesting chat on the problem of running a 'house' in a mining camp, and then she picked up her things and started to say good-by."

Puzzled, Alvarez said, "Wait a minute; we haven't yet talked about your stomach-ache."

"Oh," she said, "that's all right; it's all gone and I really feel quite well."

"But," Alvarez asked, "why are you well?"

"Because you like me!" she said.[38]

One interesting aspect of this story is the fact that Alvarez saw the woman two days in a row, for lengthy chats. He was a busy internist, yet not so busy that he couldn't sandwich in a patient who today (exotic aspects of the story aside) would be dismissed as a "middle-aged crock" and given tranquilizers. She had a chance to tell her story, and her pain vanished. Alvarez summed up the point in another of his writings: "Actually, in many cases, the eliciting of a good history will practically cure the patient."[39]

Was Alvarez exceptionally generous with his time? Not at all. The medical advice manuals of the day all commanded, Let the patient talk! "It is often very satisfying to the sick to be allowed to tell, in their own way, whatever they deem important for you to know," wrote Daniel Cathell in 1922. "Give to all a fair, courteous hearing, and, even though Mrs. Chatterbox, Mr. Borum, and Mrs. Lengthy's statements are tedious, do not abruptly cut them short, but endure and listen with respectful attention, even though you are ready to drop exhausted."[40]

Undivided attention didn't mean breaking in every twelve seconds with a question. You were supposed to *listen*, not interrogate. "Do not interrupt [the patient] in his story unless it is to gain some essential fact he has not made clear to you," advised Verlin Thomas.[41] "Make these interrogations as rare as possible." Ditto Frank Billings, a former head of the AMA, who said, "Be careful not to misdirect the story of the patient by questions which may encourage indicated replies."[42] Indeed, the same approach is understood today to be necessary for good interviewing; do not put words into the patient's mouth, lest you put in the wrong words. But few doctors today would swallow this old-style advice to listen with an unhurried air and not to interrupt. A Canadian GP, looking back, recalled how hard he found it. "This is really time-consuming. . . . I must never be in a hurry; I must not even look at my watch during an interview. A watch out of sight below my desk on the floor would have been helpful but I never did put one there."[43]

Even in the hospital, the least likely of settings, the attending physician should listen carefully and quietly. Get the patient to tell his story in detail, advised Francis Peabody, whom one cannot accuse of being a fuzzy-brained social worker. "Often the best way is to go back to the very beginning. And try to find out the circumstances of the patient's life at the time the symptoms first began." Only after this kind of long intimate chat would you, as a junior house officer (for whom Peabody was writing his little guide), be able to decide whether the stomach pain might have a psychological basis.[44]

The doctor, then, should not create the impression of haste. Said a hard-nosed English cardiologist, quoting an old mentor, there were "few things which a patient dislikes more than a feeling that the doctor is in a hurry." "Never go into a patient's bedroom with your overcoat on . . . this will make the patient think you mean to be off in a minute or two. However over-worked and pressed for time you may be, don't let your patient sense it." Finally the old mentor added, "Never sit on the patient's bed. . . . But if you *must* sit on the patient's bed, for Heaven's sake don't idly turn over the pages of his *Daily Mirror* while he pours forth his tale of woe."[45]

One can find similar pieties in today's advice manuals. What evidence is there that the doctor of the 1920s and 1930s actually did devote quite a bit of time to an individual patient? In an era of house calling, the number of calls the doctor might make per illness was high: 3.6 calls for the average illness at the end of the 1920s. The doctor called 2.4 times for a cold, 3.6 times for the typical case of mumps or other "communicable disease," 4.7 times for a "nervous disease," and so on.[46] It is, to our postmodern minds, quite incredible that in those days patients expected the doctor to call *virtually every day.* "In the majority of cases, unless quite trivial, the patient expects to be seen every day for several days at least. . . . Even if you stay only two minutes and talk about the weather all the time, it comforts the patient and the relatives . . . ," said an English manual in the 1920s.[47]

We get some hints that office calls, too, were of generous length. Verlin Thomas talks about the kinds of subjects the doctor might discuss with his patient. "You may always rest assured of interesting your patient if you discuss his hobby. The most successful business man will often drop everything to talk about golf or dogs or flowers or postage stamps." Pets too. "Men and women like to talk about their work, and by listening to them and showing a real interest you will often be able to obtain a fund of valuable information. . . . Every one is pleased to have an interested listener," Thomas concluded.[48] There you are with your office full of patients, talking about someone's hobbies. The consultations must have been rather long.

In the words of William Houston, an internist from Augusta, Georgia, "For every hour that the internist spends in technical examinations . . . he will spend from *one to three* [my italics] in talking with his patients, in educating them, in encouraging them, in hearing from them the story of their difficulties and struggles. . . ." Houston cited "Dr. X," a TB specialist, who claimed three hours of conversation for every hour spent looking at X-rays.[49]

For "nervous" patients the time allocated for consultation was especially long. Of every hundred neurasthenia patients, estimated the Committee on the Costs of Medical Care, ninety-five can be treated by a GP. Of these ninety-five patients, "each of sixty requires two visits of thirty minutes' duration; thirty need an average of six visits of twenty minutes. . . ." Of all these visits, nine out of ten would be at home. Weir Mitchell spoke of "daily chats" with his upper-middle-class nervous patients. Houston asked these patients to keep "daily records," which they would present to him once weekly. Thus he might say, "If I see you but once a week you will tell me what happened on Saturday when you were feeling very much down, but I will have no idea of how well you were on Tuesday. . . ."[50] Just imagine: He was interested in every day!

To get a sense of how much time a doctor might spend on a given patient, let us look at Dr. Frederick Parkes Weber's handling of "Miss X," an upper-middle-class unmarried woman in her late forties who lived in Hampstead, a suburb of London, at the turn of the century. She claimed to have a "pain in her left ovary" and to be subject to attacks of nervousness, especially surrounding her period. Because Parkes Weber was a Harley Street GP with a special interest in wealthy nervous patients and in "balneology" (sending them to spas), his experience of Miss X was typical of that whole world of middle-class suffering.

18 November 1907. Miss X wrote me that she took veronal [a sedative] or bromide powders as ordered by Dr. Fellner if she could not sleep. . . . The menstrual period is on again. Before, during and after these periods she suffers much—a feeling, "as if she could lift something awry from the left side."

Two weeks later (4 December 1907), Parkes Weber visited her at her Hampstead home in the afternoon because of the "extraordinary left 'ovarian' tender area," plus vomiting. She was getting her period again. He returned in the evening, and she said she felt sick whenever he pressed on her abdomen.

The next day she wrote to him, "I am pleased to be able to let you know I had a fairly good night. . . . Today 'the period' arrived this morning." He suggested she take some bromide powders. "I do not think beef-tea will do any harm if it mildly suits you."

Over the next month he had five further contacts with Miss X, all fiddling with her sedative prescriptions and musing about the pain on her left side. Parkes Weber wrote in his case notes on 30

January 1908, "She has pain and depression before having a [bowel] motion. A chronic colitis, with or without ulceration, might also be the cause of the neurasthenia. (One of her sisters once had a temporary nervous breakdown at about 23 years.)"

Parkes Weber now decided to order an exploration of her colon with a sigmoidoscope and enlisted several consultants for an examination, done on 5 February in Miss Jervis's nursing home on Bromptom Square. Nothing was found. He wrote to or saw her three additional times in February.

On 2 March Parkes Weber learned that Miss X's family had persuaded her to go to the seaside resort of Torquay: she did so and hated it: "The wind is so cold she cannot sit out in the open." "She cannot dine with the other people on account of nerves."

Then events took an ominous turn:

8 May 1908. I hear from her brother that Miss X is still at Torquay with a lady-companion, but she thinks that her left ovary is driving her out of her mind and that it will have to be removed.

Parkes Weber opposed the operation, but a week later she was back in London, "complaining more than ever of 'feeling' in the left 'ovary.' . . . She says her life is not worth having, and she *must* have the ovary (left side only) removed."

We shall not follow the drama past this point.[51] Clearly whatever therapy Parkes Weber was able to provide had not done Miss X any good. The point is, rather, that he had spent an enormous amount of time on her.

Why were these modern doctors willing to spend so much time on patients? Was it that they were good fellows? No, I don't think the distribution of generosity, charitableness, or general niceness has shifted much in the medical profession over the centuries, just as it has changed little in most of mankind over that time. I shall not be suggesting that a deterioration of medical character or of morality is responsible for the almost brutal brevity of many consultations today.

Moreover, let us admit that this leisureliness was partly a money-making strategy: "Playing on the [patient's] vanity," as

Thomas put it. It is not that frequent calls or long interviews necessarily ran up the bill, for the men I've been quoting had busy practices and could make more from "revolving-door"-style medicine than from taking time. But it was lucrative to attract patients and keep them over the years, and for that reason it was important for the doctor to be "a very nice man" for the sake of "an intangible something known as good-will." For that reason Cathell advised his readers to be "affable in manner," "refined and gentle"; to "wear a pleasant countenance and a sunny smile." "Manners help to make the majority of medical fortunes," he observed.[52]

Especially these nervous patients could be lashed alongside and carried for years, jollied with sedatives and attentive tête-à-têtes. Verlin Thomas, whose San Francisco practice included a number of hotel residents living out the years in a kind of neurotic daze, described a population of medical suckers.

> There are the women who imagine that they have some private ailment and who can easily be encouraged to believe this to be true. There are those who are readily frightened in an epidemic and those who believe that they have every new disease. . . . There are the weak, who can quickly be frightened into believing almost anything, and the large family of hypochondriacs and the poor, unfortunate incurables. All of these will come to you. Every one of them may be bled white.[53]

If doctors are no less noble than most of us, they are no nobler either. And many rubbed their hands in glee at the middle-class businessmen with stomach pain and the women who thought their ovaries hurt. But historians have to make judgments about the past, and my personal judgment is that doctors with this kind of motive were not preponderant.

Taking an interest in their patients and being alert to their psychology were certainly not virtues doctors had learned in medical school. Awareness of "biopsychosocial" factors—which showers medical students today, in sensitivity sessions taught by bearded psychiatrists—was slumbering then, waiting to be born. "We were taught to think of the worst things first," William Johnston

163

remembered of his own medical training in Toronto in the early 1920s. "We must never overlook an early cancer of the breast or cervix, and might succeed in detecting one every three years, whereas nearly every day some patient complained of a headache and the majority of these were tension headaches, on which little emphasis had been placed."[54]

But Johnston's memories bring us, I think, to the factor that separated the modern doctors from the traditional men who preceded them and the postmodern ones who would come after. They realized how helpless they were in the face of psychogenic disease. Traditional doctors, for the most part, didn't even recognize the concept of disease arising in the mind and in any case couldn't differentiate it from organic disease. Postmodern doctors believe that they are able to tame psychogenesis, with drugs. But modern doctors, once the placebos they spewed about them had failed, stood impotent before the ravages of the mind. Hence, even without a lot of complex theories about psychosomatic mechanisms, they had enough common sense to realize how much patients benefited from "a good chat."

Johnston continued, "As time went by I became more and more concerned about ill people themselves and relatively less about their illnesses. The patient gradually took precedence over his ailments." Johnston was puzzled about why this change in himself had occurred. "It came, perhaps, from the fact that I was seeing a lot of people who were ill but had no disease as disease was described in medical texts or had been demonstrated by my teachers, who were largely hospital instructors working among hospital patients." Thus with time, "One of the first things I learned from worried and anxious people was to listen long and carefully to what they had to say and to allow time for thoughtful answers to my questions."[55] Johnston was discovering that this sort of attentiveness has a healing power of its own.

CURING PSYCHOLOGICAL DISEASE: PSYCHOTHERAPY

What most GPs understood by "psychotherapy" in the years before 1960 was not Sigmund Freud's psychoanalysis, but rather the basic methods of making patients feel at ease, letting them tell their story, and speaking to them reassuringly, elaborated into a doctrine. It was the doctrine of psychotherapy by "persuasion," or "moral therapy," as it was sometimes known. Because it permeated medicine root and branch in the first half of the twentieth century and still exerts a profound subterranean influence today, we spend a moment on it.

The story begins, oddly enough, with someone who wasn't interested in psychotherapy at all and believed nervous disease to have a physical origin in "tired blood" and "exhausted ganglia." This was Weir Mitchell, the inventor of the "rest cure." For the upper-middle-class society ladies of his Philadelphia practice, Mitchell devised a cure with the following ingredients:

- *Isolation from the family in a nursing home or private hospital, so that all the tensions that presumably had made the patient sick in the first place would be temporarily in abeyance.*

- *Electrotherapy: applying tiny voltages to the muscles of the arms and legs in order to "restore tone" and make it possible for the patient to walk briskly again.*

- *Massage: trained masseuses would knead and roll clients for hours on end, in order to get the blood flowing to those "exhausted" nervous centers.*

- *"Overfeeding": these often anorexic patients were almost force-fed a milk diet. Milk therapy has a long history in the treatment of nervous diseases, but Mitchell elaborated a whole physiology of how it should restore fat and blood. If necessary, he would feed the patients nutrients by rectum too, especially cod-liver oil.*[56]

Although Mitchell believed that this regimen effected a physical cure of problems having an organic origin, obviously it worked by suggestion, by isolating the patient from the "countersuggestion" of her friends and relatives so that his own suggestion would have free play.

The rest cure had remarkable success. Mitchell described one of his own patients, "Mrs. B.," "brought to me on a couch from a distant New England state." She was down from 130 to 95 pounds, "had pain in the back, steady dyspepsia, and great weakness. Everything tired her," and she hadn't menstruated for three years. She had finally taken to her bed and was unable to rise, thus becoming one of the numerous female "paraplegics" who haunted neurologists before World War I.

So Mitchell went into action. "She was put in bed, and left it for no purpose. At first she was even moved by her maid when she wanted to turn in bed. She was fed and washed by others, and forbidden to read or use her hands, and even to talk." Meanwhile, her physiotherapy bounded ahead: "Exercise without exertion is what we want, and this is the way it was had. Every day she was masséed, thoroughly; and skin, muscles, and belly kneaded until they flushed. . . . Every day each muscle was made to contract by faradic currents." By the thirtieth day of this regimen she had started menstruating again, and after two months had gained thirty pounds. In a further month she was able to walk anywhere. "This sickly, feeble, wasted creature had become a handsome, wholesome, helpful [sic] woman, and so remains to this day. . . ."[57]

It tells us a good deal about the position of women in the nineteenth century to learn that Mitchell's rest cure became an enormous rage, spreading to Britain, France, and Germany, where the leading internists and physiologists raved about it.[58] The rest cure provided the launching pad for the next phase of our story: movement from physical therapy to psychotherapy.

Late in the nineteenth century a number of French neurologists had become absorbed with the nervous disease "hysteria." Joseph Babinski and Jules-Joseph Dejerine advocated the view that hysteria could be both induced and "cured" by such forms of psychotherapy as hypnosis. Other kinds of suggestion interested them as well, but what most intrigued Babinski in particular was the possibility of treating hysteria by persuasion. *Persuasion* means, more or less, a good chat between doctor and patient, in which the doctor explains the true source of the problems, and the patient, overcome by the force of his logic, is thus "persuaded" back into health. Neurasthenia, by contrast, Babinski believed should be treated by some kind of rest cure, à la Weir

Mitchell, on the principle that tired nerves had to rest.[59] Thus we have a double-barreled approach to psychological problems: rest plus the therapy of sweet reason.

Here Dejerine's friend, the Swiss Paul Dubois, rushes on stage. In 1904 he explained the benefits of gently persuading the patient there was nothing wrong with him so clearly and with such charm that he laid the twentieth-century foundations for psychotherapy, as the average family doctor would practice it. You've got to instill in the patient the "confident expectation of the success of [your] treatment," he wrote. The patient must be made to believe implicitly, absolutely, that whatever you do will succeed and thus trick his own mind into a recovery. So from the very beginning "a strong bond of confidence and sympathy" must be established between doctor and patient. The patient must see the physician as a "friend with no idea but to cure him. We practitioners ought to show our patients such a lively and all-enveloping sympathy that it would be really very ungracious of them not to get well."

This bond of confidence once established, you proceed with the kind of rational discussion that since the eighteenth century has been called *moral therapy*. Point out to the patient where he has gone wrong. "Question him about his childhood, and he will tell you episodes which show his natural impressionability and his exaggerated emotions. Start the patient upon the scent which you have picked up, and make him admit that he was a 'nervous subject' long before the actual attack."

It was, in short, little more than a good chat, or perhaps what we in the late twentieth century would dress up as stress counseling. But while it was going on, you would proceed as well with a modified version of the Weir Mitchell rest cure, minus all the hokum about "faradization." Dubois thought "overfeeding" and massage quite effective.

So you'd have daily chats. Always comment on favorable signs. "Nothing is insignificant in this domain; one must leave no stone unturned." The patient comes in "tired" and with terrible headaches. After two months there is no improvement. "Take heart," says the doctor. "At least you have lost that trembling of the feet that you had on your arrival."

What trembling? The patient hadn't even noticed it.

Dubois replies heartily, "To you the trembling of the feet means nothing, to me it is as important as the headaches; it is also one of the symptoms of your disease." If we can abolish the one, we can make the other disappear too.

The patient stays a month more and is cured.

Dubois seemed to be a miracle worker. An army officer, forty-one, came to him with neurasthenia that had been worsening steadily over fourteen years: headaches like a drill boring into his skull, night terrors, terrible fatigue. The cure begins:

"I still have, toward one o'clock in the morning," said the officer, "a most distressing feeling of anguish which lasts about half an hour." Dubois reassured him that previously the attacks had lasted six or seven hours. Try "walking about on the cold floor and drink a glass of water and go back to bed."

The next day the officer reported the success of the therapy. "I took my glass of water and I fell asleep like a child."

Thus little by little the officer was cured. Several months later he sent Dubois a photograph "which showed himself on horseback leaping over a high barrier. He had written these words on it: 'As well in the moral saddle as in the physical'!"[60]

Men like Dubois and Mitchell were psychiatrists, although they did not call themselves that, who presided over rest homes and clinics to which their wealthy patients could be admitted. For the average small-town GP what emerged from the rest cure and moral therapy was not so much symptom elimination around such behavioral approaches as the glass of water, but the notions of "authority" and of "rational persuasion." Dubois felt that the therapy succeeded in many cases because the "patient was pleased to give me his complete confidence."[61] Later, when generations of American doctors continued to harp on the "sanctity of the doctor-patient relationship," they were defending the establishment of this kind of confidence.

The psychotherapy of persuasion was in practice merely an extension of the kind of consultation we have already seen. "It is universally admitted," wrote the Edinburgh neurologist Edwin Bramwell in 1923, "that the personality of the physician" is the healing force. The minor psychological disorders "are cured by the words of the physician, the confidence he creates and the forces of nature, and not by the medicine he prescribes." Following Dubois, he wrote that you had only to *explain* to the patient why he was sick, and he would get better. For example, a businessman, forty-two, went to Bramwell in the middle of a nervous breakdown. Upset by problems at the office and dragged down by an earlier attack of influenza, he found himself unable to sleep. He awakened after a restless night, his mind still whirring, "and no more capable of coping with [his problems] satisfactorily than before. As the days went on his power of concentration, his memory, and his ability to come to decisions, instead of improving, became more impaired and his insomnia more pronounced." He started turning into a bear at home. Then "the thought gradually came down upon him like a dark cloud, 'What will happen to my business and my family if I break down?' He conceived the idea that his brain was failing, and the fear of insanity gradually dawned upon him."

What did Bramwell do? Drugs? Not at all. "When one explained to the patient the sequence of events and pointed out to him, using appropriate similes ... that it was brain fatigue and not brain disease from which he was suffering, the effect was instantaneous, and the patient left my room with an altogether different outlook on life."[62]

Thus we can see in action the psychotherapy of the good chat, or "the therapy of moral persuasion," as it was called. It spilled over into secular life in such forms as Norman Vincent Peale's *The Art of Living* (1937) and later *The Power of Positive Thinking* (1952), restoring health to many of his Fifth Avenue parishioners. And it spread into general medical practice all over the United States. When George Newsome, a forty-two-year-old traveling salesman, went to see Dr. William Houston, he was a dyspeptic wreck. For years he'd been on the road, "five days a week ... in hotels and two days at home with his family. He frequently spent the night in Pullman cars and had to take trains at unreasonable hours." Newsome had terrible stomach pains and insomnia and "had spent a large part of his income on doctors and radiologists."

"Now, George," said Dr. Houston, "you have only three

things to do, learn to sleep, to eat, and to understand that you have absolutely nothing to fear."

"Perhaps so," George hesitated. He had hoped the doctor would find something physically wrong with him.

So Dr. Houston "spent some time explaining to him the fundamentals of the physiology of digestion and the technique of going to sleep by muscular relaxation." Over the next few weeks George would send in reports of his progress, and Houston would give encouragement. "It is fatigue and worry that give you indigestion, not food," said Houston. George recovered. "The last I heard of him was from a man to whom he had been bragging on the train and who came to me to find out what was this secret of learning to eat and sleep."[63] This was persuasion by careful explanation in action, the first ingredient of moral therapy.

For the GP, the second element was ironclad medical authority. It was Weir Mitchell who gave the rest cure the stamp of relation between father and child, for in order to get his patients to stay in bed for a couple of months, "childlike obedience" was required. The milk cure, as Mitchell and Dubois conceived it, amounted to a test of will, "a means for taming his patient," Houston later said. And the patient's will would collapse in the doctor's authoritarian presence, for "into the narrow, monotonous square of the sickroom, into the long chain of hours without an incident, his visits come as the major event of the day."[64]

This medical authority did produce cures. Regular vomiting after meals, part of the often fatal disease of young women called *anorexia nervosa* that leaves doctors baffled even today, crumpled in front of William Houston's steely gaze. Miss Nannie Peters, twenty-one, the eldest of a farmer's ten children, had dropped like a rock from 124 to 84 pounds because she vomited her food after every meal. Doctor Houston first had a nice talk with her, and then at the next sitting explained that she had developed bad habits.

"But," she said, "sometimes the food comes back of itself, it just runs up into my mouth and I have to spit it out."

He told her, "You can help spitting it out. . . . If it rises in your throat, do not spit it out. Swallow hard and force it down." Problem solved.[65]

"A girl of twenty-one" had lost the use of her left arm since dislocating her wrist a year and a half previously. Dr. R. S. Bruce Pearson, of the Hampstead General Hospital, finally lost patience with her and insisted "that she could use it quite well if she only made the effort; full power and movement returned immediately and no relapse has occurred two months later."[66] Thus insistent suggestion, as this kind of abrupt demand was called, could have a therapeutic value.

Keep in mind, however, that authority succeeds only as long as its subjects are willing to accept it. The modern patient was willing to tolerate, indeed expected, a kind of medical tyranny that today would produce shocked exposés in the press. Although Weir Mitchell's rest cure left the feminist Charlotte Perkins Gilman fuming with rage after she had been subject to it (see her thinly fictionalized autobiographical account, *The Yellow Wallpaper*), many other female patients adored him. One wrote the following poem:

> In the City of Penn, by the Schuylkill's dark waters,
> A world renowned rest-system has its headquarters. . . .
>
> Then comes Dr. Kane who will take your case history
> The questions he asks often seem quite a mystery;
> Your symptoms and trials, your ancestors' diseases
> Are poured out for him to write as he pleases.
>
> [Next Dr. John Mitchell appears.]
> He studies the case and decides they can cure it.
> At worst, they can give you some strength to endure it.
> He plans out the treatment and keeps patients to it,
> And those who don't mind him will certainly rue it!
>
> At last some bright day at your door will appear,
> The famous neurologist, great Dr. Weir . . .
> Dr. Mitchell's opinion! You quake to receive it,
> *He says you'll get well and you'd like to believe it!*[67]

It is this "patriarchal" authority that has so outraged observers of medicine in our own time. Medical sociologists today simply become blank with fury when they hear of doctors who view patients as did William Houston, who wrote, "Children they are—weak-willed, wayward, thoughtless—whom [the doctor] can find means to lead only by drawing them close to him. . . . They will not understand his explanations as to the mechanism of impending pathological disaster, but they will feel his deep concern."[68]

In the desire to maintain this authority lay the dogma that the doctor could never admit to making a mistake. The British doctor James Nicoll remembered an ear, nose, and throat specialist who was examining a child brought into the outpatient clinic by her mother.

"These tonsils must be taken out as soon as possible," he said.

"Oh, they've been taken out before."

"Well, all I can say is that it's a disgraceful job, and doesn't reflect any credit on the person who took them out."

"Oh, but you took them out, doctor, several years ago at this hospital."

The surgeon excused himself to go look at the records. In fact as a young resident he had "had a shot at guillotining the tonsils and left quite a bit in each. The small part had grown again, and that was what he had to contend with."

Thinking rapidly, he returned to face the mother. "I see what has happened," he said. "The male tonsils have been taken out, but the female tonsils have grown again."[69]

Some historians have waxed indignant at this arrogating of authority, taking it as a sign that medicine of the post-1870 years was withdrawing from the public domain and becoming "a priesthood, its knowledge a mystery." Countering that charge is the doctor's own defense that he must act with the certainty that he is right or otherwise lose the placebo effect.[70] We shall broach these questions once again before the book is done. But I can't resist mentioning here that the evening before writing these lines I was chatting in the street in front of my house with a young female doctor who had just returned from her *first day* at the office as a general practitioner.

How'd it go?

"Oh, fine, except I discovered there was all this stuff I didn't know. After the patient left I had to run and look it up in *Harri-*

son's [a textbook] every time to make sure I'd given them the right thing."

You couldn't check before they left?

"Oh no. You can't let the patient see you looking something up."

Weir Mitchell and Paul Dubois ingrained those attitudes very deeply.

WAS PSYCHOTHERAPY SUCCESSFUL?

Up to now we have been hearing doctors' glowing anecdotes of their successes. The record has another side, presented by those who challenged the efficacy of relentless and unquestioned authority. That critique came mainly from Freudians, proponents of psychoanalysis.

"Sally Willard Pierce" was, by her pseudonymous account, a young musician who married an older businessman in Roslyn, New York, in 1919. She had been perfectly healthy up to then, although ferociously dedicated to her playing. As the honeymoon voyage upon the SS *Pater* commenced, she suddenly turned to her new husband and "cried out that she had to get off. And then without further warning she fainted dead away." When she awakened she insisted that her head felt "queer" and that her left arm was "dying." Upon her return to her father's home in suburban Ruysdale, the decision was made to put her in a "private nervous hospital" (such as the one depicted in Plate 22). There her saga began.

An early therapeutic encounter was with the "insistent suggestion" version of moral therapy, in the person of "Dr. Cozzens." He strode into her room:

"*S-so!* Still in bed. And still wearing that sling. And still coddling that arm on a pillow. . . . After all I've said. After all the definite orders I've given. . . . After everything, here you are—still in bed."

She remembered, "His voice was dark with disdain. He despised me."

He mocked her, "Still in bed. . . . Stubborn, aren't we? *We'll* show 'em, won't we?—show 'em just how badly off we really are. No matter *what* they order, we'll just go ahead and show 'em—that we're not in any shape to obey."

She told Dr. Cozzens she wasn't trying to spite him. "I want to get up, but can't—simply can't—"

"You'd be well by now," he said. "But you won't try. You've never really tried—not once since you set foot inside this cottage. Lying round in bed day in and day out. . . . Where *is* your sense of shame, anyway? Haven't you ever had one?"

On and on he went. She was now emitting broken sobs. "I'll give you until tomorrow morning to stir yourself up out of there. Tomorrow morning, when I make my rounds, if you're not up and dressed and sitting in that chair by that window, I warn you that I'm going to take measures." He threatened to put another nurse on her case, "a regular Amazon." "I keep her for just such gratuitous play-acting as yours." The upshot was that she tried to commit suicide. What worked on twenty-one-year-olds in Hampstead had failed on Sally Pierce.

At the next private psychiatric hospital ("sanitarium") she encountered the pure version of the Dubois therapy: treatment by encouragement. "Dr. Trotter," who took charge of her, was a very nice man indeed.

"You know how anxious he is to help you, don't you, Mrs. Pierce," said the nurse after Sally Pierce had demanded a sleeping pill. "It's his one aim, the one thing he lives for—to help his patients. . . . Well then, don't disappoint him, I beg you. He feels it so, when a patient disappoints him."

In fact Dr. Trotter exulted at every tiny sign of "progress." "Remember all the nice things he said to you yesterday," chattered the nurse, "how delighted he was, and how happy over your progress. You wouldn't want to disappoint him *now*, would you? . . . No, of course not; you want to keep right *on* advancing." Thus did Sally Pierce become able to walk down the hall for her "Alpine-light treatment," finally eat in the dining room, and even play bridge with the other patients. But once she was discharged and the fear of "disappointing Dr. Trotter" was no longer present, she immediately relapsed.

I shall not detail the other therapeutic disasters on Sally's martyr's path. She tried each variation of psychotherapy going, and each failed in turn. In desperation she turned to a Freudian, a psychoanalyst, who cured her.[71] Her little memoir clearly sets us up for a psychoanalytic triumph and thus loads the dice as heavily one way as all the apostles of authority and persuasion I have quoted in this chapter had loaded them in another.

But was Sally Pierce the rule or an exception? I want to make two points.

One is that in the area of the psychoneuroses these "rational" and "moral" therapies had a good batting average. Of 850 patients treated in 1921–1929 at the Cassell Hospital in England, a clinic for the "minor neuroses," one-third were quite well five years later, and another 7 percent "improved." The others had been lost sight of; they all may have committed suicide, for all that is known of them. But as far as the staff knew, few of the 850 had failed to improve at all.[72] It will be objected that patients are anxious to please and tell investigators what they want to hear, that most psychological problems improve spontaneously whether "therapy" is given or not, and that the sheer human concern and intimacy that any psychotherapy represents would effect some betterment, even if it consisted of asking the patient to stand on his head. Of five hundred patients treated at London's Tavistock Clinic in 1928–1931 who were then followed up after three years, 55 percent were "improved" or "much improved."[73] Does this improve upon chance? Who knows? But my guess is that the psychotherapies of the day had a better success rate than the bromides, iron pills, and strychnine that represented the only alternative.

In the area of curing psychosomatic diseases, however, I think the psychotherapy of the 1920s and 1930s has something to teach us. Problems like "irritable bowel," deeply embedded in the "involuntary" (autonomic) nervous system, are less susceptible to persuasion and suggestion than are the psychoneuroses. But irritable bowel, and similar psychosomatic disorders, did surrender often in the face of leisurely counseling in a friendly setting. There were various kinds.

On 22 July 1935 a twenty-two-year-old woman was admitted to the Massachusetts General Hospital in Boston for "constipation and abdominal pain of incapacitating nature for one year." The episodes had come on six months after her recent marriage: "extremely painful attacks of cramps followed by the passage of mucoid bowel movements," then succeeded by constipation, for which she took laxatives daily. There was a flood of other psychological symptoms as well: awareness of her heart beat ("palpitations"), chest pain, weakness, dizziness, loss of appetite, and anxiety.

The doctors performed the usual tests, then inquired about her past. Her father, "a 48-year old, large, athletic, irritable, drunkard, had always treated her mother badly. He had likewise been cruel to the patient and her sister, both of whom had received many severe whippings at his hand." She was so sensitive to her classmates' comments about her father's drunkenness that she left school and worked "in a tinsel factory" until her marriage at age twenty. There had been some history of constipation up to this point, but marriage made it much worse, for her new husband was "a big, dirty man who demanded sexual intercourse three times nightly. Marriage started off with severe dyspareunia [pain in intercourse] which, in the course of a short time, developed into a feeling of gross disgust." She became phobic about catching syphilis, "to the point where she was unwilling to use the toilets at her factory and hence contributed mechanically to her faulty bowel habits." She then separated from her husband and shortly after was admitted to hospital.

The psychiatric staff of the hospital treated her for the next three years, encouraging her to undergo a course of psychoanalysis as well. And even though her fundamental attitude to men didn't alter, she "received much encouragement and help," which resulted in a "distinct improvement in her gastrointestinal and neurocirculatory symptoms."[74]

The psychoanalytically oriented physicians who reported on this case, and on fifty-nine others, generally had good results. They relied partly on the "rational" insight therapies already discussed. Patients "can often learn, when the symptoms of anxiety arise, to realize their unconscious nature and dispel them. . . . Thus their conflicts may be reduced and they may become free of symptoms, although much neurosis may remain." These doctors also tried "reassurance," and then finally deep analysis, with promising results.[75]

But it wasn't just the magic tongue of the psychoanalyst that offered success with psychosomatic digestive problems. The London internist John Ryle saw himself as rescuing these patients, who often had been told they had organic disease and needed operations, from the clutches of the surgeon by giving them "full reassurance," that is, again moral therapy. "With this must be combined a simple explanation as to the nature of the disorder and the mode of origin of the pain." He described fifty cases of "spastic colon," finding them similar to asthma and migraine in being difficult to cure. But "repeated reassurances and rational treatment will often mitigate symptoms even in bad cases. In milder cases there may be complete relief."[76]

Another internist, Chester Jones at Harvard, adopted the "simplest form of psychotherapy": he just let his patients talk about their unhappy lives and reassured them, and in case after case he obtained "an almost complete disappearance of symptoms."[77] Of fifty patients whom the Johns Hopkins internist George Canby Robinson treated in the late 1930s for "digestive complaints," thirty-eight had personality disorders of some kind. Of those thirty-eight, 60 percent responded favorably to the elementary kinds of psychotherapy these physicians were able to administer. Remember that these were specialists in internal medicine, not psychiatrists, and that when they saw patients like the fifty-nine-year-old unemployed baker with a history of chronic constipation, they didn't ask him whether he loved his father more than his mother. They gave him a chance to tell his story. His constipation began two years before, when he was thrown out of work, like so many others, in the Great Depression. He was "depressed and anxious because his savings were being used up and he feared destitution"; he felt "disturbed by a son to whom he had loaned money and from whom he could get no adequate response." So the staff of the Hopkins gastrointestinal clinic talked his problems over with him—note, *not* just among themselves. They suggested various plans of diet and so forth, and he recovered.[78]

Other psychic therapies were more at the margin: Edmund Jacobson, a Chicago internist, experimented with "progressive relaxation" for spasms of the colon and esophagus. The patients would learn to relax by following Jacobson's instruction, practice daily, and be seen in clinic three times a week.[79] It worked, possibly because it's a good idea, possibly because the patients just responded favorably to all this friendly attention and humane care. And that is the point of describing all these various "therapies": not that one particular technique was better than any other, but that the medical consultation in itself, when conducted in a friendly, leisurely way, can have a curative power. The remainder of this book centers on my belief that that curative power is being lost today.

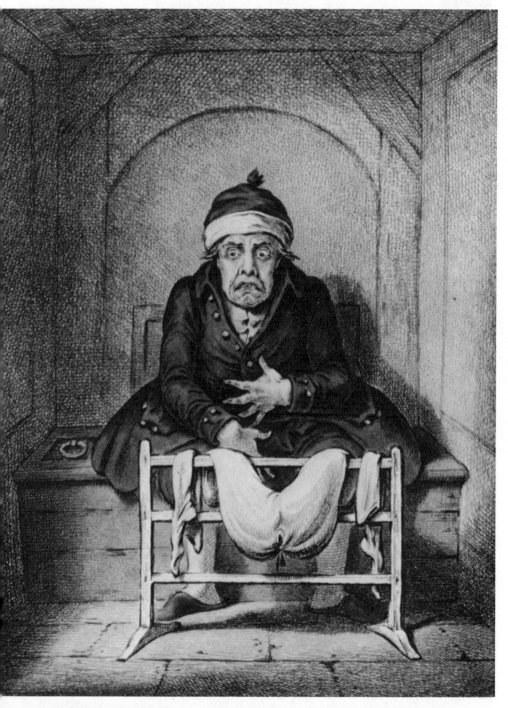

PLATE 1. "Brisk Cathartic." A caricature, possibly by James Gillray, published in London, 1804. Despite his expression, this patient imagines he's doing himself enormous good by "getting those poisons out of there."

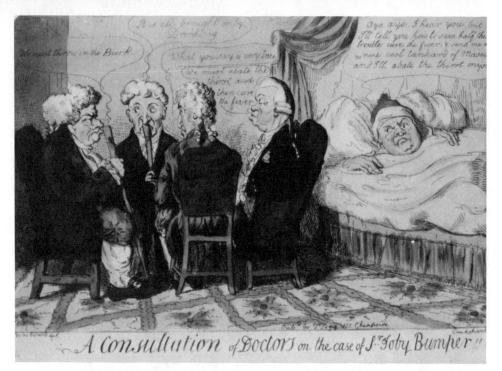

PLATE 2. "A Consultation of Doctors on the Case of Sr. Toby Bumper!" The physicians are seen as quackish fools, and the patient decides to abate his thirst himself with "a nice cool tankard of Madeira." London, c. 1809.

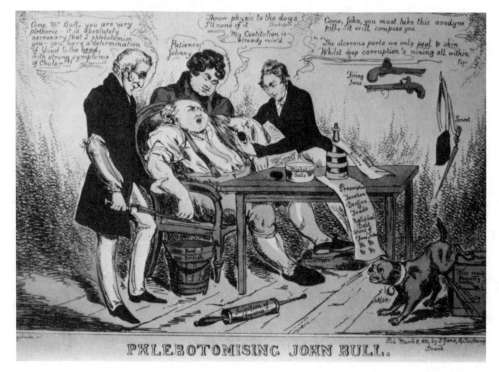

PLATE 3. "Phlebotomising John Bull." John Bull's physicians have given him enemas and medicine. Now they will bleed him by opening a vein with an oversized lancet—"phlebotomy." This caricature is a political satire, of course (the dog is urinating on a box labeled "Wise remedies—property tax"), but real patients got therapy that was very similar. Signed "Longshanks invt," the pseudonym of a caricaturist named Phillips. London, 1830.

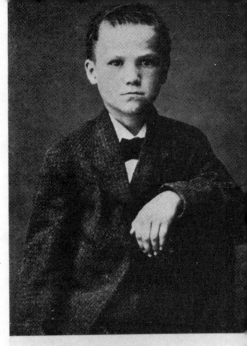

PLATE 4. Thomas Shastid, photographed after one year of apprenticeship to his physician father. He then went on to medical school at Columbia's College of Physicians and Surgeons.

MY FATHER'S APPRENTICE (1877

PLATE 5. The doctor's apprentice learns to listen to the chest.

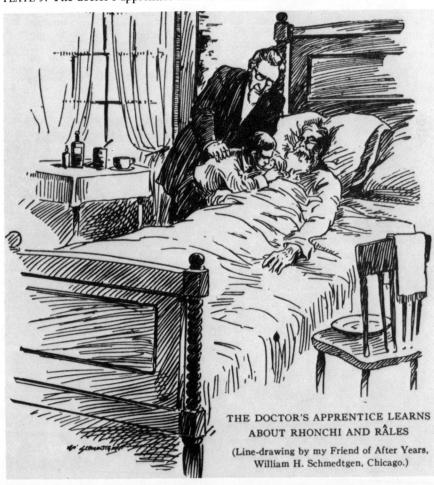

THE DOCTOR'S APPRENTICE LEARNS
ABOUT RHONCHI AND RÂLES

(Line-drawing by my Friend of After Years,
William H. Schmedtgen, Chicago.)

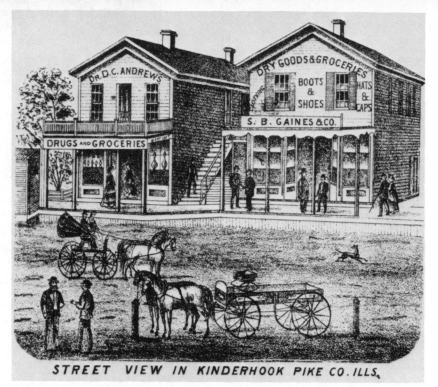

STREET VIEW IN KINDERHOOK PIKE CO. ILLS.

PLATE 6. Thomas Shastid reproduced this plate, which he took from an 1872 atlas of Pike County, Illinois, with this explanation: "An old-time doctor-druggist's store and sign—Dr. Andrews. Dr. Andrews sold in connection with his medical practice not only drugs but groceries also."

PLATE 7. Professor Nicholas Senn's surgical clinic, Rush Medical College in Chicago, sometime after 1878. Some of the physicians' new prestige was reflected luster from the surgeons.

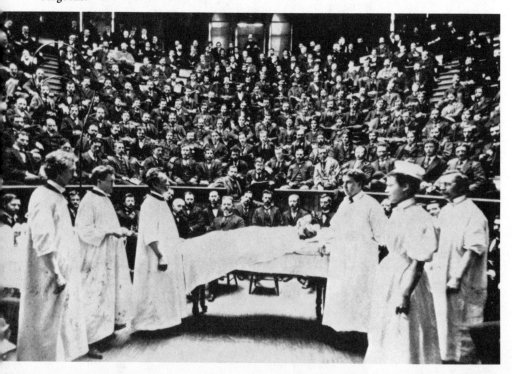

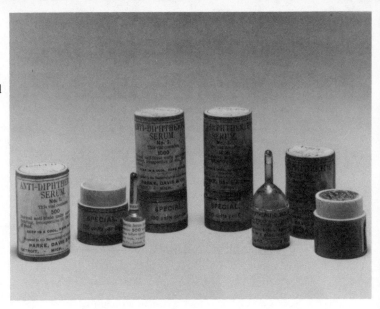

PLATE 8. The first diphtheria antitoxin packaged and sold in the United States, early 1890s.

PLATE 9. *The Doctor*, a painting by Luke Fildes, 1891. The doctor's "clinical instinct," his close observation of the little patient, together with his years of experience, will give him the correct diagnosis. Interestingly, no instruments are visible, although the doctor may well have a stethoscope in his pocket. The painting was reproduced in a booklet by Dr. Charles Gordon Heyd, former AMA president, which was issued in the 1940s as part of the AMA's campaign against socialized medicine. The booklet was entitled *Do You Want Your Own Doctor or a Job Holder?* and was sent to physicians for distribution to their patients.

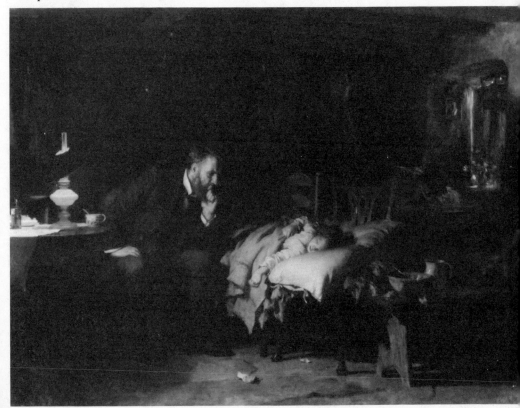

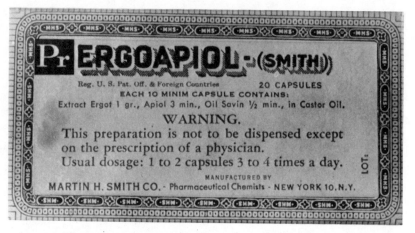

PLATE 10. The top of a box of Ergoapiol, an "ethical specialty," advertised to doctors. Although in theory it was for prescription to patients with menstrual problems, in reality it was a drug for abortion and differed from the general torrent of prepackaged medicines in being not entirely ineffective. Ergoapiol is described in more detail in my book *A History of Women's Bodies* (New York: Basic Books, 1982). This package was sent to me by a pharmacist from a small town in Ontario.

PLATE 11. The modern doctor could at least diagnose. The X-ray film assures the mother that the children do not have lung TB.

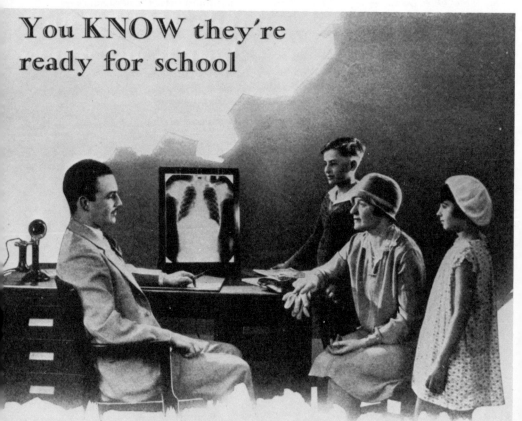

You KNOW they're ready for school

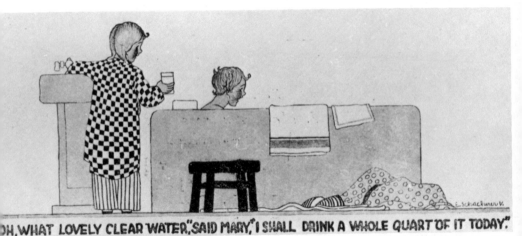

"OH, WHAT LOVELY CLEAR WATER," SAID MARY, "I SHALL DRINK A WHOLE QUART OF IT TODAY."

PLATE 12. The public health movement, which supplied all this clear water—not medical intervention—brought about the great decrease in the death rate during the 1890s and after.

PLATE 14. Not a moment to lose, but virtually none of the druggist's medicines could have cured anything (unless, of course, it was diphtheria or syphilis).

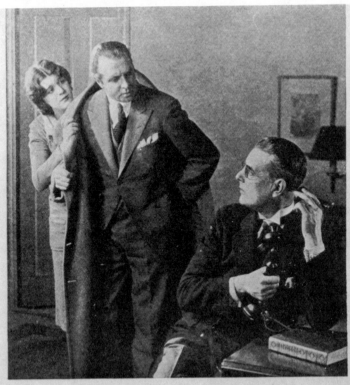

'I'll phone the prescription . . . take your car and get it!"

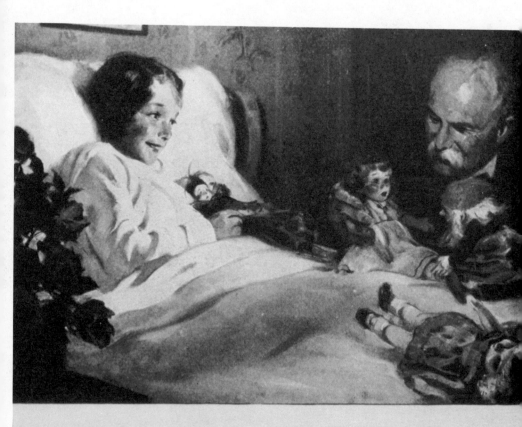

To the world—a great physician
To the child—a beloved goblin

PLATE 13. The physician is William Osler, and the message is that he could prescribe drugs that would cure your child. False, unless your child had diphtheria or syphilis.

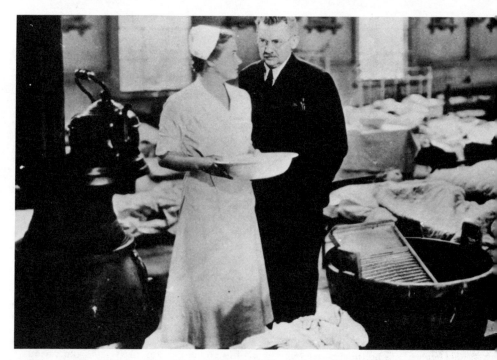

PLATES 15 AND 16. Two scenes from Twentieth Century-Fox's movie *The Country Doctor*, with Jean Hersholt as Dr. Allan Dafoe, the Ontario country doctor who delivered the Dionne quintuplets, and Dorothy Peterson as the nurse. The entire film celebrates medical nobility of spirit.

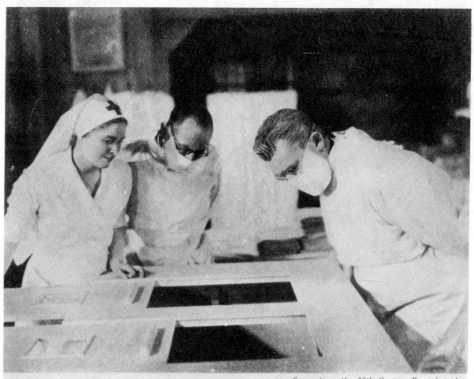

Scene from the 20th Century-Fox photoplay

"You've done something no other doctor in the world has ever done. You've kept quintuplets alive!"

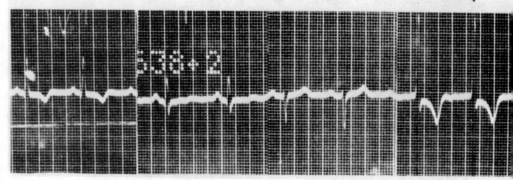

PLATE 17. Franklin Delano Roosevelt's electrocardiogram taken on March 28, 1944, just before he was given digitalis for the first time. The down-curving blips in section I represent inverted T-waves, a sign that the left side of the president's heart had swollen dangerously large.

PLATE 18. A scene from Sidney Kingsley's play *Men in White*. Dr. Hochberg, played by J. E. Bromberg, and the young, brilliant Dr. Ferguson, played by Alexander Kirkland, operate to save the life of a young victim of an infection due to an abortion (whom Dr. Ferguson had impregnated). The theme of the play is the heartburn Dr. Ferguson gets from various women because he wants to dedicate himself to medical research. The message to the theater public: medicine demands monklike dedication to "science."

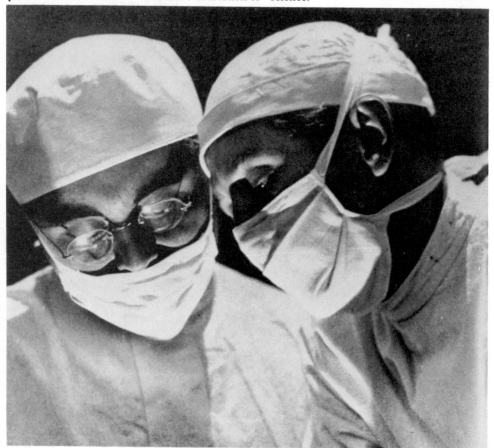

"Only a Cold"

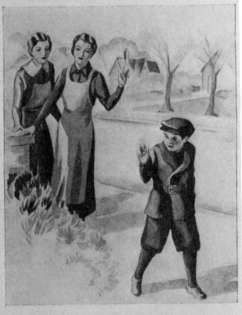

*"Junior has a cold—no, he's not sick
enough to stay home and have a doctor."*
Many a desperate illness owes
its progress to words like these.

AND YET . . . . a "cold" may be fatal. For many a serious disease, in its early stages, masquerades as a cold.

Scarlet fever, for instance, often starts with a sore throat. And diphtheria may begin with a croupy cough. A chill, a cough, and bronchitis are frequently early symptoms of pneumonia. Swelling of the neck which sometimes is present with a mere "cold" may also be a symptom of quinsy. Measles at first seems to be only a "cold in the head."

Treating these diseases as colds may mean untold suffering later, even death, or may be the cause of grave after-effects such as heart disease, rheumatism, deafness.

Then, too, even a simple cold, if not properly cared for, may bring dangerous complications—infection of the sinuses, otitis (inflammation of the ear), rheumatism, pleurisy, pneumonia.

To distinguish a cold from other diseases and to treat a cold properly require all the knowledge and skill that a physician can command.

A cold should never be neglected nor "doped" with patent medicines. If all parents called the family physician immediately when a cold afflicts their children, they would be spared the grief of many a serious illness. Moreover, the few dollars spent for a visit to the physician usually brings the quickest relief from a "common cold" and is the most economical means of caring for it.

A cold is a danger signal—one that should mean "See your doctor at once."

PLATE 19. No symptom is unworthy of the doctor's attention.

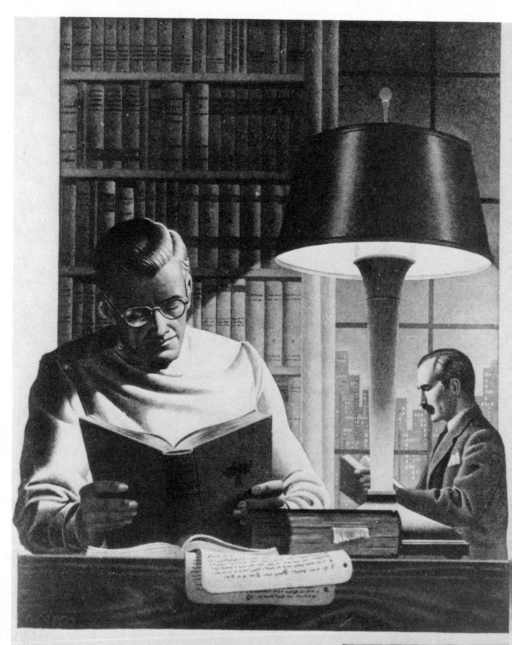

IN THE MEDICAL LIBRARY, a lamp shines on men whose schooling in the service of humanity never ends... just as at Ciba, researchers daily add to their store of knowledge from the rich resources of the Ciba Laboratory Library.

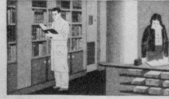

PLATE 20. While the rest of us play, the men of science work late at night.

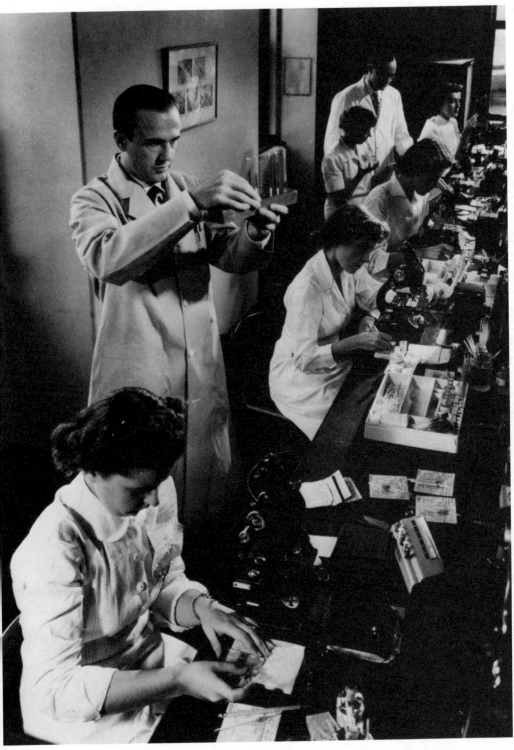

PLATE 21. The physician as man of science: those clear, noble eyes; those bowed female heads . . . (Performing blood counts and other hematological examinations in the clinical laboratory at Wesley Memorial Hospital, Chicago, 1951.)

C. JONATHAN SLOCUM, M.D.
Physician in Charge

JONATHAN SLOCUM, M.D.
Medical Director

C. L. BENNETT, M.D.
Clinical Director

DOMINICK J. LACOVARA, M.D.
Resident Psychologist

PAUL WATSON, M.D.
Gynecologist

CHARLES W. LAYNE, M.D.
Internist

GEORGE K. BRAZILL, D.D.S.
Attending Dental Surgeon

FRANCES WINTERS, R.N.
Supervisor of Nurses

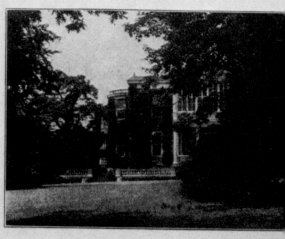

Craig House

BEACON-ON-HUDSON ♦ NEW YORK

Craig House is located at Beacon, New York, fifty-nine miles from New York City, on the eastern bank of the Hudson River in the Highlands. The hospital property covers an area of 350 acres. The grounds are well planted with a variety of ornamental trees, shrubbery and extensive gardens, while the walks and drives within the property cover several miles.

Rooms and reception rooms: All rooms are provided with a private bath. There are numerous reception and card rooms, carefully decorated and furnished. A number of single cottages are available.

Therapeutic unit: Consists of a gymnasium, indoor and outdoor swimming pool, supplied by mountain springs, a complete and modern hydrotherapy, with a trained professional in charge; a colonic irrigating room; and modern dental department with x-ray equipment. A craft shop is maintained under the direction of an expert occupational therapist.

Outside recreation: Tennis, baseball, swimming, riding, skating and winter sports are all available. We maintain our own private golf course, of 3161 yards, which course was carefully laid out several years ago by a well known architect. Our club house is located on the course i commanding position, and offers a recreation center b summer and winter. The course is at all times in cha of a professional.

The hospital is licensed by the State Department of Me Hygiene to receive 80 patients. Approved by Ameri Medical Association.

Our New York office is at 140 East 54th Street; teleph number is Plaza 5-8684. Office hours: Dr. Jonathan Slocur Tuesdays, 10 a. m. to 4:00 p. m.

Rates on Application

PLATE 22. Advertisement for a "private nerve clinic" or "neuropsychiatric institute" of the kind that Sally Willard Pierce experienced (see pp. 173–75). Note that (1) it offers a "colonic irrigation room"—this as late as 1950!—and that (2) one of the chief medical officers is a gynecologist—curious in a rest home for "nervous" patients.

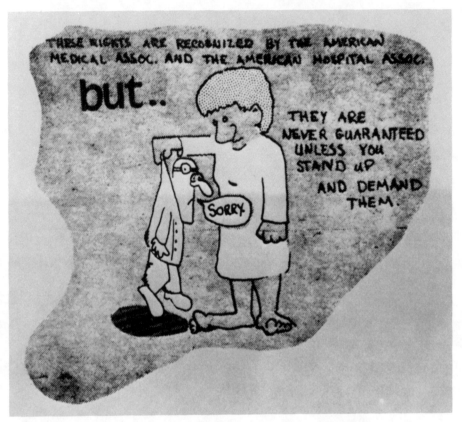

PLATE 23. Why the patient's "will to believe" in the doctor's healing hand vanishes: the "patients' rights" movement.

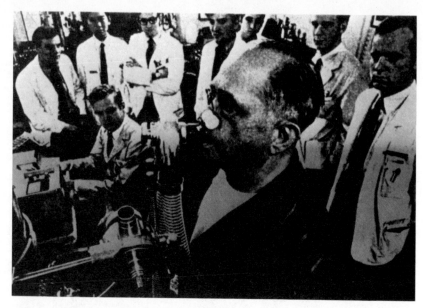

PLATES 24 AND 25. How "patients' rights" advocates create a climate of mistrust between patient and doctor. *Above:* This will happen to *you* when you go for "tests." *Below:* In the hospital you'll be treated the way these records are.

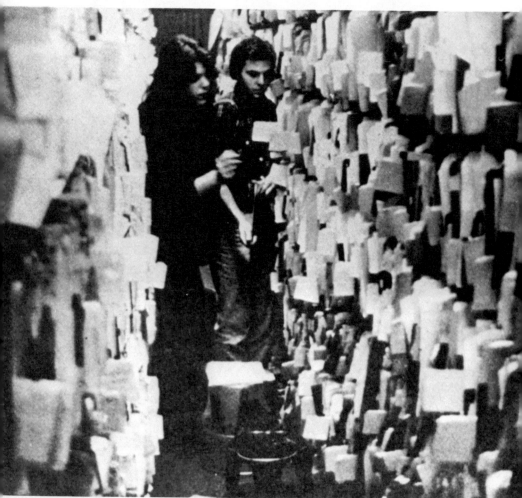

CHAPTER SEVEN
The Postmodern Doctor

*T*ODAY IT'S clear that both doctors and patients are in an epoch entirely different from the 1920s or even the 1940s. We need a label for this new epoch. Because I have used the term *postmodern* in describing the new forms of family life that have emerged since the 1960s, I'm going to try it on medicine as well. The postmodern doctor and patient: What are they like?

For doctors, postmodern medicine begins in the late 1940s, the result of a revolution in diagnosis and drug therapy. The career of the postmodern patient, on the other hand, is launched only in the 1960s and 1970s, as people become more sensitive to the emotional and physical signals their bodies give off. Together, these two events, the arrival of a new medical "style" and the turning inward of a whole generation of patients, have filled the consultation with anger and weakened the doctor's healing hand.

Lest the reader think I am about to do an axe-job on the medical profession today, let me observe at the outset that all the

179

changes developed from an impulse that was basically benign, indeed, admirable: enthusiasm about the ability to heal disease prompted by "antibiotics" and other "wonder" drugs. Who can fault doctors for their energetic implementation of this newfound ability to help others? But even the noblest of emotions can have unexpected consequences.

The Drug Revolution and the Triumph of Organic Disease

The story of the postmodern medical style begins some time before this style would actually be observed in the office of the average family doctor, just as Laennec fiddled with his stethoscope a full fifty years before the arrival of the "modern" style of bedside medicine. The first important event occurred in 1935 in Germany, where the development of a drug named *Prontosil* was announced. The essential component of Prontosil, a substance called *sulfanilamide,* had been known for years, but nobody realized that sulfanilamide would quench bacterial infections until Prontosil appeared. Sulfanilamide became the first of the *sulfa drugs.* Given a trial in 1936 at the Queen Charlotte's Hospital in London, it performed wonderfully against "streptococcal" infections and began a triumphal onmarch: never before in history had a drug worked against these particular infections.[1]

Next came a series of further discoveries. In 1938 another sulfa drug, sulfapyridine, turned out to be even more effective than sulfanilamide on some kinds of pneumonias. Sulfadiazine, sulfisoxazole, and others followed in the early 1940s. There would not be much point in listing the many kinds of infections these drugs could combat, but it would be useful to think for a moment about a typical patient with an infection, before the drug revolution. "Mrs. Annie J." had consulted Dr. William Johnston of Lucknow, Ontario, in the mid-1920s "about the end of a finger swollen and painful." While changing a tire she had cut her finger, and germs from the soil had gotten into the wound, "forging ahead into the soft tissues of this woman's fingers and hand." She had six months' treatment at home and hospital "with bathing in hot antiseptic solutions and various dressings before the infection was checked or died out. By that time not much remained of her hand except bones and tendons and it was many months later before it was useful."[2] This case was typical of millions of banal but dangerous infections before 1935. *Infection* was once a terrible word.

Then the sulfa drugs arrived in Dr. Johnston's practice. "They put an end to such severe tissue infections as that of Annie's finger and erysipelas [a strep infection marked by redness and swelling]; quinsies melted away, running ears quickly dried up, mastoid operations became almost a surgeon's lost art, rheumatic fever dwindled, bacterial endocarditis [an infection of the heart valves] was no longer an implacable death sentence...." These sulfa drugs caused a sensation far greater even than that occasioned by diphtheria antitoxin. The *New York Times* called sulfanilamide "the drug which has astounded the medical profession." In 1941 seventeen hundred tons of sulfa drugs were given to 10 to 15 million Americans.[3]

But many kinds of infections resisted the sulfa drugs. The next chapter began in 1941, the first time any patient received a drug made from a certain kind of mold: penicillin. Unlike sulfa drugs, penicillin was a substance harvested from living microorganisms, hence the term *antibiotic*. In 1942 trials of the drug on wounded soldiers began, and in the following years preliminary reports commenced. But there had been so many false starts in previous decades that no great excitement was aroused until 1945, when commercial laboratories began pouring forth massive amounts for civilian use. One can sense the enthusiasm in the pages of the staid *Journal of the American Medical Association* as the reports arrived:

3 February 1945. A group of doctors in St. Louis treated 103 patients who had pneumonia, extensive bloodstream "staph" infections, and gonorrhea. Striking results.

17 February. Fifty-four patients at Fort Bragg got penicillin for severe strep throat, a condition against which the sulfa drugs had had little success. The drug exerted a "profound effect" on the germs.[4]

On and on it went. Dozens of articles on penicillin appeared that year in the *Journal of the American Medical Association* alone. A large number of infections were now susceptible to medical treatment. In rural Ireland just after World War II, Dr. Michael Casey described the "new wonder drug accidentally discovered by an English doctor" (a reference to Sir James Fleming). "Indeed, my first experience of the use of penicillin was in the treatment of a very famous racehorse in the Curragh, before it became available for the treatment of humans."[5]

After penicillin came a deluge. There was streptomycin, discovered in 1944 by a soil microbiologist, and used four years later against TB. It was not terrifically effective for that purpose, but for the first time doctors had a drug that exerted *some* impact on the world's number one killer. (Then in 1951 came along a much better antituberculosis drug, isoniazid. Streptomycin, in the meantime, turned out to be effective against infections caused by the kind of germs found in feces, *gram-negative infections.*) Chloramphenicol appeared in 1947, effective against rickettsial infections. And typhus was blown away! Centuries of "cabin fever" and "jailhouse fever," and thousands of peasants dead in the wake of the armies of Napoleon and Gustavus Adolphus, all from the louse- and tick-borne diseases of typhus, gone! In 1948 chlortetracycline, later called *tetracycline,* was launched. It was good for just about everything, which is important because many infections soon became resistant to penicillin. Tetracycline and chloramphenicol would therefore become known as the *broad-spectrum antibiotics.*

The enthusiasm for these new drugs washed back and forth in great waves across the media. Chloramphenicol was called "one of the world's greatest medicines." Tetracycline was hyped as "God's Gift to the Doctors."[6]

And this was just the beginning. The early 1950s would see drugs that fought inflammation, either by stimulating the adrenal glands to release cortisol or by giving the body cortisone from the outside. Thus all the diseases like arthritis, in which the body's own defense system—in the form of "immune reactions" and "inflammatory responses"—wreaks havoc, would be combated. Drugs that work on the heart and lungs, on diseases of the central nervous system like Parkinson's disease, on parasites, on cancer, on schizophrenia, on hormonal imbalances causing infertility: it is pointless to review them here. The reader will easily find lists elsewhere. I want rather to discuss their impact on the doctor-patient relationship.

The effect on doctors was to imbue them with a relentless new enthusiasm about their ability to cure organic disease. When Robert Loeb, a "doctor's doctor" if there ever was one, gave the opening address to the medical students at Columbia in September 1950, he stated that these new advances "offer a degree of understanding of life processes hitherto inconceivable. . . . We have entered on a new era in the practice of medicine. . . . [The] care it offers transcends in quality and competence the fondest expectations of the physicians of the past, even the recent past." Just imagine: a new era. Not only did doctors now have "rational diagnosis," which as we have seen had been around since the late nineteenth century; they now had, in Loeb's words, "rational therapy" as well. Everywhere was talk of "vast avenues of future possibilities" and the like.[7]

How did this new excitement transform the practice of medicine? It had relatively little impact, I think, on the way men graduated before 1950 treated patients. They prescribed the new drugs, but their own bedside manner had been forged in a preantibiotic era, and there is no reason to think they suddenly abandoned the leisureliness and almost courtly good manners we have seen simply because they had a few new pills.

The transmission belt by which the drug revolution brought into being new *forms* of dealing with patients was the medical school. Medical school training had hitherto been oriented toward preparing GPs for the bedside. To be sure, previous teaching had been "scientific," but that meant developing skills in physical diagnosis. The discovery of the wonder drugs opened up an entirely new perspective. Now "science" meant letting students understand the very mechanisms of disease, because once those mechanisms were clear the appropriate drugs might be devised. Therefore, a tremendous lurch toward the "basic medical sciences," and in particular toward chemistry, took place in the 1950s. A keynote was the address to the first world conference on medical education, given in London in 1953 by Sir Lionel Whitby, the Regius Professor of Physic at Cambridge: "The challenge to our universities and medical schools is a simple one. Are we preparing our students to at least grasp the principles behind all this scientific work? . . . The doctor of the future will have to be grounded more firmly in the basic sciences." If not, he wouldn't be able to meet the "challenges of advancing knowledge," and so on.[8]

What, exactly, was this famous challenge? It lies in a discipline called *biochemistry*, the chemistry of the body. For various reasons, by the 1950s scientists had advanced to the point at which many diseases could be explained in terms of "molecular changes." Now the student could actually visualize certain molecules and see how they bump against other molecules; the student could appreciate what essential components the molecules might lack that caused disease and how they might be chemically addressed via drug therapy. All of this is extremely exciting. I remember my own sense of adventure in seeing on the page the long structure of the hemoglobin molecule, the molecule that carries oxygen in the red blood cells; or how dramatic I found the biochemistry class in which "sickle cell disease," a blood disease mainly affecting black people, was explained as the pathological, sticky adherence of hemoglobin molecules one to another because of the lack of an important amino acid. For genetic reasons the body was unable to make this amino acid, and so the red cell was pulled into a sicklelike form.

These discoveries are thrilling because they plumb the very basis, the structure, of life. One should not become a doctor without understanding them, in the way that one shouldn't become a lawyer without some feeling for the tradition of common law, or an architect without some grasp of the physical properties of construction materials. I have no wish to make an argument against biochemistry per se. However, the assumptions that justify biochemistry's place in the curriculum may carry over into medical practice in disproportionate ways, so that they come to dominate the approach to disease.

Each of the basic medical sciences, of which biochemistry is one, has a logic of its own. For example, the logic of anatomy, a traditional basic medical science, is that disease is often localized, so you have to know where things are in the body. A patient steps on a nail. You want to know what structures the nail has passed through and whether it may have severed nerves or arteries.

Biochemistry and the other newer basic sciences offered medical students a mainly *organic* picture of disease: disease arising in disorder among the molecules and correctable with appropriate drugs. It is a picture of disease that *ignores the mind.* To the extent that chemistry-oriented subjects were stressed in medical schools, medical students more and more acquired the view that disease was organic in nature and that their mission was to assail it with drugs.

Before World War II, considerable emphasis had been placed in medical schools on "treating the patient as a whole," or on "holistic views of disease."[9] By the early 1950s medical education stood at a crossroads. An old guard continued to maintain that medicine should focus on "the patient as a whole and on the patient as an individual human being." But the new subjects of biochemistry, microbiology, pharmacology, immunology, and genetics—all chemistry-oriented—required large blocks of time for mastery.[10] It was not that biochemists insisted on scrapping views of the "patient as a whole." Rather the faculty in *internal medicine,* swept away by the new therapeutic possibilities of the drug revolution, maintained that the students get a proper grounding in the chemical sciences so they could "understand" disease.

Here we encounter for the first time the internist as "heavy," striding on stage not to demand psychological treatment for stomach ulcers, but to insist that students in his hospital "service" know the enzymes involved in steroid synthesis in the adrenal glands. I would argue that this demand coming from internal medicine, the rulers of the roost in the medical establishment,[11] grew to sizeable proportions only after World War II and that it has had incalculable consequences for the practice of medicine.

A straw in the wind flew by in February 1953, in the form of a complaint from Columbia's Robert Loeb and a colleague. They had heard enough about training premeds in "social sciences" and experimental "home care programs in which medical students would participate even during their first year." "The department of medicine at Columbia has been deeply concerned with current trends," they said. They wanted "the standards of medical education in respect to internal medicine . . . maintained at the highest possible scientific level." So scrap social science. What was particularly interesting was not their dismissal of social science, but their contempt for exposing first-year students to patient care and their insistence that "basic scientific knowledge" was essential for bedside medicine.[12]

When Abraham Flexner surveyed American medical education in 1910, he described lab facilities as "wretched." Of 155 medical schools, only 14 or 15 had "any laboratory facilities definitely designed for clinical departments." How this had changed by the early 1950s! One department of internal medicine in a large private medical school had seventeen faculty members devoted to full-time research. It maintained "16 large laboratories equipped for dealing with physiological, pharmacological, chemical, and bacteriological research programs. These laboratories were staffed with 85 technicians, research fellows and faculty members." Medical school libraries had started ordering "books and journals on higher mathematics, electrical engineering, physics and electronics," said one bemused librarian.[13]

A new program, started in 1953 at Western Reserve's medical school, aimed quite explicitly at treating the medical student "more as a graduate student, giving him a home base [a laboratory desk] for laboratory work and study." Students were to be encouraged to undertake their own research projects in biochemical subjects.[14] This was wonderful for the advancement of science, but it would be hard to think of preparation less appropriate for the average family doctor, who would spend a lifetime treating middle-aged businessmen with stomach pain and upbounding female executives who in private moments felt depressed. The message was, we doctors are scientists who treat organic disease.

The skeptical reader responds, "Aw, leave those mental cases to the social workers. We want doctors who know what they're doing." This, of course, is one of the great myths surrounding medical education: the belief that because medical students cram in facts day and night, physicians who "know what they are doing" are produced. Perhaps most finally do turn out well, but it is not, for several reasons, the result of intensive training in "basic medical sciences."

For one thing, much didactic classroom instruction turns out to be mere "fact grubbing," without much grasp or retention of the larger principles that Sir Lionel Whitby was insisting on. Said George W. Pickering, professor of medicine at the University of London, in 1956, "as at present conducted, medical education in the universities is not directed to training the student's mind as a discriminating instrument but merely as a temporary storehouse for miscellaneous information collected from textbooks and lecture notes and retained for long enough to be reproduced at the moment of the examination."[15] As anyone with firsthand knowledge of a medical course will confirm, the exams are mainly five-point multiple-choice that stress minutiae. Thus one question in my biochemistry course exam was the following:

Indicate which of the following statements concerning malonyl-CoA is (are) true:
1. *It is an intermediate in ketone body synthesis.*
2. *It is an inhibitor of palmitoyl-carnitine transferase I.*
3. *It is formed by the enzyme propionyl-CoA carboxylase.*
4. *Its formation is decreased when cyclic AMP levels are high in the liver.*

Some of these points are incredibly obscure. It strikes me as legitimate to ask medical students to know something about how fatty acids are synthesized in the body, and malonyl coenzyme A is an important step in that process. But although the public imagines that "young doctors are slaving away day and night to overcome disease," what they are actually doing is memorizing the kind of arcane facts ("pickshit," as the med students call it) involved in answering the questions like this one correctly. I got it right, and for me as a humanist that represented a kind of personal accomplishment in a painful struggle to pick up the rudiments of science. But for a real medical student, the mastery of such material only invites cynicism about the usefulness of science, which in this case is serving as a sorting technique for ranking the students in class for the sake of admission to specialty programs. All students, of course, graduate from medical school and are turned loose on the public.

A second drawback of heavy emphasis on the basic sciences is that they soon are forgotten. The public expects doctors to "really learn the facts," little realizing that most of the facts not immediately relating to the doctor's practice have long vanished from his head. This process of forgetting begins even before medical school has started. Most schools require for admission an undergraduate course in organic chemistry, usually taught in the chemistry department. "You need to know this basic science," the dean intones. But most of these courses involve nine different ways to make alcohols and other facts useful in industrial chemistry. Their content has fled the mind three months after the course was taken, and med students look back bitterly on the time wasted, aware that a few weeks' study of basic principles would have sufficed for their needs.

The dean then intones, "You need to know your anatomy." So in the typical first-year anatomy course the student memorizes a staggering amount of detail about where hundreds of different muscles lie, and that means the exact point on each bone where each muscle originates and each inserts, as well as the nerve supply and blood supply for all of these muscles and organs. By the end of the first year, med students will know the names of the *cranial nerves*, the nerves of sight, hearing, and so forth, and the names of the little holes in the skull they run in and out of, as well as they know their social security numbers. These twelve nerves* become a kind of symbol of the study of anatomy: "*on old Olympus' topmost top a fat-assed German viewed a hop*" being one of the classical memory devices for their names.

I asked a distinguished obstetrician, now in his fifties, whether

---

* The twelve cranial nerves: olfactory (smell), optic (vision), oculomotor (moves eyeball generally), trochlear (moves eyeball downward and toward the middle), trigeminal (sensory nerves of the face plus the muscles of chewing), abducent (moves eyeball to the far side, away from the nose), facial (muscles of the face), vestibulo-cochlear, or "auditory-vestibular" (hearing and balance), glossopharyngeal (mainly sensations in tongue and throat), vagus (muscles in throat and many internal organs), accessory (two important neck muscles), and hypoglossal (moves tongue).

he could remember the names of the cranial nerves. He laughed at the very idea, the information having disappeared long ago. But he knew the anatomy of the pelvis extremely well.

Sometimes the disappearance of this anatomical knowledge can take on astonishing proportions. "When I was a young doctor," remembered Stanford's Russell Lee, "I saw a lady with the symptoms of appendicitis. Yet she claimed that her doctor had taken her appendix out 18 months before. We operated anyway, and we found a big, red-hot appendix. In my youthful indignation, I called her doctor and said, 'Do you remember Mrs. Curtis?' "

"Yes—an appendectomy," he replied.

"Well, we just took her appendix out," Lee said.

"My God, I wonder what I took out!" the man said.[16]

Still, because of anatomy's utility, it vanishes less rapidly than does the chemical information. Here lies one of the main problems with the basic science orientation of postmodern medical training. No matter how virtuously one may insist upon "doctors' understanding the scientific basis of X and Y," the information will inevitably be forgotten as soon as the qualifying exams are over. In the fifty-odd meetings of a weekly seminar of family doctors I attended, *not once* was any basic principle of drug action or any biochemical mechanism of disease mentioned, because it would have been meaningless to an audience that had forgotten the molecular structures for assimilating this information. Indeed, I was quite often bemused by how much had disappeared. A sixty-nine-year-old patient who showed recent loss of memory and disorientation was being discussed. Was he demented? The doctors went through the differential diagnosis of what else he might have. Some of the possibilities were straightforward: alcoholism, a recent heart attack. Others were more obscure: vitamin B_{12} deficiency, Creutzfeldt-Jakob disease. Laughter began mounting. "Academic," someone says, meaning "diseases you hear about only in medical school."

"Megaloblastic something-or-other," one doctor begins and then dissolves in laughter as she is unable to think of the rest of it. For many in the group, a command of basic medical sciences had simply vanished.

On another occasion the family doctors were talking about broken bones in the elderly. One must eat about five hundred milligrams of calcium a day to ward off osteoporosis and the like. Cheese is a good source.

So, how much cheese do you have to eat a day?

The group began buzzing with calculations. Grams and milligrams were confused. The doctors tried to go from metric to imperial. "Let's see. Two point two kilograms in a pound. Hmmmm. That works out to three pounds. We tell our patients they've got to eat three pounds of cheese a day?" Even the knowledge of these basic conversions had vanished.

This information seepage is a general problem in medicine, though one not widely discussed in public. One British physician was being unusually frank when, in a symposium on drug use in the 1970s, he confessed, "We have reached a point now where we have to guess at the similarities between drugs, and the genus of drugs to which they belong, by the sound of the name. That is really all that is left of pharmacology for many of us after we have left medical school for about fifteen years. We are groping about, hoping that the title of the brand name will give us a clue as to the action and possible chemical relatives."[17]

Still, one might argue, even if doctors do forget huge amounts, is that any reason for not trying to drum the basic sciences into their heads when they are students? Yes, in fact; it is a reason. This extreme emphasis upon the basics of science diverts doctors from the awareness that much disease arises in the mind and renders them unable even to confront this possibility as students. Remember that the whole justification for basic science was that it presumably equipped the doctor to treat organic disease effectively with drugs. Stressing the biochemical and pharmacological approaches to those diseases amenable to drug therapy subtly confirms the message that all diseases fall into this category.

This disease orientation of the American medical student had already become apparent in the 1950s. George Berry, dean of the Harvard Medical School, said in 1953 that "while the student is learning a great deal about the patient's 17-ketosteroids, undeniably important, he tends to overlook the patient's anxieties and hatreds, his attitudes in his family setting and the pressures that hem him in. . . . In brief, scientific medicine is a misnomer, I think, when it is exclusively preoccupied with the physical and chemical constitution."[18] Seen from Britain, where "scientific medicine" has always been less well established, the young American doctors appeared like lambs in their terror of the psyche. "It is not that American medical students take poor histories and make poor examinations," wrote an associate dean of the London Hospital Medical School in 1956. "It is that they appear to suffer from a lack of balance between their knowledge of medicine and their knowledge of diseased people." The American students, trained in science, were "inclined to relish cases of clear-cut organic disease and to fight shy of the more difficult problems of dysfunction." (He meant psychosomatic disorders.) When in their final year these students actually started treating patients, they found themselves "frightened away from those patients where the consideration of the 'whole man' matters most and back to those whose only complaint is one of simple clear-cut organic disease, back to 'scientific medicine.' "[19]

These trends are even more pronounced today. Incoming students are oriented more toward the sciences than ever before. The percentage of premeds majoring in the humanities fell by more than half from the 1960s to the 1970s, and the percentage of biology majors climbed from 43 to 53 percent. Because of the extreme competition to get into medical school, the percentage of first-class students has also risen: although in the 1960s only 14 percent of medical students had A averages as undergraduates, 40 percent did in the 1970s.[20]

But the personal qualities required to bring in those high marks are not necessarily the qualities that make a doctor effective in dealing with patients. Medical schools select students mainly on the basis of grades, thus indirectly giving preference "to qualities that all too often accompany a strong premed record—an intense compulsiveness, intellectual narrowness, and, sometimes, difficulties in getting along with other people." The "gruesome pressures of medical school" then deflect students even further away from the notion of the ideal doctor as "compassionate, sympathetic, perceptive and understanding." The products tend to be emotionally constricted, anxious individuals who have concentrated fiercely on grades and manipulated others to get ahead, to paraphrase one observer who was trying to figure out why the typical med student made such a poor psychiatrist.[21] *Tend* is the operative word here, for many fine physicians don't fit this picture at all. Yet the percentage of closed-off, compulsive workaholics is probably higher among physicians than in the population as a whole.

And such physicians tend to be insensitive to the human dimension of disease. Dr. Arnold Feldman remembered a student who had admitted a patient to the medical service after a suicide attempt. "The medical student's work-up included the following: 'Social history—noncontributory.' "[22]

So concerned were my own classmates about grubbing for high marks that they simply turned off every time a "psychosocial" angle was raised. In Pathology, for example, they would listen carefully to an account of amyloidosis in the kidney, because they knew it would be on the exam (even though they would seldom encounter it in real life). But the moment a technologist showed up to talk about such practical problems in kidney transplant and organ donation as comforting the relatives, they got up in massive numbers to leave or started chatting among themselves.

Courses on the psychological side of things had been introduced into the second year of study at the medical school I attended. But the students dismissed lectures on the "biopsychosocial model of disease" (a tongue-twister of psychiatrist George Engel[23]) as "bullshit":

"Hey, Jory, why weren't you at lecture today?" a fellow student asked, apropos this course.

"I don't need two hours on how I'm not supposed to brutalize my patients," responded Jory.

The problem will have become worse, not better, by the time these young men and women become interns, for in their clinical years they are exposed to the highly "disease-oriented" surgeons and internists, who are the most prestigious members of the hospital hierarchy. On the hospital floor, they are bathed in talk of "crash carts" (for cardiac arrests), and "commando" operations in head-and-neck surgery, in which removing a cancer in the mouth, for example, entails taking out many structures in the lower face and neck. What medical student can rush about with the "commando" team and retain his awareness of "the patient as a person"? The patient is a mass of diseased sinew. (*Note:* In the hospital hierarchy, *clinical clerks* are fourth-year medical students training in the hospital; *interns* are graduate M.D.'s serving a year in hospital before getting their license to practice; *residents* are licensed doctors who are doing several additional years of hospital training in a specialty.)

All this "crash" medicine carries over into students' relations with patients. The young doctors become so absorbed with disease they are unable to comprehend that patients do not understand as much as they do. At Children's Hospital of Los Angeles, for example, a resident tried to explain to a mother a possible defect in her child's heart.

MOTHER: What would cause that hole in his heart?
RESIDENT: There's a little membrane that comes down, and if it's the upper chamber there's a membrane that comes down, one from each direction. And sometimes they don't quite meet. . . .
MOTHER: Oh.
RESIDENT: It's uh . . . one thing they never get SBE from . . . it's the only heart lesion in which they don't.
MOTHER: Uh-huh.
RESIDENT (trying further to reassure): The only thing you have to worry about is other babies.
MOTHER: M-h'm.
RESIDENT: Watch your Coombs and things.
MOTHER: Watch my what?
RESIDENT: Your titres . . . Coombs titres.
MOTHER: Oh, yeah.[24]

Only a medical training in which the human dimension was completely absent could have produced this dialogue. The apparently salutary emphasis upon basic science and organic disease that followed the drug revolution turns out, then, to have some shadow sides. Let us see how they have affected the practice of medicine.

THE STYLE OF INTERNAL MEDICINE

In a major postmodern development, the style of medicine as a whole has become the style of one of its specialty branches: the specialty of *internal medicine,* which is everything from the neck to the navel. Lungs, heart, immune system, kidneys, digestion: all are the province of internists, who have trained for three or four years beyond the internship. And because internists often teach clinical skills to medical students and preside over the most feared "rotations" that the clerks and interns serve in, they have had a major impact upon medical manners in general. Many fine men and women are internists, and I hope they individually will not feel slighted by my assertion that the specialty has on the whole a quite pronounced style. Basic goodness of character may well triumph over this style. But the point is, the style itself has become a major obstacle to satisfactory doctor-patient relations.

In the beginning, internists were *consultants:* they would take on patients, referred by family doctors, who had quite specific medical problems: how to manage Mr. Jones's pneumonia, or what was the likely course of Mrs. Smith's liver disease. Then the patient went back to the family doctor. Internists were, quite appropriately for any specialty, supposed to consult: to recommend on the diagnosis and treatment of grave medical problems. This role widened dramatically with the drug revolution following World War II, as internists started to find themselves serving as personal physicians. The internists' share of all physician "visits" more than doubled from 1966 to 1980, and internists have now become the "family doctors" of as much as a third of the elderly population.[25]

The internists were equipped par excellence to know about drugs. And a public that wanted "nothing but the best" flocked to them as guardians of the new pharmacopoeia. In retrospect, it must be said that patients themselves are partly to blame for having so grossly derailed this medical specialty from its original course. But as internists took on an increasing number of people for *primary care,* which is to say, as internists became personal physicians, they brought with them the habits of mind and manners they had developed in their former incarnation as consultants. "The specialist is, by definition, called on to solve some particular problem," said Theodore F. Fox, an English internist in 1960. "And he may reasonably be reluctant to cope also with the patient as a person. It is no accident that the man who is 'Mr. Jones' to his own doctor should so often become, in hospital, 'the haematemesis [vomiting blood] in the end bed.' "[26] Thus the true problem would arise only when internists ceased being consultants, and when *family doctors* began adopting their style.

The essence of this style is a relentless persistence in diagnosis and an unbounded confidence that one is dealing with an organic disease that can be treated with drugs or surgery. This *furor therapeuticus* can be lifesaving, where it is appropriate. The historian shudders at the number of bladder cancers once dismissed as "neurasthenia" by family doctors and the metabolic disorders passed off as "nerves."

But even when one is dealing with organic disease, a human dimension is present. My argument is that internal medicine falls far shorter than family medicine in meeting the patient's expectation that he can count on an interested, sympathetic adviser. Dr. Michael Lepore was thinking of his own colleagues in internal medicine when he said that the price we have paid for the drug revolution is "the trend toward depersonalization and dehumanization of the care of the patient."[27]

How does this depersonalization appear in fact? For one thing, in clinical meetings the voices of the internal medicine people are cool and flat. There are few inflections. It is almost as if they prided themselves on who could have the flattest voice. Occasionally a colorful expression is used, such as, "Then the wheel started to fall off the wagon again," apropos a patient who had lapsed into a coma.

We are in a seminar with pathologists and internists, a *clinicopathological conference,* or CPC. A patient has died of a "leukocytic lymphoma" (blood cancer). Did he have one "diagnosis" or two? A second disease process in the brain perhaps? Back and forth flows the discussion, this finding, that finding. More data are called for. How do you diagnose this disease? Many complicated lab tests are involved: LEU 1, LEU 2, HLA DR, and so forth. A hematologist (blood specialist) is called upon to justify the diagnosis of the internal medicine team, who sit in several rows in their white coats. He has the facts down cold. Blam, blam, blam. At the end, there is no possible question.

Clearly, these are not inhumane people at the bedside. But they are intensely preoccupied with the technical intricacies of physical disease. At the end of the conference there is a flurry of excitement. In this particular lymphoma, some kind of gobbling up of red blood cells is occurring. No one had reported this finding before. This has the makings of an article.

The image these internists project to the young doctors in their charge is of a medicine stripped of its humanity. Here is another seminar session. A man in his seventies is dead of a pulmonary embolus. He came into hospital after breaking his thigh bone, which required a replacement of his hip joint. He was already quite feeble, a first replacement having been done some time ago. Then one day he suddenly developed shortness-of-breath (always referred to as *S-O-B*) and chest pain. He began calling for his daughter. The clinical clerk on duty wrote in the chart, we are told, "The approach of death seems imminent."

At this point the seminar begins howling with laughter. Of course they are not laughing at this old man, but at the sententiousness of the clerk. But for the other clerks and interns present, this is a lesson in restricting oneself to dry, scientific observations. Attempting literary case notes, perhaps a clumsy stab at giving death a human face, would definitely be seen as something to ridicule.

How does this depersonalization work out in practice? Remember that in the interview the experiences drawing doctor and patient together are the history taking and the physical exam, both opportunities for storytelling and the expression of concern. Internal medicine has downgraded these and emphasized instead the impersonal collection and interpretation of laboratory data.

For physicians who are filled with gleeful enthusiasm about their ability to cure, these tests make a lot of sense. Tests start from the assumption that there's no therapy without diagnosis. As most disorders leave some kind of biochemical trace in the blood or tissues, lab tests become an essential instrument of diagnosis. Table 7-1, based on a nationwide survey of American med-

TABLE 7–1

HOW FAMILY DOCTORS DIFFER FROM INTERNISTS IN INVESTIGATING THE PATIENT.[28]

	Percentage of Ambulatory* Encounters Referred for Testing	
	By Family Doctor	By Internist
Routine lab tests such as a complete blood count† or analysis of urine	20	32
Chest X-ray	4	16
Electrocardiogram	3	16
Blood chemistry	5	16
Panels of automated tests ‡	3	13

* *Ambulatory:* Patient is not occupying a hospital bed.
† *Complete blood count:* Number of red and white cells.
‡ "Chem 6," "Chem 12," and so on.

SOURCE: Robert Wood Johnson Foundation, *Medical Practice in the United States: A Special Report* (Princeton: RWJF, 1981).

icine in 1976–1978, shows the extent to which internists rely more on tests than do family doctors.

Thus specialists in internal medicine come across as considerably more test-oriented than family doctors, unsurprising in view of their generally higher estimation of biochemistry. In the 1950s one questionnaire asked various kinds of doctors how important they felt a knowledge of biochemistry to be. And on a scale from 0 to 4 (unimportant to very important) the average scores were as follows:[29]

Internists	2.7
GPs	2.2
Interns	2.1

It would be presumptuous for a historian like me to argue that much of this testing is unproductive or unnecessary. The testing has been criticized, however, by other internists. David Rogers, in his 1975 presidential address to the Association of American Physicians, maintained that not only were the tests expensive; they also encouraged physicians to hive themselves off into ever tinier subspecialties. And some tests could be dangerous to patients: "It is not unusual to find a fragile elder who had been able to walk into the hospital, but is now slightly confused, dehydrated, and somewhat the worse for wear on the third hospital day because his first 48 hours in the hospital were spent undergoing a staggering series of exhausting diagnostic studies. . . ." But Rogers's main criticism, from our viewpoint, concerned the dehumanizing aspect of this extensive testing. "Our relentless approach to diagnosis feeds the feeling that modern physicians are cold or impersonal."[30]

The acme of impersonal testing, however, is testing to satisfy the academic curiosity of the staff, rather than to aid in therapy for the patient. Many tests will pinpoint the diagnosis, yet make little difference in outcome. Dr. David Reuben questioned, for example, the usefulness of many invasive "endoscopic" procedures, in which long tubes are lowered through the esophagus and stomach to see where the bleeding is coming from. Despite extensive use of these in upper gastrointestinal bleeding and peptic ulcer, "for neither disorder has the superb diagnostic yield been shown to alter the outcome in general."[31]

In my own experiences at Big City Hospital, I noticed with interest this search for knowledge for its own sake rather than for the patient's benefit. A female resident in internal medicine is reporting on a woman in her late fifties who died of cancer. First we have the details: the tumor in her right iliac bone spread to her lungs. So large did it grow in the lungs that it compressed the spinal cord, giving the patient neurological symptoms. She had tumor everywhere and finally died. Even in her final days, however, the medicine service continued to investigate. They did C-T scans (a cros-sectional way of viewing the body) and other X-rays. The woman was shipped from test to test.

Question from the audience: "What possible additional information could the C-T scan have provided?"

RESIDENT: We wanted to find the primary [the original tumor].
QUESTIONER: Would it have made any difference?
RESIDENT: No. I guess it was sort of academic.

Later on, other doctors in the audience return to this point and the resident, now a bit exasperated, explains: "Well, we wanted to know if the primary was in colon or in breast. There are different treatments for them, you know" (a skillful one-upping shot).

A QUESTIONER: Listen, for a patient like this in end-stage C-A her chances are zero anyway. [*C-A* is shoptalk for cancer.] Treatment isn't going to make any difference. All you can do is palliate the symptoms. Maybe relieve pressure on the cord.

The resident by this time is quite defensive. She shrugs. "The patient refused treatment anyway. She said she didn't want it. So after that we stopped the investigation." But even before, it's clear that the resident's main interest was in the disease.

If this fiercely inquisitive style remained confined to treatment of hospital patients, that might be justifiable. But it has spread throughout medicine. The style of internal medicine is becoming the style of the profession as a whole.

I asked a young family doctor, the recent product of a high-powered medical training, what she would do about stomach pain in a young person. If it sounds like an ulcer, why not just give Tagamet (the brand name of an antiulcer drug generically called *cimetidine*) and then see what happened?

FAMILY DOCTOR: Because it could be gastric CA. Cimetidine can mask the symptoms of CA, so that it eats through the stomach mucosa and before you know it you've got a CA two feet long.

She explains that a doctor should do an "upper GI [gastrointestinal] series" on patients he suspects have an ulcer. This involves the patient's fasting the night before, going to see a radiologist, and having a "barium meal" to let the X-ray stand out. It's also expensive.

So you do an upper GI series on all stomach pains you think may be ulcer?

FAMILY DOCTOR: Yup.

It's not my affair to comment on the diagnosis of "epigastric pain." But I did get a wide range of answers from other doctors of whom I asked the same question. Some would give a tranquilizer and see what happened, others Tagamet. In general, older practitioners did not undertake these "upper GI series" at the drop of a hat. The point is that younger physicians, having been more thoroughly immersed in the internists' *furor therapeuticus*, are far more activist.[32]

The price paid for this intensification of testing is the downplaying of history taking and the physical exam, steps of the consultation that can have therapeutic power in and of themselves. Already in the early 1950s, taking the history was being treated as "a routine to be carried out rather than an individual analysis of a patient's illness." After World War II the practice of interviewing patients from a written outline began to infiltrate, so that rather than deriving the cathartic benefit of telling their story, they would answer a series of yes-no questions. Some internists tried to shuck entirely the task of interviewing patients. Addis C. Costello, who in 1970 was chairman of the American Society of Internal Medicine's practice management committee, said in an interview that "patients must be persuaded not to insist on talking with the doctor himself when a paramedic could just as well take their medical histories." He wanted state laws on paramedics eased up. More recently—I find it astonishing that this could even be contemplated—histories are being taken by computer, so that no human exchange of any kind is required.[33]

Hand in hand with this new confidence in the chemical sciences goes greater reliance on drug therapy. The United States is not necessarily the worst offender in this area, for a World Health Organization survey of selected cities in 1968–1969 found that in Lodz (Poland) and Buenos Aires (Argentina) a whopping 78 percent of all patient visits ended with a prescription. In the American communities of northwest Vermont and Baltimore, only around 50 percent of all visits saw medication prescribed. Internationally, then, American doctors aren't the most prescription-happy in the world. In some countries that are medically less advanced, it seems that more patients expect a prescription. In other words, many factors enter into prescribing aside from the doctor's enthusiasm for prescribing.[34]

But among American doctors, internists are the worst offenders. In a nationwide survey in 1976–1978, 56 percent of all visits to internists ended with a prescription, as opposed to 51 percent of the visits to family practitioners, and 30 percent of visits to psychiatrists.[35] But whatever the specialty, the willingness of American doctors to prescribe pills is staggering, in view of some of the complaints they're treating. In 1980, for example, 94 percent of all visits for colds ended with a prescription, a good deal of this medication useless.[36] It is the internists who have pointed the way toward this cascade of drugs, a cascade that deforms medical practice by substituting placebos for the healing power of compassion.

The upshot of all these changes has been a growing distance between internist and patient. One study of twenty-one internists showed that they were quite poor at identifying patients suffering from emotional distress: three thousand patients in Denver were seen by the internists and then assessed independently by psychiatrists. Some of the patients were alcoholic, had thought of suicide, and so forth. "It is evident," the psychiatrists found, "that the internists in this study did not recognize several potentially very important psychiatric diagnoses ... although the patients were willing to reveal at least some of the problems if they were asked." What's worse, "the internists did not know when they had insufficient information to make accurate assessments" and so proceeded as though the emotional problems didn't contribute to the patient's symptoms, although they might in fact have been the reason for the visit in the first place. Such failures can have grave consequences: for example, it turns out that 80 percent of suicide victims have seen a doctor within six months of their death.[37] An alert physician might have helped such patients.

The inrush of "science," it becomes clear, has crowded out some of the doctor's former empathy and ability to communicate concern. Michael Lepore, an old-style internist, places the blame right at his colleagues' feet. "Foot-of-the-bed" rounds and "chart" rounds, during which only the patient's file is discussed, "have all too often replaced bedside teaching and the laying on of hands, with the student seldom being brought into contact with the patient. The person as a whole is neglected, while his heart, his lungs, his kidneys, or his liver receives maximal attention."[38]

The "Decline of the Family Doctor": Myth and Reality

If patients are to be cured of psychological disease, they might do better to see a family doctor. But what is a family doctor? How many of them exist? Are they keeping their heads above the water? There are a number of misunderstandings in this area.

The Family Doctor Has Long Been "in Decline"

First, the "good old family doctor," or "general practitioner," was already in decline in the 1920s and 1930s. His precarious status today has nothing to do with the drug revolution that followed World War II. Of American physicians practicing in 1928, 74 percent were GPs, 14 percent were GPs "interested in but not limited to a speciality," and 13 percent were specialists. By 1942 the percentage of GPs had fallen to below half the total.[39]

Thus, long before the 1960s, the GP was under siege by the specialties. The specialist "has short hours and is seldom or never called out at night," said Daniel Cathell. "His fees are always good, *sometimes fat.* . . . And, after a much easier life, his estate generally 'cuts up' a great deal fatter after death than the general practitioner's: Yes! Educated fingers now make many a medical fortune!" Thus it is unsurprising to learn that by 1934 the old family doc had "nearly disappeared." As James Herrick, a Chicago internist, said, "Everything seemed to conspire against him. A huge volume of knowledge—bacteriology, X-rays, biochemistry, instruments of precision—suddenly poured in on him and all but overwhelmed him."[40]

By 1980, of the 403,000 physicians in the United States,

- *Only 15 percent were in family medicine or general practice.*
- *Eighteen percent were internists.*
- *Pediatrics and gynecology each comprised 7 percent.*

The other 50-plus percent of doctors was distributed among a wide variety of specialties: surgery, psychiatry, and so on.[41]

Family Doctors Still See Many Patients

Does this mean that the family doctor is now dead? Not at all. For one thing, although they are a seventh of the total number of doctors, GPs still see *about half* of all patients: 47 percent in 1980, down from 63 percent in 1966–1967.[42] Their share is so large because some physicians, such as pathologists, don't see any patients at all. Other specialists, such as surgeons, see relatively few.

Patients Personally Pick Their Specialists

Third, a number of specialists function as personal physicians. Internists have this capacity for the elderly, for example. Older people tend to choose an internist to be their personal doctor directly, without a referral. Internists get two-thirds of their patients without referral, dermatologists 70 percent, and so on.[43] Sir Theodore Fortescue Fox made a bit of fun of American patients, who make their own diagnoses and decide which expert to see. He's quoting a patient: "So I called my group this morning, told them I had a bad rash and asked to see the skin specialist. This girl on the phone tells me I've got to see my family doctor first. What kind of run-around is that when I need a skin specialist?"[44] When women need a physician, 40 percent of the time they go to a family doctor, 17 percent of the time to an obstetrician, 13 percent to an internist, et cetera.[45]

Specialists as "Family Doctors"

A final point: patients consider the doctor they're seeing at the moment as their "family doctor." They have a medical home base, and whether their doctor is an internist or a gynecologist, they go back to him for care time and again, thus assuring themselves of continuity. In a nationwide survey made in 1977, approximately 85 percent of all visits to doctors were made by patients who had seen that doctor before. When asked whether they had a "regular source of medical care," 78 percent of the men polled in 1979 said yes, as did 91 percent of the women.[46]

In short, pediatricians function as GPs for children, internists as GPs for the elderly, and "family physicians" (for whom there has been a separate Academy since 1947) as GPs for young adults. (*Note:* I have been using *GP* and *family doctor* interchangeably but strictly speaking family physicians have done a one-year residency in family medicine in addition to their year of internship. Or they may do a two-year "residency" in family medicine, one year of which counts as the internship.) Accordingly, the possibility of providing the "care of the whole patient" that we saw before World War II is still present.

Another area of misconception concerns the kind of "style" one must adopt to be effective as a family doctor. In the 1960s and 1970s the view arose that good medicine required dismantling the old patriarchal image and coming across as a democratic equal to the patient, an approach that can be quite effective. But the ingredient that is essential to successful healing, taking a genuine interest in the patient and his problems, may be conveyed through a number of styles.

The "old-time family doctors" who project a patriarchal image of authority form a kind of gentle rear guard in postmodern medicine. I visited one in his basement office, which is done over in fake pine and is cluttered with files and free drug samples. Around the desk piled high with papers stand four chairs, and in the next room an examining table, a sink, a small table with scissors and scalpels, and the disused instruments from forty years of past medical fads. A receptionist is in the outer office.

In the three hours I spend with him he sees only seven patients: five are retired, one close to retirement, and one a hypochondriac young man of thirty-eight. The doctor is extremely personable with them. "How are you today?" he asks, rather than, What seems to be the problem? He listens carefully as they explain, not interrupting, and at the end of the consultation asks, "Is there anything else?"

It is astonishing how eager he is to please. A sixtyish woman who works as a hairdresser had bruised her thumbnail and now has a black pocket of dried blood beneath it. He looks at it carefully, speculates about whether drilling a hole in the nail would do any good, and when she avers that a friend told her it would, he goes ahead and makes a small hole. Nothing comes out. All this takes about twenty minutes.

An elderly immigrant woman comes in with her daughter. The

woman has multiple problems: from her joints, all of which are painful, to a sore throat, to ear wax. He takes *twenty minutes* to try to syringe out the ear wax, which is so hardened it won't come out. He tells the daughter to have her mother soak her ear with a peroxide solution and return the next week.

The thirty-eight-year-old postal clerk exasperates me after two minutes. He has a pain here, one there; he's been gaining weight and "can't seem to get it off." He's unmarried, lives with his mother, and because of the shift work "has no social life." The neck hurts, the back hurts, the tummy hurts, and he has gas. The doctor considers each complaint in turn, nods sympathetically at the man's own explanations (all of which involve "pinched nerves"), and examines the abdomen. He has other complaints too: "burning" head, burning ears, and on and on. The doctor gives him a couple of prescriptions, and the fellow leaves, avid to have a "general checkup" as soon as possible. Some practitioners would have done anything to get rid of the guy in the first five minutes, but the doctor heard him out, and the patient seems quite pleased on departing.

There are some fairly serious medical problems: a man with a recent thirty-pound weight loss; a woman in severe pain from a stone in her ureter; an elderly man with blood in his urine. Of the seven patients, only this last is referred, to a urologist for consultation.

At the end I ask him two questions:

First, why did you prescribe tetracycline (an antibiotic) for the old woman's sore throat? He immediately divines the intent of my question and concedes that at Big City Hospital they would have given aspirin and had the patient come back once the lab tests were available. Then he tells several stories about seeing children die because they hadn't been treated quickly or aggressively enough. These stories, which involve meningitis and infected teeth, aren't exactly relevant to the woman's sore throat, but he's making the point that he doesn't like to wait. If you can reduce risks even a tiny bit by acting now, he prefers to act now.

Second, how do you make any money? After all, he's invested more than three hours on seven patients, for all of whom he is paid the standard Canadian health insurance fee. Indeed, for the twenty-minute earwax job he receives an extra $3.50. He shrugs. "All my friends ask me that too," he says. "I'm not all that interested in making money."

On the way out, his receptionist assures me that Dr. X is "very popular with his patients. They come from all over to see him."

Dr. X, who graduated from medical school in 1945 and stands perhaps on the line between "modern" and "postmodern" is a somewhat "patriarchal" figure. He wears a tie, always has a white coat buttoned about him, and does not expect to be addressed by his first name.

A different kind of presence, completely democratic yet nonetheless effective, is projected by a young family doctor in his early thirties, who wears neither white coat nor tie and feels at ease on an equal level with his patients. I watch a number of interviews. "How are things?" he asks in an open-ended way and then waits. He makes the diagnosis and writes out a prescription. "Anything else you want to ask?" he says. There usually isn't, but a listener has the impression of a friendly ear, always available, never judgmental.

A woman of fifty comes in, depressed because of a heart attack she had five months ago. "In your own mind," he asks, "is this something you expect to get better?"

And then, "What can we do to help you? What would you like us to do?"

Then later, "How much time do you think would be normal for you to recover? Can you be gentle enough with yourself to give yourself the time to heal?" This sounds corny, but she brightens when he asks it.

Now he takes time to hear how she's coping with the accident that touched off her depression. She's divorced, and we hear a long tale of how insensitive the ex-husband has been.

The young doctor asks, "Do you wonder why you're a little angry in the face of all this?"

He invites her to come back and talk more about her anger. "You've got to put on the table how you're feeling."

Now a quick change of tone indicates that the interview is over. He adds, however, "Let me say from my point that I think you've confronted this with courage and dignity. A heart attack is difficult to bear psychologically." He gives her a hug.

On another occasion he explains to me the difference between family practice and internal medicine, as he sees it.

> The family practitioner doesn't have the "rule out" syndrome that exists in internal medicine. On a patient's chart you'll see the diagnosis along with about ten other differential diagnoses that have to be ruled out. Family practice is much less interested in diagnosis. We don't find it absolutely necessary to put a label on "fatigue," for example. We're much more interested in *prognosis* than diagnosis.

This is another way of saying that these family doctors are more interested in the patient than the disease. It is a distinctive style.

I have dwelt at length upon the style of family practitioners because it shows they are still capable of supplying one of the preconditions of curing psychological disease: expressing genuine interest in the patient. Why should this distinguish family medicine, just as the relentless diagnosis of organic disease defines the style of internal medicine? Is it because family doctors are nicer people? Not at all; merely that they have not been deformed by spending four extra years of specialist training. A native sensitivity to the vicissitudes of the human condition has not yet been occluded by a wall of biochemical testing.

In some ways, to be sure, these two family doctors *are* creatures of their time. For one thing, they have a great confidence in drugs. Also, although they accept easily the notion of *psychogenesis*, or disease arising in the mind, they feel uncomfortable the moment "psychiatric" is plastered on the patient. We will discuss this matter in the last chapter.

But in one respect these two men are *not* typical of postmodern family doctors, indeed of postmodern medical practice generally. They are unhurried. An important reason most doctors today are having so little success coping with psychological disease is the press of time.

THE PRESS OF TIME

When one New York doctor covered for a colleague on vacation, he jotted down each call he received in a little book. When the colleague got back, the doctor suggested lunch so they could sit down and discuss the patients. "But when I got through with the first three or four names I closed the book because it was obvious that he doesn't remember the patients. He works fantastically fast in the office. He can see double the number of patients of anyone else in the office because he didn't involve himself with anything."[47]

One of the great plagues of postmodern medicine is the speed at which many doctors work. Even though patients say in some surveys that they don't mind these blitz interviews, this speed does reduce the amount of time in which they can tell their stories.[48] For Dr. John Burnum, an internist in Tuscaloosa, Alabama, the press of time was a great concern. "I must face the fact that the greatest tension in my life as a practitioner internist comes from the nearly insoluble dilemma of taking care of thirty to forty people per day and being forced to turn away many new patients every day. . . . Good medicine is sorely tried by the relentless patient overload."[49]

How great is the press of time? The average consultation with a family doctor in America today lasts eleven minutes; with an internist, eighteen minutes. Internists, who in the words of Dr. Burnum like to "practice reflective and scholarly medicine," take longer partly because they have more tests to perform: performing diagnostic tests on 59 percent of their patients versus the family doctor's 40 percent.[50] They also take longer partly because their list of differential diagnoses is longer: they have more to "rule out." (Given that a great majority of their patients are "walk-ins" rather than referrals, it's not necessarily because their patients are sicker that they take longer.)

In Britain this press of time is positively insensate: the average GP interview lasts only six minutes! Indeed, in some practices there, the typical patient is seen for only three or four minutes. Some British physicians have earned from their patients such nicknames as "Two-minute Todd." One practitioner would start writing out the prescription while the patient was still talking![51] But the GP's role in the British system, really that of a "medical travel agent," is different from that in the American system. In North America, GPs admit their own patients to the hospital and make much less use of consultants, so they need every second of their eleven minutes.

What evidence is there that the pace of American medicine has accelerated over the years? It's difficult to get hard statistics from before World War II because so many doctors made house calls. Around 1930, 56 percent of all GPs made them. Today virtually no doctor does.[52] And even if the house calls were brief, they were frequent during an episode of illness and accumulated to an impression of caring. A sample of GPs interviewed in 1942 saw an average of 104 patients per week. A similar sample in 1977 saw 110. That represents a slight increase in workload of 6 percent.[53]

What matters, however, is that today not enough time is available to most patients for the kind of "good chat" we saw in the last chapter. There are two issues here.

One is whether patients are happy with the amount of time they get. The answer seems to be yes, for patients are willing to declare themselves happy with the most appalling medical service; so much do they hope they've been given good care that they are seldom able to face the prospect that they haven't. Under the speed-of-light pace of the National Health System in Britain, of course, there are more than a few discontents. Gerald Stimson and Barbara Webb described patients who would rehearse their questions to themselves before the consultation, hoping they would have time to remember everything they wanted to say. When one British survey asked whether your GP takes time, "not hurrying you," 14 percent said no. Did he "explain things to you fully"? Twenty-three percent said no.[54]

There is some evidence that in the United States, as well, the percentage of patients who feel they haven't had enough time has been growing. The World Health Organization survey found in 1968–1969 that 96 percent of American patients who'd seen their doctor within the last two weeks felt he had spent enough time with them. The patients surveyed lived in northwest Vermont and Baltimore. But in 1980 when a sample of fifteen hundred patients in midtown Manhattan were asked whether their doctor "explained the reasons for all tests"—which is something of a proxy for spending enough time with them—36 percent said no, and a further 24 percent "weren't sure."[55] So perhaps patients are increasingly feeling rushed.

Second, whether the patient consciously felt hurried or not, did the consultation last long enough to give some kind of therapeutic benefit? As we know, the telling of the story can be cathartic; the laying on of hands can heal; the very act of bathing oneself in medical attention can be restoring. As I write these lines I have just returned from another seminar of the family doctors. A patient was there this time, or rather, the wife of a gravely ill patient in a hospital. She reported her husband's words from his bed of pain: "After each one of Dr. P's visits I always feel so much better." Can a consultation that lasts only eleven minutes achieve this kind of therapeutic benefit? The eleven minutes may be enough to make an organic diagnosis and write a prescription, but are they enough to heal?

Norman Cousins, in his inspirational book *Anatomy of an Illness*, describes what a tightly rationed commodity time is in American medicine today. "Time is one thing that patients need most from their doctors—time to be heard, time to have things explained, time to be reassured, time to be introduced by the doctor personally to specialists or other attendants whose very existence seems to reflect something new and threatening. Yet the one thing that too many doctors find most difficult to command or manage is time."[56] Postmodern doctors clearly feel they can give less time and still cure disease, because of the mastery over unruly nature that biochemistry has granted. I believe they're wrong. Biochemistry has not let them master the unruly mind that lies behind many of the symptoms they attempt to treat. Only the patient's faith in them will permit that, and the argument of the next chapter is that this faith is dissolving.

CHAPTER EIGHT
The Postmodern Patient

*T*HE GREAT paradox for patients today is that as they acquire a postmodern sensitivity to their bodies, their attitudes toward the medical profession are becoming once again *traditional*. This chapter tries to make sense of two events. First, people in the 1980s are far more sensitive to symptoms and more willing to seek care for them than ever before. Whatever the reason for this sensitivity, it has become a troubling factor in their relations with doctors. Second, patients in the 1980s are showing the classic signs of alienation from the medical profession, namely, diagnosing and treating themselves independent of physicians, using doctors merely as conduits for "drugs that really work," and consulting nonmedical practitioners: "quacks" in those days, "alternative healers" in ours. It is this growing desperation of patients about their own health, combined with increasing mistrust of official medicine, that sets the stage for a crisis.

DOING BETTER AND FEELING WORSE

In fact, there have been striking improvements in our health since the beginning of the drug revolution. Death rates in the United States have declined by one-third during the last three decades: from 841 per 100,000 population in 1950 to 556 in 1982.

Heart disease, the number one killer, is down 33 percent. Stroke deaths are down by one-half. In 1950, the life expectancy of the average American at birth was sixty-eight years. In 1982 it is seventy-four-and-a-half years. Nor is this decline entirely due to lower infant mortality; people sixty-five and older now have 20 percent more years to live than people of that age in 1950.[1]

Skeptics may respond that these improvements owe much to people's stopping smoking, jogging, eating well, and so forth—all undeniably important. But medical care has played a big role. In the United States, deaths in childbirth declined by 72 percent between 1968 and 1980; deaths from influenza and pneumonia are down by 53 percent, diabetes by 31 percent: all diseases "in which medical care can clearly be lifesaving." Doctors are forgetting what tuberculosis, meningitis, polio, rheumatic fever, and lobar pneumonia look like. The average GP might now wait eight years to see rheumatic fever in a child under fifteen, wait sixty years to see a case of typhoid fever, wait four hundred years to see a case of diphtheria. Thus, the assertion of some observers that "health care hardly affects health" is a gross distortion of the real improvement in people's welfare.[2]

Yet despite these historic improvements, people today are sick much more often than before World War II. As Table 8-1 shows, Americans in the 1920s reported eighty-two episodes of illness annually per 100 population; which is to say, the average person was sick less than once a year. Illness was defined as any disorder, either acute or chronic, "which wholly or partially disables an individual for one or more days," or which requires medical service, or drugs "costing more than fifty cents." People in the 1980s, by contrast, report 212 "acute" illnesses per 100 population annually, a 158 percent increase! (The chronic illnesses are not even

TABLE 8–1

HOW THE ANNUAL INCIDENCE OF ILLNESS HAS INCREASED FROM THE *1920s* TO THE *1980s*

	CCMC Survey 1928–1931 "Illness from All Causes"	NSHC Survey 1981 "Acute Conditions"	Percentage Increase, 1920s to 1980s
All ages			
Conditions annually			
per 100 population	82	212	+158 percent
Males	72	202	+180
Females	92	222	+141
Juveniles only			
Conditions annually			
per 100 population	83	276	+233
Males	84	277	+230
Females	82	274	+234

SOURCES: 1928–1931; Selwyn D. Collins, "Cases and Days of Illness Among Males and Females, with Special Reference to Confinement to Bed," [U.S.] *Public Health Reports*, 55 (January 12, 1940), 53, table 1, data on "illness from all causes . . . among 8,578 canvassed white families in 18 states during 12 consecutive months, 1928–1931," all ages, rates age-adjusted. Data on "juveniles" an average of the rates for 5–9 and 10–14 years.

1981: National Center for Health Statistics, B. Bloom, *Current Estimates from the National Health Interview Survey, United States, 1981.* Vital and Health Statistics, series 10, no. 141, DHHS pub. no. (PHS) 83-1569 (Washington: GPO, October 1982), p. 11, table 1, "Incidence of acute conditions." Data on juveniles, 6–16, p. 12.

counted.) And the definition of illness in the 1980s is substantially the same: any disorder lasting fewer than three months involving medical attention or "one day or more of restricted activity." Thus, the average person today is "sick," which means he seeks care for symptoms, more than twice a year. What is the reason?

The explanation is not that in the 1920s people were less willing to take time off from work, since illness rates for children under sixteen have increased by 233 percent. Nor can one argue that women have become somehow "softer." Illness rates for men rose in that fifty-year period by 180 percent, for women only by 141 percent. Nor can this massive increase in the number of times people define themselves as ill be the result of some statistical quirk. The survey taken in the 1920s went back to people's houses to question them three or four times over the year, whereas the 1981 survey merely asked them about "acute" illnesses within the last two weeks; nonetheless, many more postmodern patients felt they had been acutely ill in that brief span of time than did patients in the 1920s over a whole year.

No, the explanation is that people are now more willing to define their various symptoms as illness, to take care of them, and to report them to investigators. The symptoms that people notice have probably not themselves changed greatly over the ages.

Some specific points:[3]

- *Noninfectious diseases that cause considerable pain, such as an inflamed gallbladder, have not changed over the years. People in the 1920s would take time off work and buy drugs for things like gall pain, just as they do today.*

- *Some serious infectious diseases seem to be rising, despite antibiotics. Pneumonias, for example, have increased statistically from 0.7 per 100 population in the 1920s to 1.3 per 100 in 1981. That probably means that in the 1920s lots of people kept on functioning with mild pneumonias. They didn't ask help for them, and so they were never diagnosed, whereas today people go to the doctor, and the pneumonia is uncovered. Unlike in the 1920s, however, these episodes of pneumonia today are rarely fatal because of antibiotics, hence the improvement in our mortality statistics.*

- *Women today who have genitourinary problems are much more likely to seek help than women in the 1920s, for the apparent rate today is more than five times higher.*

- *The ordinary problems a GP sees have all apparently undergone staggering increases: colds have increased fourfold in frequency; sinus problems more than thirteenfold; urinary tract disease has doubled, digestive problems tripled, "accidents and injuries" quadrupled.*

- *The only common disease that has declined in frequency is tonsilitis (down about a quarter), probably as a result of aggressive antibiotic therapy plus a high rate of tonsil removals.*

In no other domain have antibiotics greatly reduced the statistical incidence of illness episodes, because people today are so much more sensitive to the episodes they *do* have and thus are more inclined to attend to them and call them illness. The average episode of illness today also lasts longer. If you had a "disabling" illness in the 1920s, you'd be out an average of 15.6 days; today it lasts 19.1 days.[4] Thus, although antibiotics have had an enormous impact on life-threatening illnesses, they have not reduced at all the incidence of run-of-the-mill illnesses.

The reason is, of course, that the whole notion of being ill is so subjective. In the last fifty years the symptom pyramid has undergone an enormous expansion. Not only are people more willing to define their various bodily twinges as illness; they're also more willing to seek help for them. Whereas in the 1920s the average person consulted a doctor (as we saw in Chapter 5) 2.9 times a year, in 1981 that figure had risen to 4.6.[5] Three Americans out of four now see a doctor annually, and a quarter of all men—and a third of all women—will see a doctor more than twice a year. In Britain, the number of people who thought they would consult a GP for "a constant feeling of depression" for three weeks or more rose from 54 percent in 1966 to 69 percent in 1977, again, evidence of rising sensitivity to internal signals.[6]

Individuals genuinely believe themselves to be sick. We aren't talking about "fakers" or "wimps." "When I've got anything, all I know is how I feel," said one woman.[7] What is interesting for us is the simple fact that patients today are so much more worried than ever before. How is your health? asked a U.S. nationwide survey in 1979. Sixteen percent of the men and 17 percent of the women thought it was fair or poor, and if they had fewer than twelve years of education, more than one-third of the respondents said fair or poor. Of the *young* men in this survey, 26 percent said they'd been worried about their health over the past year, as did 30 percent of the young women.[8] Thus despite the objective improvements in people's real health, they're more worried about it, more preoccupied and internally sensitive, than ever before.

Here we have the explanation for one of those puzzling problems in medical economics: Why don't doctors run out of patients? The supply of physicians in the United States has increased from 1 for every 714 people, in 1950, to 1 for every 508 in 1980. If current trends continue, by the year 2000 there'll be one doctor for every 370 people! Yet the supply of patients shows no signs of exhaustion. The average patient must wait 4.5 days for an appointment with the doctor, and in communities in north central Florida, where one study was done, a quarter of the younger doctors were accepting no new patients at all.[9] Therefore, despite high costs, long waits for appointments, and eleven minute-visits, the avalanche of symptoms has been so overpowering as to bury even today's legions of doctors.

A direct consequence of this avalanche for doctor-patient relations has been the burgeoning of doctors' resentment at being deluged with "trivial" symptoms. They spend four years in medical school learning about diseases like renal amyloidosis and phenylketonuria. They spend two years in a family practice residency learning to manage high blood pressure. Then they "treat" an endless procession of colds, *treating* in quotation marks, of course, because there's nothing a doctor can do about a cold save let it run its course. Colds are the most common disease seen in family practice, and most people come within a week of the cold's onset, which helps to explain why doctors believe themselves swamped with trivia.[10] When 248 doctors were surveyed in California they thought, on the average, that one patient in five had only trivial problems. Tuscaloosa's Dr. Burnum, the internist we met in the last chapter, considered 27 percent of his patients to have "only minor complaints, or no disease whatever." Among the minor problems were "dry ears," "hands asleep," "weak ankles," and "gas." He even coined a phrase, *benign dystopism,* to avoid disappointing them when they had nothing wrong with them. One Welsh physician said, "We doctors can't really treat the vast proportion of conditions that are brought to us—they're not illnesses at all."[11]

The point is that doctors tend to become short-tempered at patients' newly lowered thresholds of illness. I asked a young physician doing "doctor's replacement" (night and weekend calls for other doctors) what percentage of the symptoms she sees she herself would call a doctor for, if she were a patient?

"Oh, maybe 15 percent."

What do you see that isn't minor?

"Mainly middle-ear infection in kids. They get a cold, maybe two weeks later they've got a lot of pain. [The Eustachian tube has closed, and bacteria are growing in the middle ear.] You have to treat them."

And the adults?

"Oh, most of it is just garbage. Their stomach hurts."

Despite the best will, physicians who see their responsibility as the treating of organic diseases, like this woman, become curt and uncommunicative in coping with an onrush of medical trivia.

But before we dismiss the postmodern patient as a silly goose, two points should be made. One is that patients don't regard what they have as trivial. In a study of twelve thousand patients in twenty-four emergency departments throughout the United States, 73 percent believed they needed care "immediately" or "urgently." (In the doctors' opinion, only 33 percent of these patients were true emergencies.)[12] Second, apparently "trivial" symptoms are often just an excuse allowing the patient to gain his composure in the doctor's office in order to talk about the real, underlying problem, which is often psychological. More on that in the next chapter.

WHY THE NEW SENSITIVITY?

The large number of government surveys facilitates the historian's job of describing changes in behavior. But accounting for a major shift in attitude brings all the perils of writing "contemporary history" down on one's head. The true explanation for this new sensitivity to bodily sensations is obviously complicated, involving many factors. I want to call attention to three: changes in family life, media scare stories, and a genuine increase in smoking-related cancer that has nothing to do with media alarums.

Sheer emotional stress is associated with bodily sensations. As the style of life that I have elsewhere called modern breaks up, a lot of people are subject to new stress, and therefore to sensations that may also be new. I'd like to dilate for a moment upon the issue of style of life. The former modern family came into being late in the eighteenth century in the Anglo-Saxon world, somewhat later on the continent. It represented a secure little emotional nest for women and children, in contrast to the emotionally rather empty shell of the traditional peasant family. This modern family started to break up in the 1960s, giving way to a postmodern family style that exhibits a perfect symmetry with postmodern medicine. The couple in this new family are characterized by intense sexual ties, by a view of themselves more as a "relationship" than an "institution," and by a high degree of instability. For people marrying in the 1980s the risk of divorce is greater than 50 percent. And as second marriages have an even greater rate of breakup than first marriages, one may describe the postmodern couple as being in a state of almost permanent instability. We are thus acquiring a new style of intimate life in which (1) large numbers of people are, at any given time, outside the boundaries of family life entirely and (2) the people in families experience much more stress about the "relationship's" likely future than ever before.[13] These changes have certain consequences for health, not so much creating more illness as making people more *sensitive* to the symptoms they already have.

First of all, separated and divorced people are likely to be unhappier than married people, for obvious reasons. For a generation accustomed to translating human conditions into medical terms, unhappiness becomes "depression," a treatable disorder. Rates of depression are considerably higher for divorced than for married people. A government survey in 1974–1975 found that currently married people had an average depression score of 8.0, and formerly married of 11.3: thus 41 percent higher. Depression is then often converted into physical symptoms and appears in the GP's office. As London psychiatrist Michael Balint wrote in 1957, "Nowadays, with more and more of us becoming isolated and lonely, people have hardly anyone to whom they can take their troubles. It is undeniable that fewer and fewer people take them to their priests. The only person who is always available . . . is the doctor. In many people emotional stress is accompanied by, or possibly is tantamount to, bodily sensations. So they come to their doctor and complain."[14]

In the 1980s especially, people undergoing major life changes are sensitive to their bodies, inclined to interpret sensations as illness. In a family clinic in California, for example, around 40 percent of the single patients had "psychosocial problems," such as alcoholism, stress, and anxiety, as opposed to 27 percent of those married. The patients with psychosocial problems were more inclined to see the doctor often: middle-aged males in this category, for example, visited an average of eight times a year, as opposed to males without psychosocial problems who visited only two or three times a year. These psychosocial patients were almost twice as likely as other patients to have colds or digestive problems and three times as likely to have "endocrine and metabolic" problems.

Thus, there is some tendency for the "singles" life-style of California to encourage people to interpret their symptoms as illness. The same train of events held true in a study of ninety-four patients in a working-class Canadian city: the separated, widowed, and divorced were more likely to have psychosocial problems (one is obliged to adopt this horrid jargon). And patients with such problems were, in turn, three times more subject to inflammatory diseases, 50 percent more at risk of hypersensitivity problems, and twice as likely to have trouble with their urinary tracts. They had a virtual monopoly on diseases of the digestive system.[15]

Even those people within marriage are not spared some pretty high-voltage relationship stress. This observation would be banal if the casualties of marriage wars did not appear so often in the doctor's office. A man comes into the clinic with chest pain. He has a thick file. His immediate problem is reflux esophagitis (stomach contents spilling back up into his esophagus), managed with antacids. But the pain goes beyond that. A senior doctor explains, "There are layers." One layer is that his marriage is going bad. His wife comes in for migraine. "I've been doing some marital counseling," the doctor explains, "but they don't seem to get on the track. The oftener they come in for migraine and chest pain, the worse I know things are getting in the marriage."

The breakup of the family has reaped another harvest of symptoms for those "meeting people" and dating. We aren't talking about adolescents fumbling around at the drive-in but fully grown adults struggling desperately to find and stay with part-ners. One brand of "courtship" complaint concerns overweight. Of course many other adults are worried about their weight as well, for health reasons, or on grounds of simple personal pride. But to go by the editorial content of such singles-oriented publi-cations as *Cosmopolitan* and the chitchat surrounding the young urban professionals' exercise scene, at the epicenter of weight concerns are men and women in their thirties and forties who are struggling with relationships. The surveys don't permit us to pin this observation down statistically, but it is a strong impression that I believe is true.

A series of surveys does, however, document the extent to which weight has become a hallucinatory obsession of an entire society.

Do you think of yourself as overweight? asked a 1979 study. Fifty percent of the women and 34 percent of the men answered yes.[16]

Are you actually overweight, inquired another government survey, thereupon taking physical measurements to find out. Thirty percent of the women and 23 percent of the men were in-deed overweight. Therefore, the gap between thinking fat and being fat was 20 percent for the women and 11 percent for the men.[17] This is the "anxiety gap" that one might attribute in part to the sexual revolution.

Married or single, people anxious about their weight often turn up in the doctor's office. A study of who reports most symptoms found that weight was extremely important to the "high symp-tom reporters," who tended generally to "place a very high pre-mium on self-presentational concerns." A 1977 government survey asked respondents whether they had visited a doctor for obesity in the last twelve months. Four times as many women had done so as men (6.4 percent of the women, 1.6 percent of the men).[18] At some level, therefore, our explosive interest in sexual matters, the necessity in dating to preen and strut a bit, our ob-session about weight, and our sensitivity to internal states are all linked.

Finally, anxiety about sexually transmitted diseases has sent patients tumbling into the doctor's office. At the clinic I saw many uneasy young people consulting with the staff about an itchy groin or a vaginal discharge. The young doctors were easy to talk to, and the patients admitted quite readily they feared their symptoms were linked to sexual endeavors. The supreme expression of this particular theme occurred at a staff seminar on genital herpes, when two young female fieldworkers from a herpes "community group" came to talk. Both of them had genital herpes.

Does herpes interfere with your sex life? someone asked.

"Not with mine," one said. "Over the last seven years I've had quite a few partners. But I tend to want to know someone a little better before I make a proposal to them."

A fifty-six-year-old doctor exchanged glances with me and rolled her eyes. "I'm glad I'm getting old," she said. The anxieties we're discussing are definitely the anxieties of a new generation.

So far I've been making the argument that the major changes in family life and sexual behavior of the last twenty years create unhappiness, which is then translated into a host of physical symptoms, which then appear at the doctor's, augmenting the inexhaustible supply of care seekers. But, the skeptical reader responds, is the family the only institution to have eroded? How about all the stress from work, urbanization, and the general pace of postmodern life?

Don't forget that in the 1920s, and in the 1820s for that matter, there was plenty of stress. Individuals imagined their lives then, as now, to be extremely fast-paced. Indeed this perception of oneself as harried, and of life as "fast," is probably a historical constant. But the family is significant: unlike the workplace or the city bus, it is the one forum in which the individual may seek loving ties and solace from worry. Thus, the transformation of family life that we have seen all about us has exacted a far higher psychic cost than any of the other changes that observers conventionally point out. Of course this is speculative, but I do feel that much of the loving support that men and women once gave each other in the—now much despised—"Victorian family" helped reduce their anxiety about symptoms. It is the withdrawal of that support, as the nuclear family comes crashing down, that leaves us confused and frightened at the signals of our own bodies.

Stoking these underlying anxieties at every turn have been the media. A major reason for the current hypersensitivity to symptoms and the readiness to seek help for them as illness is a barrage of media scare stories about hideous ailments. These are ailments the vast majority of the population will never have; nor know anyone who has them. Yet every time a mass daily or the network evening news highlights one such sufferer, the health columnists leap on it and a sense of panic diffuses. "This year 40,000 U.S. women who take the birth control Pill will die," screeched the *Toronto Star* in 1980.[19] Of course the story was false and later retracted, but the impression left in the minds of many readers was doubtlessly indelible.

In the early 1980s spirits were flailed by a flurry of media stories on "environmental disease": people who had become "allergic to everything" as a result of all the "organic chemicals" around, who had to retreat to special asylums where all materials were "natural." Television viewers were afflicted by the spectacle of these poor individuals, clearly the victims of psychiatric ailments, dragging their oxygen tanks around with them as they pleaded their cases in court. Now such "environmental disorders" have become epidemic, as a result of suggestion by the mass media.[20]

In fairness, many health reporters try to do a responsible job. But every story must be given a "hook," if not by the reporter, then by the editor. And the hook is often a sensationalist one, that transforms a medical curiosity into an object of current concern for millions of people. Media stories over food hypersensitivities, for example, suddenly convinced many people that they had this rather unusual kind of allergic complaint. The great majority of people is not "allergic" to anything at all in the normal English or American diet, yet a rash of media stories entrenched this notion in the minds of many. Of twenty-three patients referred to a Manchester allergy clinic because of possible food hypersensitivity, only four turned out to be allergic to a dietary substance, "fish in one case, peas and beans in another, and oranges and tomatoes in the third." A fourth was allergic to aspirin. The other nineteen could not be confirmed in double-blind testing as allergic to anything. Yet, not to be detached from their beliefs, they often persisted in bizarre dietary restrictions such as limiting themselves to boiled potatoes. Those beliefs had been directly implanted in six of the people by reading a book, and in eleven others by the suggestion of other health workers, who themselves had likely become fearful after media allergy stories.[21]

The toxic shock scare, which intimidated millions of women into thinking a certain brand of tampon could give them a fatal septicemia, broke in June 1980, when the press picked up an obscure government report. Then a second report suggested, erroneously, that the Rely brand tampon was involved. By then a monster media sensation had erupted. Some of the headlines:

- *"Rely tampon causes toxic shock syndrome."*
- *"Toxic shock syndrome is really scarlet fever."*
- *"Tampons force blood into the peritoneal cavity."*

By the time the facts had become clearer, the public had been "stirred to such hysterical levels that toxic shock syndrome became a household word and Rely tampon the culprit." The product was scooped from the shelves; there were lawsuits, recriminations, and recommendations. One student of the episode concluded, "The media hyped the controversy at the expense of lingering public confusion and hysteria."[22]

The most spectacular media scare of the twentieth century, however, has been over *AIDS*, an acronym for *acquired immune deficiency syndrome*, a puzzling breakdown of the body's immune defenses that seems to occur in hemophiliacs and homosexuals. And only some homosexuals. Thus the vast majority of the population was not at all at risk. Nonetheless, in 1984 *1 Canadian in 50* believed him- or herself at risk of getting AIDS.[23] So hysterical had hospital personnel become on the subject in the hospital where I was observing, that instead of performing the requested tests on blood samples sent down to the laboratory from real AIDS victims, they threw them away unprocessed and reported the samples as "lost." All this, despite the fact that few hospital workers anywhere have ever contracted the disease from a patient.

The following encounter occurred. A male, forty-one, came in with "a list of things." He was a bachelor living with his parents. No girlfriends.

First, he had a bit of soreness around his anus and wanted to know "if it's AIDS."

DOCTOR: Have you ever had any intercourse with men?
PATIENT: No.
DOCTOR: Have you had any intercourse with women?
PATIENT: No.

Among his other complaints were the following:

- *A suspected loss of hearing, suggested to him by a hearing test he took at a county fair.*
- *A pain in his left ribs when he bends down or laughs.*
- *A crust on his eye; an "itchy eye" today.*
- *"I seem to be urinating a lot lately," up from seven times daily to nine times daily.*

On physical exam the doctor found nothing. "There's nothing wrong. You don't have AIDS. Your belly ache will come and go for a long time."

What am I suggesting, that the media stop reporting health stories? No, it's good to give health facts to people who want them, and to command journalists to reduce the hype would be like Canute's asking the tide to turn back. The reason these stories sell papers is that people are already so attuned to their internal states, so fearful of what various itches and twinges might mean, that they are ripe for exploitation by publicists whose job is to sell sensation. The media scare draws patients into the doctor's office, but one reason people are already so sensitive to their symptoms is that they genuinely fear they may have a grave disease, and that brings us to the third point.

They may well have one. We have already seen that people's health has been improving, but there's been one major exception to that picture over the last fifty years: the smoking-related cancers. Because of the epidemic of cigarette smoking that began in the 1910s and 1920s, an epidemic of lung cancer started twenty years later. By 1937 cancer had become the second leading cause of death in the United States, and the cancers caused by smoking—lung, larynx, esophagus and so on—had become the number one cancers, replacing those of breast and uterus.

I am going to describe how this particular "penny," the relation between smoking and cancer, dropped, because I think patients' awareness of the link between the two goes a long way to explain why so many anxious patients appear with "trivial" symptoms. Lung cancer was once a rare disease. James Wardrop, an Edinburgh surgeon who published a treatise on cancer in 1809, had never seen a cancer of the lung himself but quoted another doctor who had examined several and who believed the condition to be "very rare." William Osler in his 1892 textbook declared tumors originating in the lungs to be "rare." "The conditions which predispose to it are quite unknown," he said. A textbook for GPs published in 1927 in England did not even mention lung cancer, dwelling instead on stomach, colon, and breast: the cancers that historically have always been common. And in that same year Dr. Tylecote of Manchester, although somewhat alarmed about the incidence of lung cancer locally, agreed the disease to be rare elsewhere. "It must be quite 17 years ago that a well-known professor of pathology at the end of his first week's work in Manchester remarked to me, 'We have had two P.M.s [autopsies] on cancer of the lung this week, and during all my time at _____ hospital I only saw a couple.' " Dr. Tylecote added, "I think that in almost every case I have seen and known of, the patient has been a regular smoker, generally of cigarettes."[24]

One is struck, from the perspective of today, at the sangfroid with which an earlier generation of physicians encouraged their patients to smoke. Lois Vidal, a young English gentlewoman who, after three years off smoking, felt she needed something to calm her nerves, said around 1920, "My renewal of smoking had been endorsed by the doctor." An article in 1924 in *Hygeia*, the health magazine of the AMA, declared cigarettes "comparatively harmless to a mature person." In 1940 a scientist said that she was quite puzzled about "the excess of cancer of the tongue, mouth and lip in males; it is certainly not due to the habit of smoking a clay pipe today [early documented as a risk factor]. Why should cancer of the thorax be so very largely a male disease?" This medical befuddlement left the public in obscurity, too. One British survey in 1966 found that "laypersons commonly [think] that the prognosis for lung cancer is good."[25] In fact, only 7 percent of lung cancer patients are still alive five years after the disease has been diagnosed.

All of this is history. Nobody today believes the prospect for lung cancer to be "good," and the dawning of that realization has played a major role, I think, in the making of the postmodern patient. The penny began to drop for the public early in the 1950s, with the publication of a flurry of studies on smoking and health. Indeed, the early 1950s saw a brief dip in cigarette smoking as a result, although the rate soon climbed back up again. In 1959 the Royal College of Physicians in London set up a committee to study the subject, and their 1962 report, *Smoking and Health*, delivered the first hammer blow against the complacency of the public. They concluded, "Cigarette smoking is the most likely cause of the recent world-wide increase in deaths from lung cancer, the death rate from which is at present higher in Britain than in any other country in the world."[26]

Now one blow followed the next. In 1964 the Surgeon General of the United States found that the mortality for men who smoked was 70 percent higher than for nonsmokers. And in 1979 another, massive report from the Surgeon General announced that the number one risk of smoking was not even cancer but heart disease! Cancer was just number two.[27]

These reports had an immediate impact. In 1964, the year of the first Surgeon General's report, 53 percent of all American males and 32 percent of females still smoked. The percentage of male smokers then started dropping at once, and the percentage of females followed shortly thereafter. By 1980 only 38 percent of men and 29 percent of women smoked. If, however, one adds the number of former smokers together with current smokers, in 1980 they amounted to 68 percent of the male population (two-thirds!), and 45 percent of the female population.[28] My purpose in writing this bitter news is not to set readers in panic. After all, the likelihood of getting lung cancer recedes with the number of years one has stopped. But it doesn't vanish. And that means that a huge number of Americans today are intently concerned with whether the little wheezes, coughs, pains, and weight fluctuations they perceive might not signal the onset of one of the smoking-related cancers.

Already back in the 1950s many patients had started putting two and two together. Men would hem and haw about and then casually say to the doctor at the last minute:

"Then you don't think that these symptoms mean that there is anything seriously wrong with me?"

"No," London physician Kenneth Walker would reply. "What were you frightened that they might mean?"

"Oh, I don't know—something really serious."

"What did you think you might be suffering from?"

"Some sort of growth, perhaps?"[29]

So I think this dim apprehension of tumors did begin to infiltrate the culture, even in the minds of those who don't read Surgeon General reports. A man born in 1923 would be fifty in 1973, and in that year his risk of dying of lung cancer would be more than twice as high as that of a man who had reached fifty around the time of World War II.[30] People pick up on this kind of thing. Around 1960, for example, observers began to hear, as explanations of why doctors should make house calls, that it would be nice if someone could visit the home, so that the doctor "could see people who may really be dying and not know it. And not going to the doctor—they may think they just have a cold or something."[31] This is almost certainly a subterranean reference to lung cancer.

In the 1970s and 1980s the cancer fears have become less subterranean. A 1976 survey commissioned by the television network ABC found that, for example, "Californians are more afraid of cancer than of any single danger in the world, including violent crimes and atomic war."[32] My own conviction, therefore, is that part of this flood of "trivia," the minor chest complaints appearing in the doctor's office, represent a real need for reassurance about specters that even today many find too difficult to discuss.

Let me wrap up this section rather tentatively. Many circumstances, linked to the countercultural revolution of the 1960s, the pop-psyche movement and the increasing interest in "fulfillment," have probably made the mind more susceptible to bodily symptoms. But if we ask how, exactly, does social life in the 1980s differ from the 1920s, I think an important answer must be the family and sexuality. If we ask what symptoms, precisely, would suggest menace in the 1980s more than in the 1920s, it is probably those of cancer, especially lung cancer. And if we try to discover why we, as a nation, sit perched night after night on the brink of alarm, I think it is probably because we watch television, as in the 1920s people sat on their front porch swings. Thus we fearfully seek attention for far more symptoms than ever before.

THE REVOLT AGAINST MEDICAL AUTHORITY

The events just mentioned have made patients more dependent on doctors than ever before. Yet, paradoxically, patients are also more alienated from medicine than they were in the 1920s. In their mistrust they resemble the traditional patients of the eighteenth century. This new alienation expresses itself as a revolt against "medical authority," an authority that the modern doctor had so painfully acquired.

At some point after World War II the entente cordiale between doctor and patient began to break down. Exactly when is unclear. "Something went awry," recalled internist Michael Lepore. "Why did the profession of medicine, riding high on a crest of popular admiration and respect, its members returning from services in World War II to the well-earned plaudits of the people, witness a shift in position? It was soon to be placed on the defensive by a consumer-oriented nation of people, suspicious and critical of its doctors...."[33] Some observers date the crumbling of trust to the twin attacks on psychiatry and obstetrics that began in the 1960s under the influence of the counterculture: Thomas Szasz's *The Myth of Mental Illness* (1961), Ken Kesey's *One Flew Over the Cuckoo's Nest* (1962), and the meetings of a Boston women's health collective that began in 1969 and from which emerged the million-best-seller *Our Bodies, Ourselves* (1971). Obviously these books did not create the initial discontent, but they became popular because of it. The fire of consumer discontent, so goes this view, then spread from these outbuildings to consume the medical profession as a whole.[34]

An alternative account makes high doctors' bills, and the tendency of the profession to draw the wagons into a circle when attacked for malpractice, the take-off point of the revolt and sees as landmarks such now-forgotten works as reporter Richard Carter's exposé, *The Doctor Business* (1958).[35]

Whenever the revolt started, by the end of the 1960s doctors noticed they were dealing with a new kind of patient, one unwilling to accept the doctor as priest, or medicine as a series of secret holy rites. One English physician said in 1972, "Our patients . . . no longer fall neatly, as they did until recently, into the demanding and oh-so-satisfying rich and the grateful and very satisfied poor. The discomforting reality of twentieth century democracy is that these people have disappeared. . . ."[36]

Indeed, these formerly accepting patients were disappearing. Dr. Russell Lee, who had directed a medical clinic in Palo Alto, California, for forty years, recalled the doctor's former authority. "It was exactly like Papal infallibility; the doctor is supreme, and anything he chooses to do is all right." He told the apocryphal story of the doctor at "Henry's" bedside:

The doctor looked at Henry and said, "Marian, Henry is dead." Henry then rose up indignantly and said, "I am not dead. I'm alive." Marian replied, "Henry, lie back down; the doctor knows best." That time, Dr. Lee concluded, "is past."[37]

Thus, half a century of patients accepting authority, of Paul Dubois's doctrine of a therapeutic coalition, was going down the tubes. Dubois in 1904: "In these treatments the patient and the physician seem to work to obtain the same result—the one by his confidence and good sense, the other by his clear and convincing explanation of the matter."[38] Dubois would have fainted had he been in the living room in the New York area where, in the early 1970s, a GP remembered the following scene:

"It was . . . a youngster they were having difficulty with, and he wasn't coherent and they told me he was a diabetic . . . and there was a question of whether he was in insulin shock, a diabetic coma, or whether this was unrelated, or epilepsy. . . . They refused to bring the kid into the Emergency Room and demanded a house call, which I finally made." So when the doctor got there he couldn't tell what the problem was, and decided, just to forestall complications if it was insulin shock (meaning too little sugar circulating in the blood), to start the child on an intravenous sugar solution. "We started giving him some glucose in water, about 50 cc [cubic centimeters]. After I had given about 5 cc, she let go his arm and she said, 'You've given him enough.' So she pulled the needle out...."[39] When the mother pulled the needle out, she was acting like a traditional patient: not necessarily irrationally, although the furious doctor reproached her for that, but with contempt for his "authority."

Just as in the eighteenth century patients suspicious of the doctor sought out the herbalist and the medicine man, so in the late twentieth they are once again seeking out alternative medicine. There is a wide range of this medicine, from what is labeled *holistic medicine*, and rather uncomfortably accepted as an adjunct by official medicine, to downright quackery, which includes such practices as drilling holes in people's skulls to "let in more oxygen," diagnosing ailments by the shape of the iris ("iridology"), and the giving of consultations by such paraprofessionals as "Judy the Holistic-Health Lady" and "Anna the Body-Wrap Lady."[40] What is positive about these therapies—some of which are themselves ludicrous—is that they reestablish an intimate relationship between the patient and an authority figure he can trust, restoring the benefits of the placebo and the act of consulting. Sadly, however, the authority figure is outside of medicine proper and often makes worse the problems that are basically organic, as opposed to psychological, in origin.

My purpose is not to criticize alternative medicine, but merely to indicate how widespread it has become. In the area of alternative cancer therapies, for example, there are at least a dozen nationwide organizations, such as the Committee for Freedom of Choice in Cancer Therapy, the Cancer Control Society, and the International Associations of Cancer Victims, which have meetings, hold local symposiums, explain cancer as a result of "protein imbalance," and recommend Laetrile, a substance derived from apricot pits, one of whose active ingredients is cyanide.[41]

I pick up the *Alternative Health Services Directory* for Toronto, which is eighty pages long and lists over five hundred practitioners and clinics. It includes ads for the following:

- *"Thuna's Wholistic Centre," which features "reflexology," "iridology," and "colonics" (remember get-those-poisons-out-of-there?).*
- *"Canadian Ion Center," which offers for sale "negative ion generators," on the logic that we're driven crazy by too many "positive ions" around us.*
- *"Atlantean Harmonistics Clinic," featuring "polarity" and "Vita-flex" ("Harmony through reflexes is the idea").*
- *Also reflex therapy; the "reflexologists" go on for pages. They are the unknowing spiritual heirs of those old nineteenth-century theories about "reflex neurosis" already mentioned (pp. 152–54).*[42]

On and on it goes. Some of these alternative types are reputable, in that they have university degrees. Others are lunatics. It is a sign of the breakdown of medicine's authority that all of them are able to heal. The troubled mother who commanded the New York GP to stop after he had administered a minute amount of glucose to her son will sooner or later end up in the hands of people like these and there will probably find peace of mind.

The alternative healers reach out today to a far wider percentage of the population than the quacks of the 1920s and 1930s ever embraced. Of 133 cancer patients under treatment at the University of Pennsylvania Cancer Center, 78 percent knew of at least one other alternative treatment in addition to Laetrile, and at least 10 percent were receiving "unorthodox therapy." Of 98 rheumatology (arthritis and the like) patients in Birmingham, Alabama, 93 had tried some alternative remedy. Most common were liniments (68 percent), copper and other jewelry (41 percent), and special diets, such as honey and vinegar (39 percent).[43] The mushrooming of these therapies since the 1960s constitutes a clear sign of patient alienation.

A second indication is the recent increase in self-dosing: patients diagnosing their own ailments and prescribing their own remedies. That too was common in the eighteenth century, when local herbs were gathered and made into teas on the basis of folk wisdom about bursts and fluxes, the self-diagnoses of the day. Today, of course, people consume far more drugs than did these traditional peasants and dose themselves not just with spring and fall tonics but virtually every day. In a 1969 survey of medicine use in Britain, it was found that 86 percent of the women and 73 percent of the men had taken something within the last two weeks. Americans turn out to be even more medicine-oriented, for a 1965 cross-national survey discovered that 48 percent of the Americans, as opposed to 38 percent of the British, had taken drugs within the last *two days*.[44]

People have lots of drugs on hand, too, whether they've recently taken them or not: the average British medicine chest contains ten different items, most often pain killers. All except 6 of the 686 households surveyed had some medicines on hand, but what distinguishes these 1960s patients from the prewar variety is the great increase today in drugs that act on the central nervous system: a fifth of the British had some kind of "sedative, sleeping tablet, or tranquilizer." These were, moreover, the main kind of prescribed drug that people had on hand.[45] One contrasts this with the "modern" patient, whose home remedies were most often laxatives and tonics.

A special new theme in self-dosing is the rise of "megavitamin" supplements. Popular culture has somehow been infiltrated by the "holistic" view that if a few vitamins do one good, a lot of vitamins must be life-giving. A big boost to this kind of "orthomolecular" practice, the taking of from twenty to six hundred times the recommended daily allowance, was Linus Pauling's 1970 book on vitamin C and the common cold. In the 1970s and 1980s vitamin "megadosing" has become common coin everywhere. A 1979 nationwide survey found that 42 percent of men and 58 percent of women took vitamin supplements of some kind, much of this money thrown down the drain.[46]

It's clear that patients see a good deal of self-treatment as an alternative to the doctor. The 1969 survey of Britain found the more that patients medicated themselves, the less they visited the doctor. And they took three times more drugs purchased over the counter than prescription-only drugs.[47]

What gives postmodern drug taking a particular poignancy, however—and what clearly links it to traditional manners—is that many patients today are obliged to get the only drugs in which they have confidence *via the doctor*. They are thus quite like the eighteenth-century patients who visited a physician, not because they had any particular confidence in his knowledge or skills, but because only he knew how to write prescriptions for compounds that were truly powerful, in other words, that would purge the bowels drastically. Thus, one factor troubling doctor-patient relations in our time is that many patients show up with their own diagnoses and prescriptions. They are merely obliged to go to the doctor so that he can write it out for them. (The drugs invariably require prescriptions.)

Using the doctor as a conduit for the drugs that are truly powerful results in a tug-of-war in the doctor's office that is frustrating for both sides. Some elements of this tug-of-war are continuous with the past; some are a recent departure. Patients' expectations of ending the consultation with a prescription are as old as the hills: traditional patients wanted some complex compound, modern patients expected a slip of paper for an often useless "proprietary" drug, and postmodern patients expect a "script" at the end as well. Two British studies found that, on the whole, two-thirds of all patients expected the consultation to end with a prescription.[48]

The new feature is that, unlike the tonics and laxatives of the 1920s, the drugs patients now want are very powerful and potentially dangerous, and they have the ability to create addiction. The tug-of-war is over two kinds of these new drugs.

Since coughs and colds are the major complaint today, the major drugs patients want are antibiotics. Penicillin, tetracycline, and erythromycin have become household words because of their triumphs in the 1940s and 1950s over the terrible bacterial infections of the past. But most colds, sore throats, and lower airway infections aren't caused by bacteria but by viruses, which antibiotics will not touch. This fact has been duly repeated in the media for the past thirty years. Nonetheless, many patients expect the doctor to prescribe an antibiotic for their cold. "Patient pressure is one of the most important factors that leads physicians to over-prescribe in office practice," said Dr. Calvin Kunin, in an AMA forum on antibiotics. "This is by no means subtle and often comes from the most articulate and best-educated people including health professionals." Precisely these pressures lead to the flood tide of antibiotics that now sweeps across pharmacy counters: they are the single largest category of drug prescribed today and amount to 13 percent of all prescriptions. Up to a third of all hospital patients receive them, and many of these patients show no particular sign of infection.[49]

The powers people ascribe to antibiotics make them almost a fetish, a magic wand to wave at illness, and patients insist that the doctor co-operate. Florida patients, for example, tend to stalk out if their doctor refuses them penicillin for a cold. "I'll go see a *real* doctor who knows what he is doing," they say.[50]

The fetishizing of antibiotics may grip even sophisticated day-care workers. "Four-year-old George had a low-grade fever. After a thorough physical examination, it was concluded that he was suffering from a mild viral illness." Because his mother had already been off work three days and was anxious to get back, she and the doctor agreed he should return to day care. "However, George's day-care center had a policy that children with fevers had to be on antibiotics [day-care workers' idea of good medicine]. The mother was given an empty bottle labeled 'Panamycetin, take one teaspoon four times daily.'

"She was instructed to fill the bottle with chocolate milk and send it along with George to the day-care center. The con was a resounding success."[51]

Thus when patients with colds show up demanding penicillin they pose a real problem for the doctor. A young woman of seventeen comes into the clinic with a sore throat and a headache. As she sits down, she lets the doctor know why she's there. "I have a sore throat and I came to get some pills for it."

Several doctors who are watching the consultation from another room laugh. Doctors hate it when patients request specific drugs. "This sort of thing makes my hair stand on end," they say.[52]

So the doctor takes her temperature, listens to her chest, examines her ears, and then looks into her throat, taking a swab.

"When this comes back, we'll know whether you have an infection or not," he says: No drugs until the tests are done.

She obviously doesn't like this but goes along. This young doctor is practicing good medicine as taught in medical schools and in the best medical journals. After the consultation a senior doctor comes along and says, "I would have given her a prescription, just to calm her down." "Good medicine," in other words, bends in the wind of patient expectations.

One encounters this tug-of-war again and again between what physicians have been taught and their patients' expectations. In one course in medical school the professor posed the following scenario: "It's five o'clock on Friday afternoon. The parents of a nine-year-old bring her in with a painful sore throat and demand a 'shot of penicillin' so that she won't have to miss ballet class Saturday morning. Do you prescribe or don't you?"

The medical students all chorus, "No," having dutifully learned that two-thirds of all sore throats are viral and that even if it's "strep throat" there's no harm in waiting a day or two to treat it.

"Wrong," the professor says. "You prescribe. Because if you don't, those parents will just keep going from doctor to doctor to emergency room until they find someone who will."

In the real world of practice such patients are almost impossible for a doctor to resist who (1) doesn't want to lose his practice and (2) feels a professional instinct to seem to be "doing something." Dr. Kunin, whom we have already heard, posed his own scenario:

> Visualize the telephone calls to a busy physician requesting and sometimes even demanding that an antibiotic be prescribed for a febrile child, an irritated bladder, a nagging sore throat, a persistent cough, or recurrent diarrhea. Imagine the 'cost-benefit' analysis going on in the physician's mind—Should I demand that the patient come into the office and be seen, when I'm really already overloaded with appointments?[53]

When doctors go along, they do so grudgingly, vexed at being forced to practice bad medicine. What could alienate them more from their patients than being viewed as some kind of conduit to the big drug warehouse?

An even more intense tug-of-war takes place over tranquilizers, antidepressants, and sedatives ("psychoactive drugs"), even though they are prescribed less frequently than antibiotics. In 1980 these psychoactive drugs represented 8 percent of all prescriptions.[54] Many patients feel that they need them. But unlike for penicillin, the "indications" for drugs like Valium are vague: "I feel anxious, I feel uneasy." Ditto for the antidepressants: "I feel depressed." Thus, whether the doctor writes the prescription is even more a matter of negotiating with the patient than it is for antibiotics. One American in six uses these drugs today, so the issue is not a trivial one.[55]

Pulling and tugging over these mood-altering drugs occasion much heartburn on both sides. The family-medicine resident is describing her case: a "little man" in his late fifties, an emigrant from Eastern Europe. His wife has had a stroke. His life is miserable. "He comes in, and it's like the same tape recording every time. He hurts here, he hurts there. Every time he shows me the scar on his head where he's had an operation."

What do you do?

"Well, we started out giving him things, like Valium and other drugs. And none of it seemed to do any good. Today he wanted meprobamate [another tranquilizer]. He'd heard about it somewhere. Or some Valium. We didn't give him anything." One might imagine what this "little man" now thinks of postmodern medicine.

A woman in her late fifties, a refugee from the Middle East, comes in with her daughter. The woman wants relief from a terrible headache. It aches day and night without stop, for months. She's dizzy and sometimes fears her heart will stop. Also, she "feels bad all over."

It turns out she has a long history. A number of doctors have seen her, including a psychiatrist, whom she stopped seeing after a single visit because he asked her "too many questions." She's also been on tranquilizers and a single course of an antidepressant drug.

She very obviously wants relief, today and fast. The doctor

leaves for a moment and has a long discussion outside about what to do: give her another antidepressant? Treat her symptoms, which means, tell her to lie down in a dark room when she feels her headache? But that's not going to help much because she feels pain all the time. Give her something really powerful, like Demerol, a trade name for a synthetic narcotic? Refer her to a psychiatrist?

"We could call in the psych [psychiatry] resident," says one senior family doctor, "and that way he could give her something stronger."

But in fact they elect to treat her symptoms. "Lie down in a dark room," the doctor says when he goes back. She and her daughter are obviously unhappy at this advice but accept it anyway with a tight smile.

As these drugs are prescribed for millions of people, many such encounters go on across North America every year. The doctors feel under siege and abused, the patients feel "screwed around" and denied something that "modern science" has devised for their relief. Is it any wonder that the two sides start to become estranged from each other?

There is some evidence that, even apart from the tug-of-war, doctors and patients are becoming mutually soured. Do you think "medical practice today is still personal?" a sample of patients in New York City were asked. Three-quarters said they were not sure or no. If your doctor says a test is necessary, do you have it? Again, 34 percent said not sure or no.[56] These sound like fearful patients in helter-skelter withdrawal from the doctor-patient relationship.

A British survey asked patients whether they were willing to discuss personal problems with the doctor. Barely half said yes, and many of those said, "Yes, but I would rather go to the social services as they are more helpful," or "Yes, but I wouldn't waste his time." The younger patients in particular quite definitely resisted the idea of exposing their personal lives to the doctor.[57]

Doctors, similarly, are pulling back from involvement in their patients' personal lives. A survey in 1981 of 430 "primary care" physicians in Massachusetts found them quite uninterested in any kind of "life-style" counseling. The percentage "very prepared" to counsel patients about smoking, for example, was only 58. Only 46 percent were willing to offer advice about alcohol use, only 35 percent about diet; only 29 percent would volunteer counsel about stress.[58] These figures testify to a massive uninvolvement of doctors with patients.

Why this mutual retreat in opposite directions, this withdrawal of both physicians and patients from the intimate relationship that once offered such promise? In addition to the many circumstances we've already touched on, I want to add just one observation. This withdrawal of trust by clients—and of enthusiasm by professionals—afflicts not just medicine but virtually every institution in American society. Doctors are not the only professionals to experience an onslaught of malpractice suits from the 1960s onward, as architects and lawyers can readily testify. It is not just medicine that has been attacked in the press for the betrayal of public good for private gains, as politicians well know. Relationships of every kind that involve some kind of "patriarchal" authority and some bestowal of implicit confidence have been breaking up. But, just as each of the other institutions has been assaulted in particular by some "spearhead" group—the investigative reporters leading the assault on politicians, student "course unions" leading the assault on academics—so medicine in particular has been assailed by a spearhead group: the "patients' rights" movement.

Hospital patients received in 1972 their "Bill of Rights" from the American Hospital Association, and since then a profusion of patients' advocates, hospital ombudspersons, and the like have made it their business to see that the patient is "protected" from the doctor. The underlying assumption of the movement is that the doctor is the patient's natural enemy, rather than natural ally, as doctors themselves tend to believe. Boston's Medical Committee for Human Rights prefaced its 1975 guide for patients by saying, "If the American health care system were really working in the interests of the patient, this book would not be necessary. It is our feeling, however, that the system is not working for the patient."

The Committee advocated that patients speak up for their "rights" at the following junctures:

238

- *In the ambulance: If you feel the ambulance is "exceeding legal speed limits and traffic laws . . . you should complain loudly."*
- *In the emergency room: If you are obliged to wait for more than fifteen minutes—a standard, they tell us, recommended by the American College of Surgeons—"you should be aggressive and demand to be seen."*
- *Once in bed: "If some questions seem unrelated to your medical problem, ask their purpose. Don't tell the doctor anything you don't want in your record [because he's out to get you]."*
- *On being wheeled around for tests: "Remember your rights. If you feel you are being badly treated, complain and refuse to allow procedures."[59]*

Et cetera: On and on goes the complaining that "you" are urged to conduct. Now, taken singly, each one of these proposals has merit in its own terms: after all, who wants to be in an ambulance accident, to wait unnecessarily, or to suffer other mistreatments? But taken together, they put doctor and patient absolutely at each other's throats. At every step the patient suspects sinister intent and withdraws defensively. In addition to denying oneself the psychological benefits that accompany the consultation, any patient who rigorously defended his or her rights in the way the booklet suggests would be branded "hysterical." And the investigation of the patient's symptoms at that point would probably come to an end, the case being dismissed as "functional" or referred to a psychiatrist, especially if the complainer were a woman.

In the course of doing the research for this book, I often noted how bitterly doctors react to certain patients' rights "safeguards," which now have become meaningless bureaucratic routine. Take, for example, the signing of "informed consent." A young female radiologist was explaining:

"I had to give this woman an injection for the IVP [an intravenous pyelogram, for visualizing the kidneys with X-ray], and the nurse said, 'Aren't you going to tell her the risks?'

"The risks? Well, there are lots of risks. One in every hundred thousand dies, and then there are hot flushes and so forth. So you have to work out something to say. Because if you use the word 'die,' the patient immediately says [and here the radiologist mimicked a secretary turning down onions on her cheeseburger] 'Oh no I don't want it.'

"Later in the day we had a Russian patient who didn't speak English. Giving *him* informed consent . . . oh boy. So I clutched at my throat to indicate risks of death. And I fanned myself rapidly to show hot flushes. I don't know whether he got it or not. That just shows you what a lot of bullshit this informed consent business is."

I am not against rights for patients; I think it is ghastly when their ready good humor and willingness to cooperate are abused by cynical practitioners and impersonal hospital routines. But we have to consider the costs we pay for the benefit of reducing the "abuses." Is one of the costs the increasing inability of doctors to heal psychological disease? That is the theme of the next chapter.

CHAPTER NINE

Psychological Disease and Postmodern Medicine

*A*NYONE WHO has read this book as an argument in favor of medical authority is right. In this last chapter I want to show what doctors and patients are giving up in abandoning that authority. An increasing problem in postmodern medicine is the doctor's growing helplessness in the face of disease that arises not from organic causes but from the mind.

THE INCIDENCE OF PSYCHOLOGICAL DISEASE HAS NOT INCREASED

The view has established itself that mental illness has somehow greatly increased over the years.[1] I find this very unlikely. It may be that the social wraps have come off somewhat, so that individuals now feel less constrained in admitting to depression or anxiety. The real levels of depression today are probably the same as the real levels of neurasthenia in the 1920s and 1930s. The difference is that more people today are inclined to call themselves, or to be called by their doctors, depressed. (Remember that unhappiness is not automatic depression.)

If we extend psychological diseases to include psychosomatic disorders and psychogenic pain, again I don't think there's any more around than formerly. A "disease of modern life," for example, is thought to be peptic ulcer. And yet it turns out that ulcers of the stomach and duodenum are just as common in Africa as in western society. The Africans merely report it less often.[2] Readers of this book know how common it once was for young women not to be able to get out of bed and walk. Yet that particular symptom has virtually disappeared, its place now taken by stomach pain or tension headaches. Overall, the level of psychological disease has probably stayed the same.

Doctors' own estimates of the amount of "emotional" disease they see in their practices are no higher today than they were in the 1920s and 1930s. The estimate depends partly on the kind of patients one sees. The Tuscaloosa internist Dr. Burnum, for example, who had a stable practice with many elderly patients, put the number of "emotionally ill" patients he saw at only 10 percent and two-thirds of those had some coexisting organic disease.[3]

At the opposite end of the scale would be a hospital outpatient clinic, serving a restless clientele without family doctors. All kinds of things just drift in from the night. The doctors at the outpatient medical clinic at Chicago's Mt. Sinai Hospital, felt that two-thirds of their clients had some kind of psychological problem. Of these "functional" problems (as they put it):

- *Sixty-three percent were outright psychiatric disorders.*
- *The other 37 percent were psychosomatic diseases affecting stomach, heart, and so forth.*[4]

The estimates of typical family doctors steer a midcourse between these extremes. Their figures sound much like those quoted in Chapter 6 for the 1920s to 1940s. "Primary care" doctors in Rochester, New York, in the 1960s estimated that 14 percent of their patients had "mental or emotional disorders": one out of seven. One British study put at 13 percent the GP patients with a psychiatric or psychosomatic problem, two others at 20 percent.[5] On the whole, then, one-seventh to one-fifth of one's medical practice will likely concern patients whose problem is frankly psychological. For a further group, the uneasy mind will in some way exacerbate physical disease. Given a billion-plus patient contacts every year in the United States, that means millions and millions of encounters with disease of psychological nature.

The number of Americans who have some kind of psychological problem is far higher than these figures suggest. How many people feel depressed, anxious, highly distressed? As many as one American in four experiences symptoms that might qualify for a "psychiatric diagnosis." Thus, a major nationwide survey in 1979 found 5 percent of Americans to be experiencing a "major depression," 6 percent anxiety neurosis, and so on. One Englishman in five believes him- or herself to be suffering from "nerves." A third of a sample of the population in Florida had digestive problems, one in seven had diarrhea or high blood pressure, and so forth, leading the authors of the survey to exclaim—quite incorrectly in my view—"psychosomatic illness is reaching epidemic proportions in the Western world."[6] These figures are no higher than they've always been, as a part of the eternal twinges and twitches to which humankind is heir but are cast now as formal psychiatric ailments.

Because people today are more sensitive to symptoms in general, they are also more sensitive to psychological symptoms in particular. The incidence of these symptoms may be the same as always, but people's desire to do something about them has increased. In this regard the 1960s and after differ from past times. Take, for example, women aged twenty-five to thirty-four. Today, one out of every seven visits a doctor annually because of neurosis.[7] It is a distinctively postmodern phenomenon that many more patients, agitated about internal states, are now seeking help. The crisis of postmodern medicine is that the kind of help they get is probably inferior to that of fifty years ago.

The Doctor Faces Psychological Disease

I insist on putting in quotes the word "*psychiatric,*" as people tend to think of psychiatric disorders as fearful conditions that only specialists in "insanity" could treat. Patients feel anxious; they feel gloomy; they can't sleep and their blood pressure suddenly goes up; their bowels won't work, or work too well. These are, if you will, "psychiatric disorders," or even better, "mental illness"! But in fact they are the quotidian lot of us all, as common as the common cold. Hence the great majority of psychological disease is treated by family doctors. Of the 30 million people having an expressly "psychiatric" problem annually:

- *Fifteen percent see a psychiatrist.*
- *Fifty-seven percent see a family doctor or internist.*
- *Six percent see first a family doctor, then get a psychiatric referral.*
- *Twenty-two percent muddle through or "seek help outside the system."*[8]

When a family doctor encounters a patient with disease of psychological origin, he has several options. The point I want to make in this section is that today, he tends to choose the worse ones rather than the better.

Probably the worst option is surgery. You laugh, thinking surgery for disturbances of the mind a far-fetched notion indeed. Yet many people whose problems are psychological get operated on, and a number of times too. It is not uncommon to find, for example, that a patient with chronic abdominal pain and depression has had surgery ten or fifteen times. A woman might have had a (normal) appendix out at seventeen, a series of operations in her twenties on tubes and ovaries, a hysterectomy at thirty-five, perhaps an operation on her spine at some point, her gallbladder removed, and all her teeth pulled out. Although these individuals are suffering from an illness of the mind called *Briquet's syndrome,* they tend to be treated as organic cases by their medical attendants, who accede to the patient's request for operation after operation. No organic problem is ever found, and the pain is just as bad afterward.[9]

The operations on the "Briquet's" patients are the modern counterpart of the ovariectomies for "hysteria" in the 1870s and 1880s. When successful, they amount to surgical cure by suggestion. Just as in the late nineteenth century doctors and patients both thought the ovaries should come out to cure an organic problem causing the "hysteria," in today's Briquet's patients both doctor and patient are convinced the operation will effect an organic cure. But of course it never does, since the pain, as well as the compulsive seeking out of surgeons, arises in the mind. Then as now, there was never any shortage of surgeons willing to operate. This is admittedly an extreme case, but it shows that surgery done unwittingly for suggestion is still much alive today.

(*Note:* If the operation does suggest the patient into a cure, she gets off the treadmill and therefore does not become classified at age fifty as a case of Briquet's syndrome. The syndrome is, by definition, applied only to patients whom operations have failed to suggest into improvement. The patients continue the phantom search for surgical cures of their supposedly organic disease.)

A second option of the family doctor is to treat the psychological condition with placebos, another form of suggestion. Although doctors do not readily discuss this fact in public today because of the deception of the patient implied, placebos are essential in the practice of medicine. As one Welsh doctor explained, "If they are elderly, or not very bright, to explain to them that the medicine that you are giving them is not really doing anything, and that they are being given it because you don't think anything is wrong with them, would destroy them. So, as a matter of course, you diagnose and prescribe."[10]

Yet the former placebos are fading fast. Patients are now unimpressed by vitamin injections, and doctors too feel ever more uneasy with the old stand-bys. An elderly family doctor said, "We don't prescribe them any more because it's unethical. But we used to use them quite a bit." They would write on the prescription simply *Placebo.* "But now the young pharmacists don't know what it means. They won't dispense them anyway for ethical reasons. Stopped giving them in the mid-1960s."

Then his face brightened. "We used to give calcium gluconate. And ever hear of autochemotherapy?"

I hadn't.

"We'd take blood out of one arm and put it back into the other." Both treatments have now been discontinued.

A younger family doctor was unwilling to go beyond vitamins, but he talks vitamins when he sees a patient who needs a placebo. "I think this will really help you," he says in a very positive voice.

But the patients know they're getting vitamins?

"Yeah," he says with a shrug. He grants it's not a real placebo, yet he feels very uneasy about the ethics of deliberately lying to them and saying that a sugar pill is a powerful drug.

But that doesn't mean doctors have stopped using placebos, merely that the kinds of placebos have changed. They are now using *powerful drugs as placebos*, especially the psychoactive drugs: tranquilizers and antidepressants. These drugs can have a real effect on psychological conditions, as we shall see in a moment; but in small doses antidepressants in particular work mainly as placebos, because the drug takes several weeks to build up in the body sufficiently for the patient to begin deriving a pharmacological effect from it. Tranquilizers and sedatives can also serve as placebos. One study showed that Valium and the barbiturates were much more effective in treating anxiety if accompanied by much enthusiasm by the doctor.[11]

The antidepressants and tranquilizers are, thus, often used to cure by suggestion. A British psychiatrist noted that among GPs, "these agents . . . are not prescribed with careful attention to their pharmacological action and are often used in very small doses. They are nowadays really the stock placebos. 'Librium' has virtually replaced liniment."[12]

The family doctors are discussing a depressed man, twenty-seven. What to do? There is a need to act quickly or he'll lose his job.

Amitriptyline (an antidepressant)? That's no good, says someone, because it doesn't start to act until about three weeks.

"Oh not at all," says another doctor, burlesquing a maniacal grin. "Give him amitriptyline. It'll start to act on the *first day*." He waves his hand as though he were brandishing the bottle. "Placebo effect."

Here we have one reason why these psychoactive drugs are prescribed at such astonishing rates. They have replaced tonics and vitamin B_{12} as the new placebos. But they represent a poor solution to the problem of psychological disease. Like the old tonics, they may bring mental relief by suggestion. But unlike the tonics they can lead to unwelcome problems: mainly, addiction. What starts out as a one-shot effort to get a troublesome patient off a busy GP's back can become, with time, a serious pharmacological addiction. Especially with the antidepressants, patients return for more and more and finally become hooked on them without necessarily getting a long-term solution to their problems.[13] The tonics didn't necessarily bring about long-term solutions either, but at least they weren't dangerous.

The family doctor's main line of defense against psychological illness is to use psychoactive drugs not for their placebo effect but for their real chemical value, just as penicillin is prescribed for its chemical value in killing bacteria. The drugs, in other words, may bring about a genuine organic cure, a concept with which doctors feel comfortable. These drugs are thought to right the chemical balance in the brain, whose unpredictable synaptic clefts and unreliable serotonin receptors have made the mind ill. Or so the thinking goes.

These psychoactive drugs have had a capital impact upon the practice of medicine. The "old" psychoactive drugs, available since the midnineteenth century, did in fact sedate anxious people and help them sleep, but not terribly well, and moreover they produced lots of "daytime" sedation. The new drugs exert a specific, pharmacological effect on moods of two kinds: anxiety and depression. The minor tranquilizers calm anxiety; the antidepressants elevate the mood of those who are thought to be depressed not so much from life's tribulations as from long-standing biochemical disorders in their brains (thus *primary depression*, or *endogenous depression*, as opposed to *neurotic depression*, for which the antidepressants are less effective).

The first of the new psychoactive drugs, Miltown (meprobamate), was introduced in 1955. A downpour then burst five years later with the marketing of the first of a family of drugs called the *benzodiazepines*: Librium, the trade name for chlordiazepoxide. In 1963 followed what has probably become the best-selling prescription name in history, Valium (diazepam). Thereafter new tranquilizers fell in a steady rain: Dalmane, Tranxene, Ativan, and so on. By the 1980s some 70 million prescriptions a year were being written for them.

Simultaneously, a shower of antidepressants had begun. The first of the tricyclics—so named after their chemical structure— was tried clinically in 1958. Elavil (amitriptyline) and Sinequan (doxepin) would emerge to dominate the market. For these mood elevators, over 25 million prescriptions a year were being written in the 1980s.[14]

These drugs dramatically changed the experience of many patients with emotional upset. There should be no doubt about this: we are not talking about placebos or smelling salts for fainting fits. The risk of a seriously depressed person committing suicide, for example, is about 15 percent. And it is unquestionably the availability of antidepressants that reduced the suicide rate of middle-aged American men from 1970 to 1979 by 56 percent, and of middle-aged women by 13 percent.[15] A GP in small-town England said,

> I have examined my records of patients from 1946 to 1949 and in those days the average duration of a depressisve episode was about ten months. I had to boost up their morale all the time, and keep seeing and encouraging them. The only thing that gave them any real relief was their barbiturate at night.
>
> That same kind of depressive episode now lasts about seven months, and of course they are made to feel a lot more comfortable after two or three weeks on tricyclic antidepressant drugs.[16]

Naturally doctors became enthusiastic about these drugs. Not only did they cure some kinds of depression and anxiety; they also saved time talking to patients.

Thus, drugs slowly began to replace a "good chat" in the treatment of emotional upset. And I use a word like *upset*, instead of clinical expressions like *depression* and *anxiety*, because most patients whose underlying problem is emotional come with some kind of bodily symptom rather than solely with neurosis. Of prescriptions for minor tranquilizers, only one-third are for "emotional disorders without a somatic component. The remainder is for a wide variety of physical disorders in which stress is assumed to play a . . . role."[17]

Family doctors would accordingly turn to these drugs for a wide range of problems whose underlying cause was psychological. Of the patients with psychosocial problems in a California clinic, 18 percent got antidepressants, 16 percent pain killers, and 11 percent tranquilizers. Of the 330 patients whom a British GP discovered to have psychological problems in a five-week period of his practice, two-thirds received Valium or something like it.[18]

In the treatment of neuroses in particular, GPs after the 1960s would reach overwhelmingly for drugs. Of the neurotic patients whom forty-six London doctors saw in the early 1960s, 33 percent received sedatives and a further 20 percent tranquilizers and antidepressants. Only one-quarter got "reassurance, discussion and counseling," and 5 percent were referred to psychiatrists. A nationwide study of American medical practice in 1977 found that 58 percent of neurotic or depressed patients received drugs from their family doctors, and only a third received counseling. That was on the first visit. On subsequent visits the percentage receiving drugs was even higher. Moreover, the first visit by these upset patients lasted on average only fourteen minutes, the follow-up visits only twelve minutes.[19] Thus, the family doctors had neither inclination nor opportunity for anything even remotely resembling a good chat, to say nothing of psychotherapy. What do you give neurotic or depressed patients? asked a government nationwide survey in 1980:

- *Of visits by men, 46 percent received a drug of some kind.*
- *Of visits by women, 56 percent were given a drug.*
- *The older the patient was, the more often drugs were prescribed, so that depresssed or neurotic patients under twenty-five received drugs only a third of the time, and patients over sixty-five received them 85 percent of the time.*[20]

The main thing family doctors want to know about psychiatry is how to prescribe drugs. A survey of 160 GPs in small-town Missouri asked them what they thought to be the most important aspect of psychiatry for medical students. They put psychopharmacology at the top of the list. Among the *least* important aspects: "long-term psychotherapy."[21]

Drugs have been substituted for the kind of informal psychotherapy family doctors used to do. Patients sense this acutely. A group of English patients were asked whether they would have liked "more information" from their doctor. Those who said yes were also likely to agree that their doctor was too inclined to write out prescriptions. Of the patients who "would like ten minutes uninterrupted conversation with a sympathetic doctor," many more felt their own doctor was prescription-happy than prescription-shy.[22]

Some patients explode in anger at this casual drugging: "I'd been feeling tired, rundown and very weepy. It seemed relentless, and, although I rarely go to the doctor, I felt it wise to get a good physical and checkup. He listened for about 2 minutes (not even looking at me), suddenly said, 'You're depressed,' handed me a prescription and walked out. I was so angry I slammed his office door as I left and rushed home in tears. I could have been a bit of furniture for all he cared—and I didn't even get a physical."[23]

I am not arguing that most family doctors are brutes. I'm arguing that the organic orientation of their training has made them afraid of diseases arising in the mind. This fact struck me on numerous occasions when dealing with the family doctors of the Clinic. A resident presents the case: a woman, twenty-eight, with a history of smoking, comes in complaining of coughing up blood and large amounts of mucus. This is pretty routine. Then the bombshell drops: this patient has a long record of split personality, talking alternately in a deep "evil" voice and a high "nice" voice. The deep voice knows about the nice one, but the nice voice doesn't know about the deep voice. Moreover, she has a history of dropping bricks on her foot and such in order to be admitted to the hospital.

Then another bombshell bursts. She's being seen now, not because of her psychological problems, but because her tuberculin test was *positive*, suggesting she might have TB. So, does she really have TB, or did she somehow induce a positive test in order to be admitted to the hospital once again? A fascinating psychological case, but that's not what the family doctors want to talk about. They want to discuss the technical issues of screening for TB, when to repeat tests, how many X-rays you order, and which drugs you prescribe.

An unfair example? Doctors really need to know more about TB? Here is another case the whole seminar agreed was frankly "mental." A woman patient of twenty-eight is flirting with anorexia nervosa. She now weighs 95 pounds (down from 110) and is determined to drop even more by using laxatives and limiting herself to one meal a day, which, moreover, she permits herself only if she has lost weight the previous day. She is desperate to "get rid of these flabby thighs" and has not had a period in nine months. Otherwise no complaints.

What to do, given the imminence of a potentially fatal tip toward emaciation? The resident presenting the case duly consulted with psychiatrists expert in anorexia and received lots of impressive talk about "family therapy" and "intervention on the dynamic level." The resident, intimidated by this, is now uncertain about her ability to cope and recoils when "psychotherapy" is proposed to her in the seminar. The word falls like a cow pie. The senior doctors maintain an uneasy silence, and it is not brought up again that meeting.

Another resident has a male patient, twenty-seven, who is "very depressed." How to proceed? In fairness to these physicians, who generally impressed me with their humaneness and concern for the emotional side of patients' lives, no one urges massive drugging. What alternatives are left then? The resident vaguely proposes psychotherapy. Someone asks her what she understands by the term. What would she do?

She is completely disoriented by the question. "Ummmm, I think there's something about supportive as opposed to intervention. Oh yeah, and I think I remember something about neurosis. I don't really know a lot about it."

She will probably pick up some commonsense solutions to depression over years of practice, but trust herself ever to do "psychotherapy," as opposed to prescribing pills? Never.

THE DECLINE IN THE HEALING POWER OF THE CONSULTATION

I am not blaming family doctors for not attempting formal psychotherapy. It involves specialized skills that one learns only in the specialty of psychiatry, or in training programs entirely outside medicine. I am blaming them for ignoring the informal psychotherapeutic power of the consultation itself. As we saw in earlier chapters, the healing power of the consultation lies in the catharsis that the patient derives from telling his story to someone he trusts as a "healer." We have already discussed the extent to which patients now generally trust their "healers" less and less. Here I want to make the point that doctors, by their concentration on the "chief complaint," are further diminishing the potential of the encounter.

One consequence of the organic bias of postmodern medicine has been to steer the consultation toward a single, identifiable physical problem, the "chief complaint." Many patients, as they walk into the doctor's office, don't yet have a chief complaint. They have a collection of ill-defined symptoms and anxieties and desires for reassurance, all simmering together in an inchoate pot. The doctor sees his job as distilling this ill-assorted collection into one clearly defined problem that he can investigate systematically and prescribe for rationally. "When the patient begins to talk, many doctors immediately go down a form of clinical check list." A doctor is speaking. "They have been trained that way and this technique quickly creates recognizable patterns that can be pigeonholed and dealt with." The check list, he says, will point to a likely chief complaint. The doctor then asks a series of yes-no questions to confirm his working hypothesis, which he has early made in the consultation. Now he is able to prescribe.

"The consequence of this approach," the author continued, "can be one of the greatest faults in modern general practice. This is the organization of vague symptoms into categories, then labeling these producing a disease that can be approached in the traditional medical manner. Having created a disease in this way, it becomes difficult to unmake."[24] Thus the Procrustean bed of the chief complaint can squeeze a riot of symptoms like diarrhea, sleeplessness, and worry about a daughter's divorce into the diagnosis of depression, treatable with Elavil.

This exaltation of the chief complaint accelerated in American medicine after World War II, part and parcel of training young doctors to be "scientists." As an article on medical history taking complained in 1952, "By forcing a patient to express his 'chief complaint' in a few fully quotable words, they often failed to get on the right track. Often the chief complaint as recorded by the student contained a plausible excuse for the hospital visit, but did not reflect the patient's real reasons for seeking help." The students would thus investigate irrelevant symptoms, the real cause of the visit remaining undiscovered.[25]

By the 1980s pursuing the chief complaint had become an absolute fetish in many institutions and doctors' offices. The patient's chart would have a big black box in which the "CC" was to be entered. To simplify things for the doctor, a nurse or receptionist would inquire about it in advance so the doctor would have to do as little inquiry as possible.

> Thus, the search for the chief complaint has moved to the office desk, located near or within the waiting area, where the patient is asked to divulge (either publicly or over the telephone) this often sensitive and complicated information or to simplify falsely by answering "pain" or "rash" or "checkup" as the reason that he or she wants to see the doctor. . . . When it is discovered that the chief complaint is wrong, credibility and rapport crumble; patient and physician may even fall into an argument over whether the symptom or sign is present.[26]

Here is a typical encounter, in which a disease-oriented young doctor investigates the chief complaint. The patient comes in, an older man. The doctor doesn't shake hands. "I'm Doctor X," he mumbles. "What's the problem?" (Thus, what's the chief complaint?)

During the consultation the doctor looks at his own hands, rubbing first one finger and then another. The patient has an infection in his throat. The doctor does a competent enough physical examination and asks the appropriate questions, concerned mainly with whether the infection is spreading to the lungs.

But this is the second time the patient has been in the clinic this month, the last time for a stomach disorder. One might well ask, "Is there a hidden agenda? Does this man really want to talk about something else?"

The doctor has no interest in that. "You'll be OK after a few days," he says. "These things take a while to go away." The medical care was professional. But the doctor's total lack of interest gave the man no opening for bringing up anything else that might have been on his mind.

Perhaps there was nothing. But one Dutch study showed that a *majority* of patients had some reason for seeing the doctor other than their "chief complaint."[27] Mothers take children with "coughs" into a pediatric clinic. The CC is simple. But a mother's question, "Don't you think he's too thin, doctor?" is a tip-off to the real problem: a conflict with the mother-in-law about rearing the boy. Another mother wants to be reassured that her son's night sweats don't mean TB. Another mother wants to send her daughter on a "convalescent holiday" in order to gain a few days of personal freedom. Thus under many of the "coughs" lies a second diagnosis that a series of yes-no questions would not have uncovered. "It is important to listen rather than to ask," the author realized. "What the doctor should really be trying to do is to help the parents to talk."[28]

Now it is clear that the endless parade of "flus" we saw in the last chapter may conceal deeper problems requiring careful *listening* rather than careful questioning to uncover.

DOCTOR: Come in. What can I do for you?
PATIENT: Well, I have got flu, doctor. I have got all pains in my arms.
DOCTOR: When did you start to feel not so well?
PATIENT: The week-end. It started Saturday afternoon, shivering with cold. . . .

Then in midstream the patient dropped a reference to her husband hitting her with a shoe when he came home drunk Saturday night. The doctor, happily, grabbed the reference and steered the consultation toward the husband's drinking, which she had clearly wanted to talk about. Her flu was unimportant.[29] But a scientific hotshot would have ignored this clue to a hidden agenda and resolutely investigated the chief complaint.

The hidden agenda may just be reassurance for a kind of complaint one would be embarrassed to tell the receptionist over the phone. A young woman of seventeen went to see a doctor in Cambridge, England. "She said she had terrible abdominal pains for at least three months." The doctor's antennae went up at *terrible*, which is often a code word that the patient wants to talk about something else. He asked about her periods and then said, "Is there anything else you would like to mention?"

"Not really," she said, which is code for *yes*.

"Well, perhaps you would like me to examine you down below?"

"I don't mind," which is a young Englishwoman's code for *yes*.

So he examined her and found nothing and then asked a few vague questions about sex ("How are you getting on with intercourse?") that encouraged her finally to talk.

It turned out that in petting with her the night before the boyfriend had somehow scratched her, making her bleed. He had insisted she go to the doctor. Thus careful listening had picked up what a yes-no investigation could not possibly have, and she was spared the rigors of a systematic investigation of "lower abdominal pain" postmodern style, with barium enema, colonoscopy, and the rest.[30]

The erosion of careful listening and the concentration upon organic symptoms mean that several things of value are lost from the consultation. One we have just seen: patients with a hidden agenda are denied an opportunity to say what is really troubling them. Some disease-oriented doctors will shrug their shoulders at this, but for patients it is a major loss causing the doctor-patient relationship to deteriorate. Second, the patient is denied the cathartic value of telling his story, a very real therapeutic benefit to which no doctor can be indifferent. I think earlier chapters in this book have established that value, and I will not further illustrate it here.

All of this reminds us that the interaction between doctor and patient, in and of itself, represents the much-feared "psychother-apy." Listening is the main kind of informal psychotherapy the family doctor is able to conduct. Listening, rather than drugs, is his major ally against disease arising in the mind. The doctor must, as Michael Balint put it, use *himself* as a drug.[31] It is his own concern, expressed in willingness to listen attentively, that may produce a cure.

PROGNOSIS AND CRISIS

I think the best demonstration of the fallacious-ness of the disease-oriented, organic approach is that the pros-pects today for some of the diseases that arise in the mind are significantly worse than they were forty years ago. Although therapy of the psychosomatic diseases remains pretty much a puzzle, it is clear that some of them can be helped precisely by the techniques we've been discussing. I want to talk briefly about the experience today of patients who have "irritable bowel syn-drome," not because it is numerically as important as the com-mon cold, but because its worsening prognosis shows how much we give up as postmodern medicine turns its back on the tradi-tions of the past.

Irritable bowel, the reader will recall, is abdominal pain com-bined with diarrhea, or constipation, or the one alternating with the other. Among the problems that a gastroenterologist (a sub-specialist in internal medicine) sees, it is perhaps second, sur-passed only by various inflammations of the bowel.[32]

When gastroenterologists today treat irritable bowel, their long years of organic training in internal medicine stand behind them: drugs are the treatment of choice, mainly anticholinergics to slow the bowel down, plus tranquilizers, combined with meddling about with fiber in the diet.[33] These remedies have the poor suc-cess that one might predict. The prognosis of irritable bowel today is gloomy.

An English study showed that, despite sophisticated medical therapy, a sample of fifty irritable-bowel patients who were fol-lowed for a year or so had virtually no change in their condition.

"The nature of the symptoms remained constant in all but one patient; and two patients, who had improved at the end of one year, relapsed again." What was striking, however, was the therapeutic value of the follow-up itself, i.e., of doctors' coming round and showing an interest in the patient. "Although there was little or no change in the severity of the symptoms, most patients felt better and more able to cope. . . . Many expressed their gratitude that someone had at last made an attempt to understand them and did not regard their symptoms as imaginary." This important observation was made in passing. The authors concluded that the prospects of patients with the condition were "poor."[34]

Adopting a "psychological" approach to irritable bowel involves much courage mustering by internists, but when they have attempted it the results have been promising. A high-powered group of gastroenterologists announced in 1976, "We have found that such patients, given a few minutes each visit to complain of symptoms and discuss interpersonal conflicts with an attentive listener, do not demand symptom relief. By the next visit, the original symptom is often gone."[35] Thus a "good chat" had worked!

A group of doctors in Göteborg, Sweden, divided one hundred irritable bowel patients into two groups: fifty received only drugs, fifty had drugs plus psychotherapy, consisting of ten hour-long sessions over three months by psychiatrists. Although this is not quite the same thing as a good chat, it nonetheless was effective: the psychotherapy group did much better.[36]

In 1983 another distinguished gastroenterologist reminded his colleagues of the importance of *listening* in the treatment of "functional" digestive disorders (of which irritable bowel is chief): "The story may even seem tedious, but the physician's time is well spent in listening and interpretation. The patient will not be satisfied with the consultation or have confidence in its outcome until *the story has been fully told and the doctor has shown genuine concern.*"[37]

What is striking in all this is not the novelty of psychotherapy, although these doctors all believe themselves to be highly innovative. It is the reintroduction of a procedure that had proved its worth under modern medicine for fifty years and then had been forgotten as a result of the surge toward organic explanations of disease. That procedure is not really psychotherapy. It is relying on the healing power of the close doctor-patient relationship as such, the healing power of the good chat, although the good chat has now been dressed up as psychotherapy.

I felt an almost painful sense of déjà vu as I read Dr. Paul Latimer's account of the usefulness of psychotherapy in treating irritable bowel. His patient was an anxious middle-aged businessman, of whom we have seen many in this book, with a history of "abdominal pain and alternating constipation and diarrhea." Latimer, bristling with credentials in psychiatry, saw himself a true pathbreaker as he wrote, "The first step in treatment was to provide the patient with a comprehensible and plausible explanation of his difficulties."[38] Shades of Paul Dubois's therapy by persuasion! Shades of William Houston, and Francis Peabody and George Canby Robinson, all internists in the 1920s and 1930s who believed implicitly what doctors are only rediscovering: that letting patients tell their story to an enthusiastic, interested physician has a healing power of its own!

None of these names appears in the bibliography of Latimer's 1983 book. Indeed there is scarcely a reference more than ten years old. I write this not to criticize Latimer, who is a progressive figure in the context of his time, but to point out that, contrary to popular belief, medicine is indeed capable of forgetting knowledge. As today the giant machine grinds out ever new "findings," all kinds of old wisdom is being forgotten.

And one of the things that is being forgotten is that medicine is an art as well as a science. George Bernard Shaw wrote in 1911,

> As a matter of fact, the rank and file of doctors are no more scientific than their tailors; or, if you prefer to put it the reverse way, their tailors are no less scientific than they. Doctoring is an art, not a science: any layman who is interested in science sufficiently to take in one of the scientific journals and follow the literature of the scientific movement, knows more about it than those doctors (probably a large majority) who are not interested in it, and practise only to earn their bread. Doctoring is not even the art of keeping people in health (no doctor seems able to advise you what to

eat any better than his grandmother or the nearest quack): it is the art of curing illness.[39]

The crisis of postmodern medicine is that this art of curing illness is now being lost. It is not just because of the doctors. Their patients no longer seem able to muster the requisite faith that the doctor can cure, that his healing hand and all-knowing gaze will restore; they insist instead that he prescribe drugs. Such phrases as his "all-knowing gaze" inspire derision today, and yet that gaze will cure if one believes that it will. The patient's rights movement and the mass media have done their clients a grim disservice in insisting that it won't, and that the doctor is really out to victimize them.

But the accusing finger must jab most forcefully at the medical profession itself, a profession that presides over the $287 billion a year we now spend on health care. That is 10 percent of our gross national product, or $1,225 for every man, woman, and child in the United States annually.[40] Although postmodern medicine has done great good in the conquest of much organic disease, it has conspicuously failed to overcome much of the *illness* that assails us, illness that is ever more frequent as we increasingly interpret the eternal aches and twinges of the body as medical symptoms requiring care.

Can the profession recognize that, although its organic advances are of enormous value, they must be combined with concern for individuals' well-being—a well-being that provides psychological comfort and therefore promotes healing? Will doctors return to training students in the nearly abandoned "art of curing"? If not, despite brilliant new chemical and diagnostic knowledge, the medical profession will continue on its path of crisis and frustration. But if medicine can stretch sufficiently to be both an advanced science *and* a healing art, it will successfully fulfill its ancient aspirations in unprecedented ways.

NOTES

Chapter One: Introduction

1. David Rabin et al., "Compounding the Ordeal of ALS: Isolation from My Fellow Physicians," *NEJM*, 19 August 1982, pp. 506-509. The disease is known medically as *amyotrophic lateral sclerosis* (ALS).

2. Linda Ballon, *NEJM*, 23 December 1982, p. 1650, letter.

3. David W. Swanson et al., "The Dissatisfied Patient with Chronic Pain," *Pain*, 4 (1978), pp. 374-375.

4. For data on the total number of physician visits per year in the United States, as well as the average per person, see National Center for Health Statistics, J. G. Collins, *Physician Visits, Volume and Interval Since Last Visit, United States, 1980,* Vital and Health Statistics, series 10, no. 144, DHHS pub. no. (PHS) 83-1572 (Washington: GPO, June 1983), pp. 8-9, figures 1 and 2. In 1981, 74 percent of the survey population had seen a doctor at least once in the previous twelve months; the average number of visits per person was 4.6. National Center for Health Statistics, B. Bloom, *Current Estimates from the National Health Interview Survey, United States, 1981,* Vital

and Health Statistics, series 10, no. 141, DHHS pub. no. (PHS) 82-1569 (Washington: GPO, Oct. 1982), p. 4, table D.

5. Examples from Patrick S. Byrne and Barrie E. L. Long, *Doctors Talking to Patients: A Study of the Verbal Behaviour of General Practitioners Consulting in Their Surgeries* (London:, HMSO, 1976), pp. 35, 41.

6. Ibid., pp. 75–76.

Chapter Two: The Traditional Doctor

1. I. S. L. Loudon, "A Doctor's Cash Book: The Economy of General Practice in the 1830s," *Medical History*, 27 (1983), p. 262; for an overview of medical organization in Britain in the eighteenth and nineteenth centuries, see M. Jeanne Peterson, *The Medical Profession in Mid-Victorian London* (Berkeley: University of California Press, 1978), chap. 1.

2. Anna Robeson Burr, *Weir Mitchell: His Life and Letters* (New York, 1929), p. 291.

3. According to the Boston surgeon Harvey Cushing, quoted in Richard D. Walter, *S. Weir Mitchell, M.D.—Neurologist: A Medical Biography* (Springfield: Charles C Thomas, 1970), p. 185.

4. John Gregory, *Lectures on the Duties and Qualifications of a Physician*, new ed. (London, 1772), p. 25. The first edition appeared in 1770.

5. Ibid., pp. 4–5.

6. Joseph M. Toner, *Contributions to the Annals of Medical Progress and Medical Education in the United States* (Washington, 1874), p. 106.

7. William Douglass, *A Summary, Historical and Political of the ... Present State of the British Settlements in North America*, 2 vols. (Boston, 1755), II, p. 352.

8. Ibid., vol. II, p. 351.

9. Thomas Hall Shastid, *My Second Life* (Ann Arbor: George Wahr, 1944), p. 1105.

10. This summary is based on the account of Boerhaave in Lester S. King, *The Medical World of the Eighteenth Century* (Chicago: University of Chicago Press, 1958), pp. 59–93.

11. William Buchan, *Domestic Medicine: Or, a Treatise on the Prevention and Cure of Diseases by Regimen and Simple Medicines*, 10th ed. (London, 1788), p. 151; 1st ed. in 1769.

12. Edward Baynard, *Health, A Poem, Shewing*

How to Procure, Preserve, and Restore It, 8th ed. (London, 1749), pp. 7–8; 1st ed. 1719.

13. John Howship, *Practical Observations on the Symptoms . . . Diseases of the Lower Intestines, and Anus,* 3d ed. (London, 1824), pp. 104–105; 1st ed. 1820.

14. Baynard, *Poem,* pp. 37, 39.

15. On Rush and calomel, as well as for an authoritative account of nineteenth-century American medicine generally, see William Rothstein, *American Physicians of the Nineteenth Century* (Baltimore: Johns Hopkins, 1972), p. 50.

16. Oliver Wendell Holmes, "Currents and Counter-Currents in Medical Science" (1860), in Holmes, ed., *Medical Essays, 1842–1882* (Boston, 1911), p. 193.

17. Jacob Bigelow, "On the Medical Profession and Quackery" (1844), in Bigelow, ed., *Modern Inquiries* (Boston, 1867), p. 214.

18. For a recent informed discussion of the differing routes to general practice in Britain, see Loudon, "Doctor's Case Book," and Loudon, "The Origin of the General Practitioner," *Journal of the Royal College of General Practitioners,* 33 (1983), pp. 13–23.

19. Samuel W. Gross, ed., *Autobiography of Samuel D. Gross, M.D.,* vol. 1 of 2 volumes (Philadelphia, 1893), pp. 17–28.

20. Franklin H. Martin, *Fifty Years of Medicine and Surgery* (Chicago, 1934), pp. 5–8.

21. Drake, *Practical Essays,* p. 6; italics in original.

22. Paul Starr, *The Social Transformation of American Medicine* (New York: Basic Books, 1982), p. 43. Toner, *Contributions,* says that middle-class people tended to speak of their medical attendants as "physicians"; lower-class, as "doctors," p. 60.

23. Rothstein, *American Physicians,* pp. 93, 98.

24. Arthur Hertzler, *The Horse and Buggy Doctor* (New York, 1938), pp. 38–39.

25. Harry Marion-Sims, ed., *The Story of My Life by J. Marion Sims* (New York, 1894), p. 138.

26. Daniel Drake, *Practical Essays on Medical Education and the Medical Profession in the United States* (Cincinnati, 1832), pp. 5, 11.

27. Walter Rivington, *The Medical Profession* (Dublin, 1879), p. 381, concerning candidates for the Army Medical Department.

28. Sims, *Story of My Life,* pp. 140–143.

Notes

29. W. Brockbank, ed., *The Diary of Richard Kay
... A Lancashire Doctor* (Manchester: Chetham Society, 1968), pp. 155–156.

30. Richard H. Shryock, "Selections from the Letters of Richard B. Arnold, M.D.," *Johns Hopkins Hospital Bulletin*, 42 (1928), pp. 170–171.

31. Charles Cowan, "Report of Private Medical Practice for 1840," *Journal of the [Royal] Statistical Society of London*, 5 (1842), pp. 82–83; the "average duration" he based on 523 cases in 1840.

32. Peter Tempelman, ed., *Select Cases, and Consultations in Physick by the late Eminent John Woodward* (London, 1757), pp. 62–64.

33. Frank Felsenstein, ed., *Tobias Smollett: Travels through France and Italy* (Oxford: Oxford University Press, 1979), pp. 88–102; 1st ed. 1766. Smollett was a prominent coffeehouse physician in London.

34. Hertzler, *Horse and Buggy Doctor*, p. 109.

35. Daniel Webster Cathell, *The Physician Himself and What He Should Add to the Strictly Scientific* (Baltimore, 1882), p. 93.

36. Hertzler, *Horse and Buggy Doctor*, p. 34.

37. See Buchan, *Domestic Medicine*, pp. 218–219, for a simple classification.

38. *Dorland's Illustrated Medical Dictionary*, 26th ed. (Philadelphia: Saunders), pp. 493–497.

39. Quoted in Loudon, "Doctor's Cash Book," p. 265, note 60.

40. Rivington, *Medical Profession*, p. 339; 1860s and 1870s.

41. Charles Rosenberg, "The Practice of Medicine in New York a Century Ago," *Bulletin of the History of Medicine*, 41 (1967), pp. 243–244, note 45.

42. Joseph McDowell Mathews, *How To Succeed in the Practice of Medicine* (Philadelphia, 1905), p. 133; the explanations are mine, not Mathews's. *Ipecac* is short for *ipecacuanha*.

43. The pharmacologist Eugene DuBois thought that about one-third of the 160 drugs in the *New York Hospital Pharmacopoeia* of 1816 were inert. Indeed "one third to one sixth" of the drugs in the *New York Hospital Formulary* of the 1920s were likely inert, said a committee on which he sat. Discussion in "The Use of Pla-

cebos in Therapy," *New York State Journal of Medicine,* 46 (1946), p. 1719.

44. Richard Phillips, ed., *A Translation of the Pharmacopoeia of the Royal College of Physicians of London, 1824* (London, 1831), pp. 148–153; the "infusions" continued for several more pages. Tincture of gentian violet is still medically used on the skin, but not given internally.

45. Holmes, *Medical Essays,* pp. 184, 203; he exempted from the scuttling, opium, "which the Creator himself seems to prescribe," wine, and anesthesia. Italics in original.

46. Loudon, "Doctor's Cash Book," p. 267.

47. Shastid, *My Second Life,* pp. 427–428; italics in original.

48. Hertzler, *Horse and Buggy Doctor,* p. 9.

49. Sims, *Story of My life,* pp. 170–172.

50. Ibid., pp. 149–150.

51. Worthington Hooker, *Physician and Patient* (New York: 1849), p. 33. Shortly after writing this Hooker became a professor of medicine at Yale.

52. William N. Macartney, *Fifty Years a Country Doctor* (New York, 1938), p. 41.

53. Francis Home, *Clinical Experiments, Histories and Dissections,* 2d ed. (London, 1782), pp. 351, 365–366; 1st ed. 1780. Autopsy findings specified that the patient did not have cirrhosis in the liver. "Part of the pulmonary artery was ossified," so the failure may have been primarily right-sided; the postmortem made no comment on the left side of the heart.

54. Richard Brookes, *The General Practice of Physic,* vol. 1 of 2 volumes, 3d ed. (London, 1758), pp. 300–305; 1st ed. 1751.

55. William Withering, *An Account of the Foxglove and Some of Its Medical Uses* (Birmingham, 1785). For the story of the vicissitudes of digitalis therapy, see J. Worth Estes, *Hall Jackson and the Purple Foxglove: Medical Practice and Research in Revolutionary America, 1760–1820* (Hanover: University Press of New England, 1979). Squill was underused as well. Estes notes that among the many drugs registered with the British Patent Office, 1620–1786, only five "were claimed to be effective in the treatment of dropsy. None contained foxglove or squill ..." (pp. 205, 229–231).

56. On overcrowding in the medical profession, Toner estimates that at the end of the eighteenth century there was one

doctor for every eight hundred people in cities, every twelve hundred people in the countryside. Toner, *Contributions,* p. 105.

57. Estes, *Hall Jackson,* p. 35.

58. Hooker, *Physician and Patient,* p. 405; italics in original.

59. Shryock, "Selections Letters," p. 164.

60. Rosenberg, "Practice Medicine," p. 229.

61. Cathell, *Physician Himself,* p. 188.

62. Douglass, *Summary North-America,* vol. 2, p. 351.

63. Shastid, *My Second Life,* pp. 1104–05.

64. John Brooks Wheeler, *Memoirs of a Small-Town Surgeon* (New York, 1935), pp. 293–294; the event happened sometime before Knox's death, which occurred before Wheeler began medical school in 1875.

65. Cathell, *Physician Himself,* pp. 13, 56.

66. Sims, *Story of My Life,* pp. 115–116. Much additional evidence confirms this single anecdote. See Richard Shryock, "Public Relations of the Medical Profession in Great Britain and the United States: 1600–1870," *Annals of Medical History,* n.s., 2 (1930), pp. 308–339; Peterson, *Medical Profession Victorian London,* pp. 133, 194–196; Rivington, *Medical Profession,* pp. 396–397.

Chapter Three: The Traditional Patient

1. U.S. Bureau of the Census, *Historical Statistics of the United States: Colonial Times to 1970,* vol. 1 of 2 volumes (Washington: GPO, 1975), pp. 56–57. Life expectancy for females in 1850 at birth was 40.5, at 20, 60.2.

2. Data for Adams County and Natchez from "Mortality Schedule," roll no. 2730 in the Mississippi State Archives in Jackson. The cover reads "Seventh Census of the United States, original returns of the assistant marshalls, third series: persons who died during the year ending June 30, 1850." Only 9 of the 117 adult deaths occurred to persons over sixty. These deaths are not attributable to an epidemic, for at the end of his report the marshall noted of the past year, "The city of Natchez and County of Adams have been remarkably healthy."

3. Thomas R. Forbes, "Births and Deaths in a London Parish," *Bulletin of the History of Medicine* 55 (1981), p. 387, table 9. Many additional studies of mortality are cited in Shorter, *A History of Women's Bodies* (New York: Basic Books, 1982), chap. 9. I assume that most of the "consumption" deaths Forbes reports were caused by lung TB.

4. W. Brockbank et al., *The Diary of Richard Kay, 1716-51 of Baldingstone, near Bury, a Lancashire Doctor* (Manchester: Chetham Society, 1968), p. 112.

5. Vanessa S. Doe, ed., *The Diary of James Clegg of Chapel en le Frith*, vol. 2 of 3 volumes (Matlock: Derbyshire Record Society, 1978-79), pp. 449-450; in some unnamed illness in 1728 she was referred to as "poor Anne Gee," then on the next page as "weak but more cheerful," vol. 1, pp. 25-26 and p. 29. I am grateful to Irvine Loudon for telling me of the Kay and Clegg diaries.

6. John Beresford, ed., *The Diary of a Country Parson: The Reverend James Woodforde*, vol. 3 of 5 volumes (London, 1924-1931), pp. 155ff. Entries from 25 November 1789 to 17 March 1791.

7. Joseph Mathews, *How to Succeed in the Practice of Medicine* (Philadelphia, 1905), pp. 77-78.

8. Holmes' "The Young Practitioner" (1871), in Holmes, ed., *Medical Essays, 1842-1882* (Boston, 1911), p. 382.

9. Daniel W. Cathell, *The Physician Himself and What He Should Add to the Strictly Scientific* (Baltimore, 1882), p. 146.

10. Eunice M. Schofield, *Medical Care of the Working Class About 1900* (Federation of Local History Societies in the County Palatine of Lancaster, 1979), p. 6. It is clear that many of these remedies had ancient pedigrees.

11. James Bower Harrison, *Popular Medical Errors* (London, 1851), pp. 9-10.

12. Mathews, *Succeed Medicine*, pp. 131-132.

13. Isabella Beeton, *The Book of Household Management* (London, 1861), pp. 1059, 1061.

14. Holmes' "Currents and Counter-Currents in Medical Science" (1860), in *Medical Essays*, p. 186.

15. For one illustration see David Rorie, "Some Fifeshire Folk-Medicine," *Edinburgh Medical Journal*, n.s., 15 (1904), p. 518.

16. William Buchan, *Domestic Medicine*, 10th ed. (London, 1788), pp. 162-163.

17. John Gregory, *Lectures on the Duties and Qualifications of a Physician*, new ed. (London, 1772), p. 232.

18. Thomas H. Shastid, *My Second Life* (Ann Arbor: George Wahr, 1944), p. 730.

19. Buchan, *Domestic Medicine*, p. 162.

20. Beeton, *Household Management*, p. 1065.

21. Samuel W. Gross, ed., *Autobiography of Samuel D. Gross*, vol. 1 of 2 volumes (Philadelphia, 1893), p. 152.

22. Harrison, *Popular Medical Errors*, p. 9.

23. Rorie, "Fifeshire Folk-Medicine," p. 517.

24. Ibid., p. 515.

25. Shastid, *My Second Life*, p. 890.

26. Ibid., p. 1051.

27. Alice H. Murphree, "Folk Medicine in Florida: Remedies Using Plants," *Florida Anthropologist*, 18 (1965), pp. 180, 182.

28. Arnold Krochmal, *A Guide to Medicinal Plants of Appalachia* (Washington, D.C.: GPO, 1971; U.S. Department of Agriculture no. 400), pp. 72, 104.

29. Shastid, *My Second Life*, pp. 496–499.

30. S. W. P. Holloway, "Medical Education in England, 1830–1858: A Sociological Analysis," *History*, n.s., 49 (1964), p. 312. "Twenty-four hundred" is roughly the total number of diplomas of the Royal College of Surgeons and licentiates of the Society of Apothecaries. Because many men held both degrees, the total of diplomaed medical men (excluding the handful of physicians with M.D.'s) would have been less.

31. Paul Starr, *The Social Transformation of American Medicine* (New York: Basic Books, 1982), pp. 63–64.

32. Examples from John Keevil, "Coffeehouse Cures," *Journal of the History of Medicine*, 9 (1954), p. 193; and James Harvey Young, *The Toadstool Millionaires: A Social History of Patent Medicines in America before Federal Regulation* (Princeton: Princeton University Press, 1961), pp. 5–8.

33. Buchan, *Domestic Medicine*, pp. xvii–xxi.

34. Walter Rivington, *The Medical Profession* (Dublin, 1879), pp. 93–94.

35. Peter Templeman, ed., *Selected Cases, and Consultations in Physick by . . . John Woodward* (London, 1757), pp. 1–3. On women's culture, see Shorter, *History Women's Bodies*, chaps. 8 and 11.

36. William Norman Pickles, *Epidemiology in Country Practice* (Bristol, 1939), pp. 60–61.

37. A good account may be found in William G. Rothstein, *American Physicians in the Nineteenth Century: From Sects to Science* (Baltimore: Johns Hopkins University Press, 1972), pp. 125–151.

38. Starr, *Social Transformation,* p. 99. See also Rothstein, ibid., pp. 152–176.

39. Rothstein, ibid., p. 38.

40. M. Jeanne Peterson, *The Medical Profession in Mid-Victorian London* (Berkeley: University of California Press, 1978), pp. 140–145.

41. Harry Marion-Sims, ed., *The Story of My Life by J. Marion Sims* (New York, 1894), pp. 158–160.

42. Worthington Hooker, *Physician and Patient* (New York, 1849), p. 281.

43. Shastid, *My Second Life,* pp. 226–227.

44. Irvine Loudon, "Two Thousand Medical Men in 1847," *Society for the Social History of Medicine Bulletin,* no. 33 (December 1983), p. 8.

Chapter Four: The Rise of the Modern Doctor

1. René T. H. Laennec, *A Treatise on the Diseases of the Chest,* translator John Forbes (London, 1821; French ed. 1819), pp. 300–308, 326–328. These signs are somewhat less distinctive than Laennec believed.

2. On these developments see W. D. Foster, *A Short History of Clinical Pathology* (Edinburgh: Livingstone, 1961), pp. 11–33.

3. James Harrison, *Popular Medical Errors* (London, 1851), pp. 16–17.

4. The story is told briefly in Foster, *History Clinical Pathology,* pp. 53–59.

5. See Frederick C. Shattuck and J. Lewis Bremer, "The Medical School, 1869–1929," in Samuel Eliot Morison, ed., *The Development of Harvard University Since the Inauguration of President Eliot, 1869–1929* (Cambridge, 1930), pp. 555–583.

6. John B. Wheeler, *Memoirs of a Small-Town Surgeon* (New York, 1935), pp. 37–38.

7. Franklin H. Martin, *Fifty Years of Medicine and Surgery* (Chicago: Surgical Publishing Co., 1944), pp. 30, 67.

8. William N. Macartney, *Fifty Years a Country Doctor* (New York, 1938), pp. 27–28.

9. Herbert H. Lang, ed., *Pat Nixon of Texas: Autobiography of a Doctor by Pat Ireland Nixon* (College Station, Texas: Texas A and M University Press, 1979), p. 136.

10. On these developments see Paul Starr, *The So-*

cial Transformation of American Medicine (New York: Basic Books, 1982), pp. 114–121; Rosemary Stevens, *American Medicine and the Public Interest* (New Haven: Yale University Press, 1971), pp. 41–43; Michael J. Lepore, *Death of the Clinician, Requiem or Reveille* (Springfield: Charles C Thomas, 1982), p. 25.

  11. Wheeler, *Memoirs Small-Town Surgeon*, p. 42.

  12. Silas Weir Mitchell, *Doctor and Patient*, 3d ed. (Philadelphia, 1901) pp. 39–40; the first edition was in 1887.

  13. My account of the stethoscope, as well as much of the following, is indebted to Stanley J. Reiser's splendid book, *Medicine and the Reign of Technology* (Cambridge: Cambridge University Press, 1978).

  14. William Allen Pusey, *A Doctor of the 1870s and 80s* (Springfield, 1932), p. 90.

  15. Thomas H. Shastid, *My Second Life* (Ann Arbor: George Wahr, 1944), p. 710.

  16. Quoted in W. Burton Wood, "Pulmonary Tuberculosis in General Practice," *Lancet*, 4 October 1930, p. 727.

  17. Arthur Conan Doyle, *The Stark Munro Letters* (London, 1895), pp. 251–252; his arrival is on page 208.

  18. Daniel Webster Cathell, *The Physician Himself and What He Should Add to the Strictly Scientific* (Baltimore, 1882), p. 11. This enormously popular guide went through three editions, the last published in Baltimore in 1913; a revised version, which will also be cited in this chapter, entitled *Book on the Physician Himself from Graduation to Old Age*, started to be published by the Davis Company in Philadelphia in 1889. This volume, for some reason, was labeled the "ninth edition," and it proceeded to go through a number of subsequent editions, the thirteenth, or "crowning," edition appearing in Philadelphia in 1922. It is a 1924 reprinting of that "crowning" edition that I used in this book.

  19. James B. Herrick, "The Relation of the Clinical Laboratory to the Practitioner of Medicine," *Boston Medical and Surgical Journal*, 13 June 1907, p. 766.

  20. Stevens, *American Medicine*, p. 268.

  21. James B. Herrick, "The Practitioner of the Future," *JAMA*, 22 September 1934, p. 884; osteosarcoma is a kind of bone cancer.

  22. Walter C. Alvarez, *Incurable Physician: An Autobiography* (Englewood Cliffs, N.J.: Prentice-Hall, 1963), pp. 53–54.

  23. James Mackenzie, *The Future of Medicine* (London, 1919), pp. 186–187.

24. Ibid., p. 61.

25. Charles L. Leonard, "The Application of the Roentgen Rays to Medical Diagnosis," *JAMA*, 4 December 1897, pp. 1157–1158; William Osler, *The Principles and Practice of Medicine*, 6th ed. (New York, 1906), p. 860; the first edition of this famous text-book appeared in 1892.

26. Wood, "Pulmonary Tuberculosis in General Practice," pp. 728–729.

27. Osler L. Peterson et al., "An Analytical Study of North Carolina General Practice, 1953–1954," *Journal of Medical Education*, 31 (December 1956), pt. 2, p. 107. Forty-three percent of the doctors surveyed had their own ECG.

28. Harvey Van Allen, "The Limitations of the Roentgen Method of Diagnosis," *NEJM*, 10 September 1936, p. 483. Although the X-ray gives no direct view of the heart valves, it can show calcification of the valves, and it can help demonstrate valvular disease by showing dilation of the left atrium. Dr. Van Allen was doubtless aware of this; he evidently felt the referring doctor wasn't.

29. Osler, *Principles*, p. 851; on p. 848 a discussion first appears in his textbook of hypertension as a factor in arteriosclerosis. To avoid tedium I shall avoid mentioning other such technological diagnostic aids in general practice as the clinical thermometer, the ophthalmoscope and laryngoscope.

30. Reiser, *Medicine and the Reign of Technology*, p. 106.

31. Mentioned in passing, for example, in Cathell, *Book on Physician*, p. 24; William Stanley Sykes, *A Manual of General Medical Practice* (London, 1927), p. 115.

32. James Mackenzie, *Diseases of the Heart*, 2d ed. (London, 1910; first ed. 1908), pp. 370–376.

33. *Principles and Practice of Medicine*, p. 775; in account of "heart-block."

34. Cited, for instance, in William V. Johnston, *Before the Age of Miracles: Memoirs of a Country Doctor* (Toronto: Fitzhenry and Whiteside, 1972), p. 106.

35. Roger I. Lee and Lewis W. Jones, *The Fundamentals of Good Medical Care* (Chicago, 1933; Pubs. of the Committee on the Costs of Medical Care, no. 22), p. 244.

36. Peterson, "North Carolina General Practice," p. 107.

37. Howard Robertson and S. E. T. Cusdin, "The Doctor's Surgery," *Practitioner*, 170 (1953), pp. 574–581, quote from

p. 580. *Surgery* is the British term for doctor's office; the authors of the article were architects.

38. Cathell, *Physician Himself,* p. 18.

39. Verlin C. Thomas, *The Successful Physician* (Philadelphia, 1923), p. 265.

40. Richad C. Cabot, "The Relation of Bacteriology to Medicine," *Boston Medical and Surgical Journal,* 10 May 1900, p. 481.

41. Mackenzie, *Future of Medicine,* p. 148.

42. Arthur E. Hertzler, *The Horse and Buggy Doctor* (New York, 1938), p. 52.

43. Morphine had been the subject of research since 1886. This account of drugs draws heavily upon Alfred G. Gilman et al., *Goodman and Gilman's The Pharmacological Basis of Therapeutics,* 6th ed. (New York: Macmillan, 1980); the fifth edition (1975) contains historical information on some drugs that was omitted from the sixth edition. I have also relied on Béla Issekutz, *Die Geschichte der Arznei-mittelforschung* (Budapest: Akadémiai Kiadó, 1971).

44. The tendency to assume that discoveries spread instantaneously after their appearance runs through some of the traditional history of medicine. Richard H. Shryock, for example, suggests that emetine, an alkaloid of ipecac, was used in the treatment of amoebic dysentery soon after its discovery in 1820. In fact, the rational use of emetine as an amebecide would begin only in 1912. Shryock, *The Development of Modern Medicine: An Interpretation of the Social and Scientific Factors Involved* (Philadelphia, 1936), p. 162.

45. John J. Black, *Forty Years in the Medical Profession, 1858–1898* (Philadelphia, 1900), p. 124.

46. Cathell, *Book on the Physician Himself,* pp. 226, 251.

47. Shastid, *My Second Life,* p. 1046.

48. The statistic is from George T. Welch, "Therapeutical Superstition," *Medical Record,* 8 July 1893, p. 35.

49. Johnston, *Before the Age of Miracles,* p. 58.

50. To sort out this forest of chemical names, acet-anilid (antifebrin) was first in the series. Introduced in 1886, it proved too toxic for use. Phenacetin then followed in 1887. Acetaminophen, derived from phenacetin, was first used medically in 1893 and became popular only after 1949. All three of these drugs, in contrast to aspirin, are known as the para-aminophenol derivatives, because all stem from a phenol molecule with an amino group attached (*para*) to it. See *Goodman and Gilman, Pharmacological Basis,* 6th ed., p. 701.

51. In the 1908 edition of his *Diseases of the Heart.*

52. Patricia S. Ward, "The American Reception of Salvarsan" *Journal of the History of Medicine,* 36 (1981), pp 44–62.

53. Cathell, *Book on the Physician,* p. 241.

54. William R. Houston, *The Art of Treatment* (New York: 1936), pp. 5–6.

55. The following account comes from Howard G. Bruenn, "Clinical Notes on the Illness and Death of President Franklin D. Roosevelt," *Annals of Internal Medicine,* 72 (1970), pp. 579–591.

56. Hertzler, *Horse and Buggy Doctor,* p. 177.

57. Peterson, "North Carolina General Practice," p. 43.

58. See, for example, Joseph S. Collings, "General Practice in England Today: A Reconnaissance," *Lancet,* 25 March 1950, p. 565.

59. Shattuck, "Medical School," p. 582.

60. Ibid., p. 560.

61. Cecil Kent Austin, "Medical Impressions of America," *Boston Medical and Surgical Journal,* 30 May 1912, p. 800. The author practiced in Paris.

62. Charles L. Dana, "The Doctor's Future," *New York Medical Journal,* 4 January 1913, p. 2.

63. Martin, *Fifty Years of Medicine,* pp. 112–126.

64. Joseph M. Mathews, *How To Succeed in the Practice of Medicine* (Philadelphia, 1905), pp. 117–118.

65. Thomas, *Successful Physician,* pp. 92–94.

66. Lepore, *Death of the Clinician,* p. 125; Cathell, *Book of the Physician,* p. 76.

67. Doyle, *Letters of Stark Munro,* pp. 213–215.

68. Cathell, *Physician Himself,* pp. 10, 19, 21.

69. Ibid., p. 58; Cathell, *Book of the Physician,* p. 148.

70. Lepore, *Death of the Clinician,* p. 271.

71. Ibid., p. 272.

Chapter Five: The Making of the Modern Patient

1. Jules Romains, *Knock ou le triomphe da la médecine* (Paris, 1924). Quotes from 1947 Gallimard edition, pp. 34, 96–107, 165.

2. In 1746–1748 Richard Kay and James Clegg, physicians in rural England, saw roughly equal numbers of adult patients. Including only the consultations in which the patient is mentioned by name (few for either physician), Clegg treated forty men and

fifty-three women, Kay twenty-nine men and twenty-nine women. Vanessa S. Doe, ed., *The Diary of James Clegg of Chapel en le Frith, 1708-1755*, 3 volumes (Matlock: Derbyshire Record Society, 1978-1981); W. Brockbank and F. Kenworthy, eds., *The Diary of Richard Kay, 1716-51, of Baldingstone, near Bury: a Lancashire Doctor* (Manchester: Chetham Society, 1968). Of eleven cases treated surgically by Johann H. Steger and his son Johann J. Steger over the period 1784-1811 in Lichtersteig, Switzerland, ten were males; dislocated shoulders, riding accidents and the like were the order of the day; the gravest was a leg amputation. Martin Gaberthüel, *Krankengeschichten und Operationsberichte, 1784-1811, nach den Aufzeichnungen von Johann Heinrich Steger* ... (Zürich: Juris, 1980), pp. 19-98.

     3. Selwyn D. Collins, "Frequency and Volume of Doctors' Calls Among Males and Females in 9,000 Families, Based on Nation-Wide Periodic Canvasses, 1928-31" [United States] *Public Health Reports*, 55 (1 November 1940), p. 1985, table 1. By *man* and *woman* are meant males and females of all ages. Children are under five. Data are for "illness attended by private physicians not designated as specialists: total calls by physicians per 1000 population, males and females, all causes."

     4. Shorter, *The Making of the Modern Family* (New York: Basic Books, 1975).

     5. Worthington Hooker, *Physician and Patient* (New York, 1849), pp. 384-385.

     6. Charles Cowan, "Report of Private Medical Practice for 1840," *Journal of the [Royal] Statistical Society of London*, 5 (1842) (Ser. A: General), p. 84.

     7. John Janvier Black, *Forty Years in the Medical Profession, 1858-1898* (Philadelphia, 1900), p. 246; Black, it is true, did much obstetrics.

     8. Silas Weir Mitchell, *Doctor and Patient*, 3d ed. (Philadelphia, 1901), p. 11; first ed. 1887.

     9. Charles Bell Keetley, *The Student's and Junior Practitioner's Guide to the Medical Profession*, 2d ed. (London, 1885), p. 19; first ed. 1878.

     10. Daniel W. Cathell, *The Physician Himself and What He Should Add to the Strictly Scientific* (Baltimore, 1882), p. 59.

     11. Verlin C. Thomas, *The Successful Physician* (Philadelphia, 1923), pp. 72, 142.

     12. Clegg, *Diary*, vol. 3, p. 708.

13. Hooker, *Physician and Patient*, pp. 184–185.

14. Mitchell, *Doctor and Patient*, p. 45.

15. Maurice Cassidy, "Doctor and Patient," *Lancet*, 15 January 1938, p. 177.

16. John Horder, "The Role of the General Practitioner in Psychological Medicine," *Royal Society of Medicine. London. Proceedings*, 60 (1967), p. 266.

17. David Riesman, "High Blood Pressure and Longevity," *JAMA*, 4 April 1931, p. 1105. Riesman had a number of cranky theories about the causes of hypertension.

18. William R. Houston, *The Art of Treatment* (New York, 1936), p. 451.

19. Arthur E. Hertzler, *The Horse and Buggy Doctor* (New York, 1938), p. 149.

20. See, for example, Stephen Taylor, *Good General Practice: A Report of a Survey* (London: Oxford University Press, 1954), pp. 199, 417.

21. Axel Munthe, *The Story of San Michele* (New York, 1929), pp. 33, 39–40. "Colitis" actually means inflammation of the colon.

22. Herbert P. Hawkins, "The Reality of Enterospasm and Its Mimicry of Appendicitis," *BMJ*, 13 January 1906, p. 65.

23. Robert Hutchison, "Chronic Abdomen," *BMJ*, 21 April 1923, p. 667.

24. Hertzler, *Horse and Buggy Doctor*, p. 143.

25. Thomas, *Successful Physician*, p. 267.

26. Thomas Mann, *The Magic Mountain*, Eng. trans. H. T. Lowe-Porter (New York, 1927; 1st German ed. 1924); I used the Random House Vintage edition of 1969, p. 439.

27. See on this Alden B. Mills, *The Extent of Illness and of Physical and Mental Defects Prevailing in the United States* (Washington: Committee on the Cost of Medical Care, 1929) no. 2, p. 15.

28. I. S. Falk et al., *The Costs of Medical Care* (Chicago: Committee on the Costs of Medical Care, 1933) no. 27, p. 33.

29. I. S. Falk et al., *The Incidence of Illness and the Receipt and Costs of Medical Care Among Representative Families: Experiences in Twelve Consecutive Months During 1928–1931* (Chicago: Committee on the Cost of Medical Care, 1933) no. 26, p. 274, table B-17.

30. John Pemberton, "Illness in General Practice,"

BMJ, 19 February 1949, pp. 306–307; data on six practices for one winter week in 1947 contrasted with "Dr. Calvert Holland's Analysis of 200 Cases of Sickness in Men Living in Sheffield in 1843."

31. Falk, *Incidence Illness*, p. 48, table 11. The bottom income bracket had 0.79 illnesses per year, the top 1.15.

32. Cathell, *The Physician Himself*, p. 38.

33. "1930s London suburb," Innes H. Pearse and Lucy H. Crocker, *The Peckham Experiment: A Study in the Living Structure of Society* (London: Allen and Unwin, 1943), p. 97, note 2. "Londoners, 1953–54": John Horder and Elizabeth Horder, "Illness in General Practice," *Practitioner*, 173 (1954), p. 183; includes 190 "first consultations" and 514 additional "items of illness during the same period which were not brought to any agency." "Smalltown Upper New York State, 1940s": Earl Lomon Koos, *The Health of Regionville: What the People Thought and Did About It* (New York: Columbia University Press, 1954), calculated from figure 4, p. 40. "Nationwide Survey": Falk, *Incidence Illness*, p. 106, table 23 (63 percent had seen a GP, 9 percent a specialist, 3 percent "sectarian," and so on). "Saw doctor 2.9 times a year": Collins, "Frequency and Volume of Doctors' Calls," p. 1984, table 1. The heading: "Calls by any practitioner per 1000 population: both sexes, all causes." The average "case" received 4.6 calls annually from the doctor.

34. Falk, *Incidence Illness*, p. 287, table B-32; 16 percent for cities of 5,000 to 100,000 population. Allon Peebles, *A Survey of the Medical Facilities of Shelby County, Indiana: 1929* (Washington: Committee on the Costs of Medical Care, 1930) no. 6; a Shelby County family would spend thirty dollars yearly on drugs as a whole.

35. Nathan Sinai and Alden B. Mills, *A Survey of the Medical Facilities of the City of Philadelphia: 1929* (Chicago: Committee on the Costs of Medical Care, 1931) no. 9, p. 94, table 41.

36. C. Rufus Rorem and Robert P. Fischelis, *The Costs of Medicines* (Chicago: Committee on the Costs of Medical Care, 1932) no. 14, p. 102, table 13. According to Harry H. Moore, "patent and proprietary medicine" sold to the general public in 1923 amounted to 50.3 percent of all drug sales, "ethical specialties" dispensed upon prescription another 15.3 percent. In 1923 a prescription would have been required for alcohol and narcotics. *American Medicine and the People's Health* (New York, 1927), p. 134.

37. On Listerine see *Hygeia*'s excerpt from a pharmaceutical journal, printed in July 1926, p. 407. On Konjola, Bromo-Seltzer, etc., Rorem, *Costs of Medicines*, pp. 119, 149.

38. Peebles, *Medical Facilities Shelby County*, pp. 144–145.

39. William Stanley Sykes, *A Manual of General Medical Practice* (London, 1927), p. 5.

40. Koos, *Health Regionville*, p. 89; class differences from p. 88.

41. Gladys V. Swackhamer, *Choice and Change of Doctor: A Study of the Consumer of Medical Services* (New York: Committee on Research in Medical Economics, 1939) p. 39.

42. Ibid., p. 17.

43. Paul Starr, *The Social Transformation of American Medicine* (New York: Basic Books, 1982), pp. 133–140. On the restricting of drug sales over-the-counter see James Harvey Young, *The Medical Messiahs: A Social History of Health Quackery in Twentieth-Century America* (Princeton: Princeton University Press, 1967), chaps. 8 and 12.

44. See, for example, the editorial against testimonials, "The Real Reason for the Passing of the General Practitioner," in the *Boston Medical and Surgical Journal*, 11 February 1897, pp. 142–143.

45. This was the breakdown, at least, in Shelby County. Peebles, *Medical Facilities Shelby County*, p. 86.

46. Rorem, *Costs of Medicines*, p. 114. For example, BiSoDol, which was advertised to doctors and dentists under numerous extravagant claims, contained magnesium carbonate, baking soda, and a bit of oil of peppermint. See the report of the AMA's "Council on Pharmacy and Chemistry," in *JAMA*, 29 October 1932, p. 1511.

47. *Hygeia*, August 1929, p. 830.

48. James Peter Warbasse, "State Journalism," *New York State Journal of Medicine*, 8 (1908), p. 600.

49. George Bernard Shaw, *The Doctor's Dilemma*, first produced in 1906, published in 1911. Quote from the 1946 Penguin edition, p. 110. "Paddy" is "Sir Patrick Cullen," another physician.

50. Rorem, *Costs of Medicine*, pp. 141–142.

51. For a glimpse of the countless unsanctioned patent medicines, see American Medical Association, *Nostrums and Quackery*, 2d ed. (Chicago, 1912); Arthur J. Cramp, *Nostrums and Quackery*, vol. 2 (Chicago, 1921), and Cramp, *Nostrums and Quackery and Pseudo-Medicine*, vol. 3 (Chicago, 1936).

52. Quote is by Hugo O. Pantzer of Indianapolis, in the discussion of Edwin Walker's paper, "A Further Protest Against the

Routine Use of Purgatives," *American Journal of Obstetrics*, 64
(1911), p. 755. See Houston, *Art of Treatment*, on the persistence of
these views on catharsis right through the 1930s, pp. 427–428.

53. Shaw, *Doctor's Dilemma*, pp. 67–68.

54. William Norman Pickles, *Epidemiology in
Country Practice* (Bristol, 1939), pp. 29–30.

55. Mitchell, *Doctor and Patient*, pp. 31–32.

56. Hertzler, *Horse and Buggy Doctor*, p. 100.

57. Catalogued by Morris Fishbein, *The New Medi-
cal Follies: An Encyclopedia of Cultism and Quackery* . . . (Toronto,
1927), pp. 48–57. Fishbein was the editor of the *Journal of the American Medical Association* and of *Hygeia*.

58. "Nationwide survey": Collins, "Frequency and
Volume of Doctors' Calls," p. 1988, table 1, "Percent of all practitioners'
calls that were calls by nonmedical practitioners, both sexes, all causes."
"Shelby County": *Medical Facilities Shelby County*, p. 19. Two of the
doctors and all the Christian Science practitioners were not occupied
full time. "U.S. as a whole": Peebles, *Survey Statistical Data Medical
Facilities*, p. 16.

59. Collins, "Frequency and Volume of Doctors'
Calls," p. 2001, figure 5, "Other non-medical." Osteopaths and chiropractors excluded from the 121 calls.

60. George P. Reynolds, "Hysterical Paraplegia: A
Case of Many Years' Duration, Responding Well to Treatment," *Boston
Medical and Surgical Journal*, 7 October 1926, pp. 704–707. I have
somewhat condensed this long account.

61. Joseph S. Collings, "General Practice in
England Today: A Reconnaissance," *Lancet*, 25 March 1950, p. 555.

62. Koos, *Health of Regionville*, pp. 53–54. Italics
in original.

63. Ibid., p. 61.

64. I used the edition that appeared two years later.
Cathell, *Book on the Physician Himself from Graduation to Old Age*,
Crowning Edition (Philadelphia, 1924), p. 25.

65. Stories of 26 June and 27 October 1895, the latter excerpted from the *Boston Transcript*.

66. For example, Dr. S. Josephine Baker's series in
the *Journal*, of which a sample is the March 1922 issue, on "Unnecessary Diseases of Childhood." She explains "how to fight germs" and
"the meaning of resistance," among other things, pp. 30–43.

67. Herbert H. Lang, ed., *Pat Nixon of Texas*

(College Station: Texas A and M University Press, 1979), quotes from pp. 177–178.

67. Edward W. Morris, "The Hospitals," *BMJ*, 10 July 1920, p. 43; his position was "house governor."

69. Cathell, *Book on the Physician Himself*, pp. 64–65.

70. Bernard F. Dick, ed., *Dark Victory* (Madison: Wisconsin Center for Film and Theater Research/University of Wisconsin Press, 1981), pp. 9–18, 76.

71. Sidney Kingsley, *Men in White: A Play in Three Acts* (New York, 1933), quotes from pp. 14–15, 19.

72. Ibid., pp. 35–36.

73. Max Pinner and Benjamin F. Miller, eds., *When Doctors Are Patients* (New York: Norton, 1952), p. 108.

74. Ibid., p. 26.

75. Thomas Hall Shastid, *My Second Life* (Ann Arbor: Wahr, 1944), p. 38.

76. James Thomson Bell Nicoll, *The Span of Time: The Autobiography of a Doctor* (London: Hodder and Stoughton, 1952), p. 221.

77. Shastid, *My Second Life*, pp. 1078–1079. *Y. of P.* means a doctor who had already begun practicing before the passage of the state's licensing law, thus whose medical qualification was his "years of practice."

Chapter Six: Disease of Psychological Origin

1. Paul Dubois, *The Psychic Treatment of Nervous Disorders*, 6th ed. translated and edited by Smith Ely Jelliffe and William A. White (New York, 1909), p. 388; first French edition, *Les psychonévroses et leur traitement moral* (Paris, 1904); first English edition 1905.

2. Hans Selye, *The Physiology and Pathology of Exposure to Stress* (Montreal: Acta, 1950). For Sydenham on hysteria, see his "Epistolary Dissertation to William Cole," of 20 January 1682, in R. G. Latham, ed., *The Works of Thomas Sydenham*, English translation, vol. 2 of 2 volumes (London, 1848–1850), pp. 56–118. Robert Whytt, *Observations on the Nature, Cause, and Cure of Those Disorders Which Have Been Commonly Called Nervous, Hypochondriac, or Hysteric*, 2 ed. (Edinburgh, 1765), pp. iii, vii, 88. The "first edition" also appeared in 1765.

3. J. Russell Reynolds, "Remarks on Paralysis, and

Other Disorders of Motion and Sensation, Dependent on Idea," *BMJ*, 6 November 1869, p. 483.

4. Ernst von Leyden, "Ueber periodisches Erbrechen (gastrische Krisen) nebst Bemerkungen Über nervöse Magenaffectionen," *Zeitschrift für Klinische Medizin*, 4 (1881), p. 606. The owner of the Sonneberg baths was Dr. F. Richter, "ueber nervöse Dyspepsie und nervöse Enteropathie," *Berliner Klinische Wochenschrift*, 27 March 1882, pp. 195–198. Carl Ewald, "Die Neurasthenia Dyspeptica," *Berliner Klinsche Wochenschrift*, 26 May 1884, pp. 322–324, 342–344. Ottomar Rosenbach, "Die Emotionsdyspepsie," *Berliner Klinische Wochenschrift*, 25 January 1897, pp. 70–75, continued 1 February 1897, pp. 97–101. Walter B. Cannon, "The Influence of Emotional States on the Functions of the Alimentary Canal," *American Journal of the Medical Sciences*, 137 (1909), p. 482.

5. The "Bible" of the American Psychiatric Association, the *Diagnostic and Statistical Manual of Mental Disorders*, 3d ed. (Washington: American Psychiatric Association, 1980), has ceased using *neurosis* as an official diagnostic category, pp. 9–10.

6. Edwin Holmes Van Deusen, "Observations on a Form of Nervous Prostration (Neurasthenia), Culminating in Insanity," *American Journal of Insanity*, 25 (April 1869), pp. 446–461; "Supplement to Annual Report for 1867 and 1868." George Beard, "Neurasthenia, or Nervous Exhaustion," *Boston Medical and Surgical Journal*, 29 April 1869, pp. 217–221.

7. Joseph Collins, "The General Practitioner and the Functional Nervous Diseases," *JAMA*, 9 January 1909, p. 89.

8. For a recent introduction, see Edward Shorter, "Les Désordres Psychosomatiques: sont-ils 'Hystériques'? Notes pour une recherche historique," *Cahiers internationaux de Sociologie*, 76 (1984), pp. 201–224.

9. The current doctrine, summarized by Fred O. Henker, is that "practically any illness may be significantly influenced by mental processes. . . . We now include standard medical conditions such as pneumonia, or even cancer, when a comprehensive work-up discloses significant psychological involvement." "Psychosomatic Illness: Biochemical and Physiologic Foundations," *Psychosomatics*, 25 (1984), p. 20.

10. John Gregory, *Lectures on the Duties and Qualifications of a Physician*, new ed. (London, 1772), pp. 23–24; 1st ed. 1770.

11. Thomas Arthur Rose, *An Enquiry into Prognosis in the Neuroses* (Cambridge, 1936), p. 71.

12. "82 percent": J. Richard Wittenborn, "Somatic Discomforts Among Depressed Women," *Archives of General Psychiatry*, 36 (1979), pp. 465–471, interested in "a distressing level of somatic discomfort." The special number of the *Journal of Nervous and Mental Disease* was 170 (7) (July 1982); see especially Dietrich Blumer and Mary Heilbronn, "Chronic Pain as a Variant of Depressive Disease: the Pain-Prone Disorder," pp. 381–406. Joseph Collins, *Letters to a Neurologist . . . Reprint from the Medical Record 1908* (New York, 1908), pp. 93–99.

13. "If you would only": Walter C. Alvarez, *Nervousness, Indigestion, and Pain* (New York: Hoeber, 1943), p. 322. "200 patients": John W. Macy and Edgar V. Allen, "A Justification of the Diagnosis of Chronic Nervous Exhaustion," *Annals of Internal Medicine*, 7 (1934), p. 863. "1000 unstable colon": Sara M. Jordan, "The Unstable Colon and Neurosis," *JAMA*, 31 December 1932, p. 2235. Dubois, *Psychic Treatment Nervous Disorders*, p. 249.

14. Dubois, *Psychic Treatment Nervous Disorders*, p. 258. Arthur Hertzler, *The Horse and Buggy Doctor* (New York, 1938), p. 154.

15. Margot Jefferys, et al., "Consumption of Medicines on a Working-Class Housing Estate," *British Journal of Preventive Social Medicine*, 14 (1960), pp. 71, 74.

16. Michael Balint, *The Doctor, His Patient and the Illness*, rev. ed. (New York: International Universities Press, 1972), pp. 48–50; 1st ed. 1957; the events occurred sometime in the 1950s.

17. Ibid., p. 50.

18. Frank N. Allan and Manuel Kaufman, "Nervous Factors in General Practice," *JAMA*, 18 December 1948, pp. 1135–1138.

19. "Ontario": William Victor Johnston, *Before the Age of Miracles: Memoirs of a Country Doctor* (Toronto: Fitzhenry and Whiteside, 1972), p. 73. "75 percent": Israel Strauss's comment, in the discussion of Peter G. Denker, "Results of Treatment of Psychoneuroses by the General Practitioner: A Follow-Up Study of 500 Patients," *A.M.A. Archives of Neurology and Psychiatry*, 57 (1947), pp. 504–512, comment on p. 511. See also Horace K. Richardson, "Psychopathy and the General Practitioner," *NEJM*, 24 October 1935, who felt 50–75 percent of all GP cases to be "functional disorders of the nervous system," p. 790.

20. Maurice Cassidy, "Doctor and Patient," *Lancet*, 15 January 1938, p. 176. "174 patients": George Canby Robinson, *The Patient as a Person: A Study of the Social Aspects of Illness* (New York,

1939), p. 27. Francis Weld Peabody, *The Care of the Patient* (Cambridge, 1927), pp. 23–25, 29.

21. "Nervous problems 1917": I. S. Falk et al., *The Costs of Medical Care* (Chicago: Committee on the Costs of Medical Care, 1933), no. 27, pp. 31–32, citing a survey by the Metropolitan Life Insurance Company. James L. Halliday, "Psychoneurosis as a Cause of Incapacity Among Insured Persons," *BMJ*, Suppl., 16 March 1935, pp. 85–87, 101.

22. The classic "sham" operation, a fake ovariotomy which marked the beginning of the end of the removal of ovaries to cure "hysteria," was done by James Israel in 1879. "Ein Beitrag zur Würdigung des Werthes der Castration bei hysterischen Frauen," *Berliner Klinische Wochenschrift*, 26 April 1880, pp. 243–244.

23. Hertzler, *Horse and Buggy Doctor*, p. 241. He rationalized that her "tumor of the uterus" would sooner or later have to come out anyway.

24. Henry O. Marcy, "The Causal Relation Intra-Abdominal Diseases Bear to Nervous Disturbances Recognized by Gynecologists, Ignored by Neurologists," *JAMA*, 1 September 1900, p. 536.

25. Ibid., p. 536.

26. William R. Houston, *The Art of Treatment* (New York, 1936), pp. 479, 507.

27. For a review of some of this needless surgery, covering the *Transactions* of the American Surgical Association, 1880–1942, see Benjamin A. Barnes, "Discarded Operations: Surgical Innovation by Trial and Error," in John P. Bunker et al., eds., *Costs, Risks and Benefits of Surgery* (New York: Oxford University Press, 1977), pp. 109–123.

28. Alvarez, *Nervousness, Indigestion, and Pain*, p. 424.

29. "Sugar pills": Gilbert Honigfeld, "Non-specific Factors in Treatment, I. Review of Placebo Reactions and Placebo Reactors," *Diseases of the Nervous System*, 25 (1964), p. 151; much fascinating evidence on placebo use turned up at the roundtable discussion among Cornell's medical faculty, "The Use of Placebos in Therapy," *New York State Journal of Medicine*, 46 (1946), pp. 1718–1727; for material cited in this and following paragraphs, see in particular the contributions by pharmacologist Harry Gold.

30. Examples cited by John T. G. Nichols, "The

Misuse of Drugs in Modern Practice," *Boston Medical and Surgical Journal*, 14 September 1893, p. 263.

31. "Calcium": Cassidy, "Doctor and Patient," says that "Calcium is for some inscrutable reason the fashionable one at the moment," p. 178. Wheeler, "Use of Placebos in Therapy," p. 1725.

32. Cornell's Eugene F. DuBois, "Use of Placebos in Therapy," p. 1719.

33. William N. Macartney, *Fifty Years a Country Doctor* (New York, 1938), pp. 235–236.

34. According to Charles Brown-Séquard, "Remarques sur les effets produits sur la femme par des injections sous-cutanées d'un liquide retiré d'ovaires d'animaux," *Archives de physiologie normale et pathologique*, 22 (1890), p. 456.

35. Banks's contribution to a dicussion at a BMA meeting, *BMJ*, 2 October 1869, p. 378.

36. On nitroglycerin see Dale G. Friend et al., "Action of Triethanolamine Trinitrate in Angina Pectoris," *American Heart Journal*, 48 (1954), pp. 775–779 (the authors studied nitroglycerin too). Of the arthritic-pain patients, 52 percent were relieved by aspirin, 46 percent by placebo. Robert C. Batterman and Arthur J. Grossman, "Effectiveness of Salicylamide as an Analgesic and Antirheumatic Agent," *JAMA*, 24 December 1955, pp. 1619–1622. "Finnish ulcer study": Heikki Bäckman et al., "Placebo Effect in Peptic Ulcer and other Gastroduodenal Disorders," *Gastroenterologia*, 94 (1960), p. 15, table 2.

37. Gold, "Use of Placebos in Therapy," p. 1723.

38. Walter C. Alvarez, *Incurable Physician: An Autobiography* (Englewood Cliffs, N.J.: Prentice-Hall, 1963), pp. 59–60.

39. Alvarez, *Nervousness, Indigestion, and Pain*, p. 116.

40. Daniel Cathell, *Book on the Physician Himself*, crowning edition (Philadelphia, 1922), pp. 63–64. Italics in original.

41. Verlin C. Thomas, *The Successful Physician* (Philadelphia, 1923), p. 261.

42. Frank Billings, "The Resourceful General Practitioner of Modern Medicine," *JAMA*, 24 February 1923, p. 520.

43. Johnston, *Before the Age of Miracles*, pp. 80–81.

44. Peabody, *Care of the Patient*, pp. 35–43.

45. Cassidy, "Doctor and Patient," p. 176.

46. Selwyn D. Collins, "Frequency and Volume of Doctors' Calls Among Males and Females in 9,000 Families, Based on

Nation-Wide Periodic Canvasses, 1928–31" [*U.S.*] *Public Health Reports*, 55 (1 November 1940), table 1, p. 1985; table 4, p. 2004.

47. William Stanley Sykes, *A Manual of General Medical Practice* (London, 1927), p. 3.

48. Thomas, *Successful Physician*, pp. 106–107. "The patient has had that for which he craved: an opportunity to be completely heard. You have had an opportunity to study your patient while he was telling his story" (p. 262).

49. Houston, *Art of Treatment*, p. 73.

50. Roger I. Lee et al., *Fundamentals of Good Medical Care* (Chicago: Committee on the Costs of Medical Care, 1933) no. 22, p. 279. Silas Weir Mitchell, *Doctor and Patient*, 3d ed. (Philadelphia, 1901), p. 58. Houston, *Art of Treatment*, p. 519.

51. The papers of Frederick Parkes Weber are at the Contemporary Medical Archives Centre in the Wellcome Institute in London; quotations are from the volume of "Medical Notes" from 20 August 1907 to 31 December 1908.

52. Cathell, *Book on the Physician Himself*, pp. 60–61, 65.

53. Thomas, *Successful Physician*, p. 16.

54. Johnston, *Before the Age of Miracles*, p. 73.

55. Ibid., pp. 72, 80–81.

56. Mitchell presented an early, succinct account of his "rest cure" in "Rest in Nervous Disease: Its Use and Abuse," in Edward C. Seguin, ed., *A Series of American Clinical Lectures*, vol. 1, no. 4 (New York, 1876), pp. 83–102.

57. Ibid., pp. 95–96.

58. William S. Playfair introduced the rest cure to England, "Notes on the Systematic Treatment of Nerve Prostration and Hysteria Connected with Uterine Disease," *Lancet*, 28 May 1881, pp. 857–859, continued 11 June 1881, pp. 949–950. Rudolph Burkart was an early advocate in Germany, "Zur Behandlung schwerer Formen von Hysterie und Neurasthenie" [*Volkmann*] *Sammlung Klinischer Vorträge*, no. 245 (1884), pp. 1771–1818.

59. Joseph Babinski, "Définition de l'hystérie," *Revue neurologique*, 9 (1901), pp. 1074–1080.

60. Dubois, *Psychic Treatment of Nervous Disorders*, pp. 226–228, 243, 245–247.

61. Ibid., p. 388.

62. Edwin Bramwell, "A Lecture on Psychotherapy in General Practice," *Edinburgh Medical Journal*, n.s., 30 (1923), pp. 55–56.

63. Houston, *Art of Treatment*, pp. 416–417.

64. Mitchell, "Rest in Nervous Disease," p. 84; Houston, *Art of Treatment*, pp. 512, 514.

65. Houston, *Art of Treatment*, p. 407.

66. R. S. Bruce Pearson, "Psychoneurosis in Hospital Practice," *Lancet*, 19 February 1938, p. 456.

67. Quoted in Anna Robeson Burr, *Weir Mitchell: His Life and Letters* (New York, 1929), pp. 186–187. Italics in original.

68. Houston, *Art of Treatment*, p. 70.

69. James Thomson Bell Nicoll, *The Span of Time: The Autobiography of a Doctor* (London: Hodder and Stoughton, 1952), p. 105.

70. M. Jeanne Peterson, *The Medical Profession in Mid-Victorian London* (Berkeley: University of California Press, 1978), p. 282. On certainty, Thomas Preston, *The Clay Pedestal: A Re-examination of the Doctor-Patient Relationship* (Seattle: Madrona, 1981), pp. 85–86.

71. S. W. and J. T. Pierce, pseud., *The Layman Looks at Doctors* (New York, 1929), pp. 26–27, 63–71, 81–87.

72. Ross, *Enquiry Prognosis Neuroses*, p. 79. The average stay was 4.1 months. Of the 1,320 patients discharged by 1933, 10 percent were "known to have relapsed in the whole period."

73. Mary C. Luff and Marjorie Garrod, "The After-Results of Psychotherapy in 500 Adult Cases," *BMJ*, 13 July 1935, pp. 54–59. A variety of therapies were used, including psychoanalysis.

74. Benjamin V. White et al., *Mucous Colitis: A Psychological Medical Study of Sixty Cases* (Washington: Committee on Problems of Neurotic Behavior, 1939) Psychosomatic Medicine Monograph no. 1, pp. 42–44.

75. Ibid., pp. 87–90.

76. John A. Ryle, "An Address on Chronic Spasmodic Affections of the Colon," *Lancet*, 1 December 1928, p. 1119.

77. Chester M. Jones, *Digestive Tract Pain: Diagnosis and Treatment* (New York, 1938); see, for example, "patient R. T.," a widow, forty-four, pp. 129–130.

78. George Canby Robinson, "Personality Disorders Causing Digestive Tract Complaints," *Johns Hopkins Hospital Bulletin*, 68 (1941), p. 216, case 12.

79. Edmund Jacobson, "Spastic Esophagus and Mucous Colitis," *Archives of Internal Medicine*, 39 (1927), pp. 433–445.

Chapter Seven: The Postmodern Doctor

1. On the discovery of the sulfa drugs and antibiotics, see Harry F. Dowling, *Fighting Infection: Conquests of the Twentieth Century* (Cambridge: Harvard University Press, 1977), chaps. 8–10.

2. William V. Johnston, *Before the Age of Miracles: Memoirs of a Country Doctor* (Toronto: Fitzhenry and Whiteside, 1972), p. 69.

3. Ibid., p. 112. Dowling, *Fighting Infection*, p. 122.

4. Carl G. Harford et al., "Treatment of Staphylococcic, Pneumococcic, Gonococcic and Other Infections with Penicillin," *JAMA*, 3 February 1945, pp. 253–259, 10 February, pp. 325–329. Norman Plummer et al., "Penicillin Therapy in Hemolytic Streptococcic Pharyngitis and Tonsilitis," *JAMA*, 17 February 1945, pp. 369–374.

5. Michael Casey, "Fifty Years of General Practice," *Irish Medical Journal*, 74 (1981), p. 155.

6. Dowling, *Fighting Infection*, p. 187.

7. Robert F. Loeb, "Medical Education at Mid-Century," *Journal of Medical Education*, 26 (1951), p. 347. Melvin Casberg, "Medical Education Takes an Inventory," *Journal of Medical Education*, 25 (1950), p. 311.

8. Lionel Whitby, "The Challenge to Medical Education in the Second Half of the 20th Century," *Journal of Medical Education*, 28 (November 1953), p. 30.

9. See, for example, George S. Stevenson, "Why Patients Consult the Gastro-Enterologist," *JAMA*, 1 February 1930, pp. 334–335; George Canby Robinson, *The Patient as a Person: The Study of the Social Aspects of Illness* (New York, 1939), pp. 410–414.

10. The dilemma is summed up in an editoral note on "General Medical Education," *Journal of Medical Education*, 27 (January 1952), pp. 44–45.

11. It is especially portentous that internal medicine became a model for medical students because, next to neurosurgery, internal medicine has the highest prestige among doctors of any specialty. See Allan M. Schwartzbaum and John H. McGrath, "The Perception of Prestige Differences among Medical Subspecialties," *Social Science and Medicine*, 7 (1973), p. 367, table 1.

12. Robert Loeb and Dana W. Atchley, *Journal of Medical Education*, 28 (February 1953), p. 87–88, letter.

13. John E. Dietrick and Robert C. Berson, *Medical Schools in the United States at Mid-Century* (New York: McGraw-Hill, 1953), pp. 175–176. "Libraries": William D. Postell, "Trends in

Medical Education and Their Implications for the Medical Library," *Journal of Medical Education*, 30 (September 1955), p. 491.

14. On Western Reserve, Thomas H. Ham, "Current Trends in Medical Education: A Research Approach," *Journal of Medical Education*, 33 (March 1958), p. 298.

15. George W. Pickering, "The Purpose of Medical Education," *BMJ*, 21 July 1956, p. 115.

16. See the discussion of "PSRO's," in *Medical World News*, 3 May 1974, p. 26.

17. Dr. J. T. Hart, in "The Medical Use of Psychotropic Drugs: A Report of a Symposium . . . ," *Journal of the Royal College of Practitioners*, 23, suppl. no. 2 (June 1973), p. 73.

18. George P. Berry, "Medical Education in Transition," *Journal of Medical Education*, 28 (March 1953), p. 32.

19. John R. Ellis, "The Medical Student," *Journal of Medical Education*, 31 (January 1956), p. 45.

20. Davis G. Johnson, *Physicians in the Making* (San Francisco: Jossey-Bass, 1983), table 10 on p. 51, p. 105. This improvement is not the result of "mark inflation" either, for average MCAT scores have risen, too.

21. Donald Light, "The Impact of Medical School on Future Psychiatrists," *American Journal of Psychiatry*, 132 (1975), pp. 607–610.

22. Arnold Feldman, "The Family Practitioner as Psychiatrist," *American Journal of Psychiatry*, 135 (1978), p. 730.

23. The phrase became popular after George Engel's article "The Need for a New Medical Model: A Challenge for Biomedicine," *Science*, 196 (8 April 1977), pp. 129–136.

24. Barbara M. Korsch and Vida F. Negrete, "Doctor-Patient Communication," *Scientific American*, 227 (2) (August 1972), p. 68. *SBE* is subacute bacterial endocarditis, also called *infectious endocarditis. Coombs titre* is a reference to R. R. A. Coombs's test for the presence in the blood of antibodies to one's own red blood cells.

25. National Center for Health Statistics, J. G. Collins, *Physician Visits: Volume and Interval Since Last Visit, United States, 1980.* Vital and Health Statistics, series 10, no. 144, DHHS pub. no. (PHS) 83-1572 (Washington: GPO, June 1983), p. 25, table J.

26. Theodore F. Fox, "The Personal Doctor," *Lancet*, 2 April 1960, p. 750.

27. Michael J. Lepore, *Death of the Clinician* (Springfield: Charles C Thomas, 1982), p. 3.

28. Robert Wood Johnson Foundation, *Medical*

Practice in the United States: A Special Report (Princeton: RWJF, 1981), pp. 52–53. Although the report distinguished between "general practice" and "family practice," I have taken data only for the latter.

29. Report of the First Teaching Institute, AAMC, "The Teaching of Physiology, Biochemistry, Pharmacology," *Journal of Medical Education*, 29 (July 1954, pt. II), p. 107, table 2. Members of the "Society for Clinical Investigation" scored 2.7; teaching members of the American College of Physicians, 2.6.

30. David E. Rogers, "On Technologic Restraint," *Archives of Internal Medicine*, 135 (1975), pp. 1394, 1396.

31. David B. Reuben, "Learning Diagnostic Restraint," *NEJM*, 1 March 1984, p. 592.

32. In a reanalysis of the 1976–1978 U.S. nationwide survey financed by the Johnson Foundation, Roger A. Rosenblatt and colleagues found the younger, hospital-trained family physicians more test-oriented than the older GPs. "The first group was more likely to order a culture or an x-ray examination. . . ." But the family doctors also did more "patient education." "The Structure and Content of Family Practice: Current Status and Future Trends," *Journal of Family Practice*, 15 (1982), p. 711.

33. "A routine": Stewart Wolf et al., "Instruction in Medical History Taking," *Journal of Medical Education*, 27 (July 1952, pt. I), p. 251. "Outline": Stanley J. Reiser, *Medicine and the Reign of Technology* (New York: Cambridge University Press, 1978), pp. 180–181. "Costello interview": Arthur Owens, "Financial Success Story: The Internists," *Medical Economics*, 22 June 1970, p. 163. "Computer": Herbert Benson and Mark D. Epstein, "The Placebo Effect: A Neglected Asset in the Care of Patients," *JAMA*, 23 June 1975, p. 1226.

34. Robert Kohn and Kerr L. White, eds., *Health Care: An International Study. Report of the World Health Organization* (London: Oxford University Press, 1976), p. 53, figure 7.9, "total crude rates."

35. *Report Johnson Foundation*, pp. 50–51.

36. National Center for Health Statistics, B. K. Cypress, *Medication Therapy in Office Visits for Selected Diagnoses. The National Ambulatory Medical Care Survey. United States, 1980*. Vital and Health Statistics, series 13, no. 71. DHHS pub. no. (PHS) 83-1732 (Washington: GPO, January 1983), p. 7, table 1. Data are on "upper respiratory infections."

37. Troy L. Thompson et al., "Underrecognition of

Patients' Psychosocial Distress in a University Hospital Medical Clinic," *American Journal of Psychiatry*, 140 (1983), p. 160. George E. Murphy, "The Physician's Responsibility for Suicide. II: Errors of Omission," *Annals of Internal Medicine*, 82 (1975), pp. 305–309. What percentage of nonsuicidal patients had seen a doctor in the last six months? Nationwide statistics aren't available for six-month intervals. But whereas 80 percent of all suicide victims had seen a doctor within six months, in 1981 only 74 percent of a nationwide sample of Americans had visited a doctor *within the past year.* National Center for Health Statistics, B. Bloom, *Current Estimates from the National Health Interview Survey, United States, 1981.* Vital and Health Statistics, series 10, no. 141, DHHS pub. no. (PHS) 83-1569 (Washington: GPO, October 1982), p. 4, table D.

        38. Lepore, *Death of the Clinician*, p. 17.

        39. Allon Peebles, *A Survey of Statistical Data on Medical Facilities in the United States* (Washington: Committee on the Cost of Medical Care, 1929) no. 3, p. 25. In larger cities specialists were 19 percent of the total. On 1942: Bernhard J. Stern, *American Medical Practice in the Perspective of a Century* (New York: Commonwealth Fund, 1945), p. 50.

        40. Daniel Cathell, *Book on the Physician Himself from Graduation to Old Age*, crowning ed. (Philadelphia, 1922), p. 31. James B. Herrick, "The Practitioner of the Future," *JAMA*, 22 September 1934, p. 881.

        41. Johnson, *Physicians in the Making*, p. 139, table 25.

        42. NCHS, *Physician Visits*, p. 25, table J.

        43. *Report Johnson Foundation*, pp. 26–27.

        44. Fox, "Personal Doctor," p. 750.

        45. National Center for Health Education, *Office Visits by Women. The National Ambulatory Medical Care Survey. United States, 1977.* Vital and Health Statistics, series 13, no. 45. DHEW pub. no. (PHS) 80-1796 (Washington: GPO, March 1980), p. 6.

        46. National Center for Health Statistics, *The National Ambulatory Medical Care Survey: 1977 Summary: United States, January–December 1977.* Vital and Health Statistics, series 13, no. 44. DHEW pub. no (PHS) 80-1795 (Washington: GPO, April 1980), p. 4. "Regular source": National Center for Health Statistics, *Highlights from Wave I of the National Survey of Personal Health Practices and Consequences. United States, 1979.* Vital and Health Sta-

tistics, series 15, no. 1. DHEW pub. no. (PHS) 81-1162 (Washington: GPO, June 1981), p. 13, table 2.

47. Eliot Freidson, *Doctoring Together: A Study of Professional Social Control* (New York: Elsevier, 1975), p. 148.

48. When Barbara Korsch and collaborators studied a pediatric clinic in Los Angeles, they found "no significant relationship . . . between the time of interaction and the percent of patients who were satisfied." "Gaps in Doctor-Patient Communication," *Pediatrics*, 42 (1968), p. 860.

49. John F. Burnum, "What One Internist Does in His Practice," *Annals of Internal Medicine*, 78 (1973), p. 440.

50. *Report Johnson Foundation*, data on length of "ambulatory encounters," p. 24; on "diagnostic tests," p. 50.

51. First to pinpoint the six-minute interview were T. S. Eimerl and R. J. C. Pearson, "Working-time in General Practice," *BMJ*, 24 December 1966, p. 1552. More recently, John Fry, ed., *Trends in General Practice 1979* (London: Royal College of General Practitioners, 1979), p. 28. In her study of GPs around Manchester in the mid-1970s, Freda Fitton found Dr. X to average nine minutes per patient, Dr. Y four minutes. *The Doctor/Patient Relationship: A Study in General Practice* (London: HMSO, 1979), p. 41. Gerry Stimson and Barbara Webb, from whom the "Two-minute Todd" and "still talking" anecdotes come, timed the average consultation in "practice A" at four minutes. *Going to See the Doctor: The Consultation Process in General Practice* (London: Routledge, 1975), pp. 1, 27, 60.

52. "Around 1930": Selwyn D. Collins, "Frequency and Volume of Doctors' Calls among Males and Females in 9,000 Families, Based on Nation-Wide Periodic Canvasses, 1928–31" [U.S.] *Public Health Reports*, 55 (1 November 1940), p. 1983. "Today": NCHS, *Physician Visits*, 1980, p. 24, table H. In a sample of 1,036,000 physician visits, 0.6 percent were at home.

53. 1942: Stern, *American Medical Practice*, p. 75, a sample of white male GPs in Maryland and Georgia, office and home visits. 1977: National Center for Health Statistics, *Characteristics of Visits to Female and Male Physicians: The National Ambulatory Medical Care Survey. United States, 1977.* Vital and Health Statistics, series 13, no. 49. DHHS pub. no. (PHS) 80-1710 (Washington: GPO, June 1980), p. 5, table C, male doctors only in general and family practice. Office visits only but presumably they made few or no home visits. Note that the average number of patients seen by internists weekly declined from 84 in 1942 to 58 in 1977, assuming the two surveys are com-

parable. In 1942, however, it is likely that a number of these visits were *to the same patient.*

54. Stimson and Webb, *Going to See the Doctor,* p. 34. One survey: Ann Cartwright and Robert Anderson, *General Practice Revisited: A Second Study of Patients and Their Doctors* (London: Tavistock, 1981), p. 7, table 3.

55. WHO survey: Kohn, *Health Care,* p. 182, table 7.43.D. Manhattan: Cynthia L. Janus et al., "Lay Attitudes Toward Physicians and Medical Technology," *Mt. Sinai Journal of Medicine,* 48 (1981), p. 348, table X.

56. Norman Cousins, *Anatomy of an Illness as Perceived by the Patient: Reflections on Healing and Regeneration* (New York: Bantam, 1981; first published 1979), p. 137.

Chapter Eight: The Postmodern Patient

1. These statistics from National Center for Health Statistics, *Health, United States, 1983,* DHHS pub. no. (PHS) 83-1232 (Washington: GPO, December 1983), pp. 97–99. Life expectancy at age 65 increased from 13.9 years in 1950 to 16.8 years in 1982.

2. "Declined by 72 percent": David E. Rogers et al., "Who Needs Medicaid?" *NEJM,* 1 July 1982, p. 16. "The average GP": J. M. Last, "The Iceberg: 'Completing the Clinical Picture' in General Practice," *Lancet,* 6 July 1963, p. 30. For other statistics on the rarity of various conditions in general practice, see Keith Hodgkin, *Towards Earlier Diagnosis in Primary Care,* 4th ed. (Edinburgh: Churchill Livingstone, 1978), p. ix and passim. On the view that "health care hardly affects health," see Paul Starr, *The Social Transformation of American Medicine* (New York: Basic Books, 1982), p. 410, and the other writers he cites. The most egregious tosser-out of baby with bath water is Ivan Illich, *Limits to Medicine* (Harmondsworth: Penguin, 1977; 1st ed. 1976), pp. 21–46.

3. This analysis of specific diseases contrasts 1928–1931 with 1979, because in that latter year both acute and chronic conditions were counted. 1928–1931 morbidity data from I. S. Falk et al., *The Incidence of Illness and the Receipt and Costs of Medical Care Among Representative Families: Experiences in Twelve Consecutive Months During 1928–31* (Chicago, 1933; Committee on the Costs of Medical Care, no. 26), appendix table B-17, p. 274; column "all incomes," 8,639 families in 130 communities surveyed. Based on 33,156 illnesses among 38,668 white individuals. Trained interviewers visited each family approximately once every two months. The 1979 morbidity

data are from National Center for Health Statistics, *Current Estimates from the National Health Interview Survey, United States, 1979*, DHHS pub. no. (PHS) 81-1564 (Washington: GPO, April 1981), acute conditions on p. 13, chronic on pp. 34–36.

4. Average duration computed from the sources in table 8-1.

5. Appropriate NCHS data cited in table 8-1. Data on p. 4. The average in 1964 was 4.6 as well, so the increase in frequency of visiting occurred sometime before then. NCHS, *U.S. Health, 1982*, p. 90.

6. "Three Americans of four": National Center for Health Statistics, Charlotte A. Schoenborn, *Basic Data from Wave I of the National Survey of Personal Health Practices and Consequences*, Vital and Health Statistics, series 15, no. 2, DHHS pub. no. (PHS) 81-1163 (Washington: GPO, August 1981), p. 14, table 4. "Britain depression": Ann Cartwright and Robert Anderson, *General Practice Revisited: A Second Study of Patients and Their Doctors* (London: Tavistock, 1981), p. 52.

7. Quoted in Gerry Stimson and Barbara Webb, *Going to See the Doctor: The Consultation Process in General Practice* (London: Routledge, 1975), p. 20.

8. National Center for Health Statistics, Kathleen M. Danchik, *Highlights from Wave I of the National Survey of Personal Health Practices and Consequences*, Vital and Health Statistics, series 15, no. 1, DHHS pub. no. (PHS) 81-1162 (Washington: GPO, June 1981), p. 10, table 1. "Young" is ages 20–24.

9. "Supply of physicians": NCHS, *U.S. Health 1982*, p. 113. "Wait 4.5 days": Gerald L. Glandon and Jack L. Werner, "Physicians' Practice Experience during the Decade of the 1970s," *JAMA*, 5 December 1980, p. 2518. "North Central Florida": Richard A. Henry, "The Doctor in the Rural County," in Richard C. Reynolds et al., eds. *The Health of a Rural County* (Gainesville: University Presses of Florida, 1976), p. 69, table 1. The "25 percent" applied both to metropolitan and nonmetropolitan areas.

10. On the frequency of complaints in family practice, see Robert Wood Johnson Foundation, *Special Report: Medical Practice in the United States* (Princeton: RWJF, 1981), p. 61. Hypertension followed a close second. For other data that also place URIs no. 1, C. Richard Kirkwood et al., "The Diagnostic Content of Family Practice: 50 Most Common Diagnoses Recorded in the WAMI Community Practices," *Journal of Family Practice*, 15 (1982), p. 489, table 2.

On how long patients wait before consulting, National Center for Health Statistics, Trena M. Ezzati, *The National Ambulatory Medical Care Survey, 1977 Summary*, Vital and Health Statistics, series 13, no. 44, pub. no. DHEW (PHS) 80-1795 (Washington: GPO, April 1980), p. 9, table G. Seventy-nine percent of patients who consult a doctor for a URI come within a week of the onset of symptoms.

11. "Survey California": H. G. Gough, "Doctors' Estimates of the Percentage of Patients Whose Problems Do Not Require Medical Attention," *Medical Education*, 11 (1977), p. 381. One-third of the doctors estimated as trivial more than 25 percent of visits. John F. Burnum, "What One Internist Does in His Practice," *Annals of Internal Medicine*, 78 (1973), p. 442, table 4. He considered these complaints "minor" only after excluding major diseases. "Welsh physician": Jean Comaroff, "A Bitter Pill to Swallow: Placebo Therapy in General Practice," *Sociological Review*, 24 (1976), p. 86, "Dr. F."

12. Marilyn J. Gifford, "Emergency Physicians' and Patients' Assessments: Urgency of Need for Medical Care," *Annals of Emergency Medicine*, 9 (1980), pp. 505–506.

13. This is the argument of Edward Shorter, *The Making of the Modern Family* (New York: Basic Books, 1975).

14. "Unhappiness becomes depression": idea from Peter Tate, "Doctors' Style," in David Pendleton and John Hasler, eds., *Doctor-Patient Communication* (London: Academic Press, 1983), p. 80. Government survey of depression: National Center for Health Statistics, Rona Beth Sayetta, *Basic Data on Depressive Symptomatology, United States, 1974–75*, Vital and Health Statistics, series 11, no. 216, DHEW pub. no. (PHS) 80-1666 (Washington: GPO, April 1980), p. 9, table 2. Michael Balint, *The Doctor, His Patient and the Illness*, rev. ed. (New York: International Universities Press, 1972), p. 225. First ed. in 1957.

15. On the sensitivity to symptoms of people amidst life changes see James W. Pennebaker, *The Psychology of Physical Symptoms* (New York: Springer, 1982), p. 138. "Family Clinic California": Diane Stumbo et al., "Diagnostic Profile of a Family Practice Clinic: Patients with Psychosocial Diagnoses," *Journal of Family Practice*, 14 (1982), pp. 281–285. On a "Canadian city": Michael Brennan and Amy Noce, "A Study of Patients with Psychosocial Problems in a Family Practice," *Journal of Family Practice*, 13 (1981), pp. 837–843, especially p. 840, table 2.

16. NCHS, *Highlights Wave I*, p. 11, table 1, ages twenty to sixty-four.

17. National Center for Health Statistics, Sidney Abraham, *Obese and Overweight Adults in the United States,* Vital and Health Statistics, series 11, no. 230, DHHS pub. no. (PHS) 83-1680 (Washington: GPO, February 1983), p. 4, table B. Eighty-fifth percentile of overweight, relative to desirable weight, ages 20–74. 1971–1974 data.

18. "Psychologist research most symptoms": Pennebaker, *Psychology Physical Symptoms,* p. 144. "1977 government survey": National Center for Health Statistics, Beulah K. Cypress, *Office Visits by Women: The National Ambulatory Medical Care Survey, United States, 1977,* Vital and Health Statistics, series 13, no. 45, DHEW pub. no. (PHS) 80-1796 (Washington: GPO, March 1980), p. 13, table J, visit rates given for both males and females.

19. This was the lead in a story headlined "The Risk of Contraceptives," *Toronto Star,* 25 October 1980, p. A–12. It was retracted on 1 November, p. A–8.

20. The story provides weekly drama for a number of large dailies and TV stations. For an overview, see Carroll M. Brodsky, " 'Allergic to Everything': A Medical Subculture," *Psychosomatics,* 24 (1983), pp. 731–742.

21. David J. Pearson et al., "Food Allergy: How Much in the Mind?" *Lancet,* 4 June 1983, pp. 1259–1261. The article did not say how the other two had got the idea.

22. James K. Todd, "Toxic Shock Syndrome—Scientific Uncertainty and the Public Media," *Pediatrics,* 67 (1981), pp. 921–923.

23. Toronto *Globe & Mail,* 23 March 1984, p. M-3. The less educated the respondents, the more fearful they were.

24. "Edinburgh surgeon": James Wardrop, *Observations on Fungus Haematodes or Soft Cancer, in Several of the Most Important Organs of the Human Body* (Edinburgh, 1809), p. 165, quoting Matthew Baillie. William Osler, *The Principles and Practice of Medicine* (New York, 1893), p. 556, first published the year previously. "GPs 1927": William Stanley Sykes, *A Manual of General Medical Practice* (London, 1927), pp. 72–76. Frank E. Tylecote, note on "Cancer of the Lung," *Lancet,* 30 July 1927, pp. 256–257.

25. Lois Vidal, *Magpie* (London, 1934), p. 257. M. V. O'Shea, "Cigaret Smoking—How It Affects the Body," *Hygeia,* January 1924, p. 45. "1940 scientist": Julia Bell, "A Determination of the Consanguinity Rate in the General Hospital Population of England and Wales," *Annals of Eugenics,* 10 (1940), p. 384. "British Survey

1966": Philip Ley, "Patients' Understanding and Recall in Clinical Communication Failure," in Pendleton, *Doctor-Patient Communication*, p. 92, citing research he had published in 1966.

26. Royal College of Physicians of London, *Smoking and Health* (London: RCP, 1962), p. 43.

27. Public Health Service, *Smoking and Health: Report of the Advisory Committee to the Surgeon General of the Public Health Service*, PHS pub. no. 1103 (Washington: GPO, n.d. [1964], p. 28. U.S. DHEW, Public Health Service, *Smoking and Health: A Report of the Surgeon General*, DHEW pub. no. (PHS) 79-50066 (Washington: GPO, n.d. [1979]), pp. 1–12.

28. Ibid., smoking statistics in the Surgeon General's 1979 *Report*, p. A-9, and NCHS, *Health, United States, 1982*, p. 83, table 30.

29. Kenneth Walker, *Patients and Doctors: The Layman's Guide to Doctors and Doctoring* (Harmondsworth: Penguin, 1957), p. 156.

30. For data, see National Center for Health Statistics, A. Joan Klebba, *Mortality from Diseases Associated with Smoking: United States, 1960–77*, Vital and Health Statistics, series 20, no. 17, DHHS pub. no. (PHS) 82-1854 (Washington: GPO, January 1982), p. 11, table E, cohort 50–55.

31. Eliot Freidson, *Patients' Views of Medical Practice* (New York: Russell Sage, 1961), p. 102.

32. Cited by Terry W. Dagrosa, "Cancer in America," *Nursing Forum*, 19 (1980), p. 325, who paraphrases the conclusions of the network.

33. Michael Lepore, *Death of the Clinician* (Springfield: Charles C Thomas, 1982), p. 273.

34. Starr, *Social Transformation American Medicine*, emphasizes the attack from psychiatry, p. 409. In retrospect the attack from obstetrics has probably been more influential. The Boston Women's Health Book Collective produced *Our Bodies, Ourselves*, which was first published in 1971.

35. Scholars such as John C. Burnham represent this viewpoint. "American Medicine's Golden Age: What Happened to It?" *Science*, 215 (19 March 1982), pp. 1474–1479.

36. The English physician John Stevens, quoted by M. Lloyd, "Medical Authoritarianism and Its Effect on Health Care," *Medical Journal of Australia*, 14 September 1974, p. 413.

37. In a roundtable discussion on "PSRO's," *Medical World News*, 3 May 1974, p. 26.

38. Paul Dubois, *The Psychic Treatment of Nervous Disorders* (London, 1905; the French edition appeared in 1904), p. 388.

39. Quoted in Eliot Freidson, *Doctoring Together: A Study of Professional Social Control* (New York: Elsevier, 1975), p. 56.

40. These examples from Tony Smith, "Alternative Medicine," *BMJ*, 30 July 1983, p. 307; Faith T. Fitzgerald, "Science and Scam: Alternative Thought Patterns in Alternative Health Care," *NEJM*, 27 October 1983, pp. 1066–1067.

41. Examples from Barrie R. Cassileth, "After Laetrile, What?" *NEJM*, 17 June 1982, pp. 1482–1485.

42. Published in North York, Ontario, by "Creative Communications Consultants," n.d.

43. "133 cancer patients": Cassileth, "After Laetrile," p. 1483; "98 rheumatology patients": Summary of paper by Cody K. Wasner et al., "The Use of Unproven Remedies," *Arthritis and Rheumatism*, 23 (1980), pp. 759–760.

44. "1969 survey Britain": Karen Dunnell and Ann Cartwright, *Medicine Takers, Prescribers and Hoarders* (London: Routledge, 1972), p. 21; "half the women had taken something prescribed compared with less than a third of the men." "Americans more medicine oriented": Kerr L. White et al., "International Comparisons of Medical-Care Utilization," *NEJM*, 7 September 1967, p. 521, table 12.

45. Dunnell, *Medicine Takers*, pp. 82–83.

46. Linus Pauling, *Vitamin C and the Common Cold* (San Francisco: Freeman, 1970). "1979 survey": NCHS, *Highlights Wave I*, p. 17, table 3; "down the drain": for a skeptical look at "megadosing" of vitamins, see James O. Woolliscroft, "Megavitamins: Fact and Fancy," *DM* (*Disease-A-Month*), February 1983.

47. Dunnell, *Medicine Takers*, p. 31. Within the last two weeks 28 percent of the adults had taken at least one of each kind; 13 percent had taken only prescribed, 39 percent only over-the-counter, and 20 percent none.

48. Freda Fitton and H. W. K. Acheson, *The Doctor/Patient Relationship: A Study in General Practice* (London: HMSO, 1979), p. 69; Stimson and Webb, *Going to See the Doctor*, p. 30.

49. Calvin M. Kunin, "Comment," on a paper by

Henry E. Simmons and Paul D. Stolley; "This Is Medical Progress? Trends and Consequences of Antibiotic Use in the United States," *JAMA*, 4 March 1974, pp. 1023–1028, the comment, pp. 1030–1032, quote p. 1030. "13 percent of all prescriptions": National Center for Health Statistics, H. Koch, *Drug Utilization in Office-Based Practice, A Summary of Findings, National Ambulatory Medical Care Survey, United States, 1980*, Vital and Health Statistics, series 13, no. 65, DHHS pub. no. (PHS) 83-1726, p. 17, table 2. "Up to a third": quoted in Simmons-Stolley paper, p. 1024.

50. Alice H. Murphree, "Folk Beliefs," in Reynolds, ed., *Health of a Rural County*, p. 118.

51. Recounted in a medical column by Howard Seiden, *Toronto Star*, 14 June 1984, p. G-2.

52. The comment was reported by Comaroff, "Bitter Pill," p. 90.

53. Kunin, "Comment," p. 1030.

54. NCHS, *Drug Utilization*, p. 17, table 2. Of the 7.7 percent of all prescriptions represented by drugs for the CNS (excluding analgesics and antipyretics), anticonvulsants represented 0.4 percent, antidepressants 1.5 percent, tranquilizers 0.8 percent, stimulants 1.3 percent, and sedatives-hypnotics 3.7 percent.

55. Glen D. Mellinger and Mitchell B. Balter, "Prevalence and Patterns of Use of Psychotropic Drugs: Results from a 1979 National Survey of American Adults," in G. Tognoni et al., eds., *Epidemiological Impact of Psychotropic Drugs* (New York: Elsevier, 1981), p. 125. Sixteen percent had used a psychoactive drug within the preceding twelve months.

56. Cynthia L. Janus et al., "Lay Attitudes toward Physicians and Medical Technology," *Mount Sinai Journal of Medicine*, 48 (1981), pp. 346, 347.

57. Fitton, *Doctor/Patient Relationship*, pp. 57, 59.

58. Henry Wechsler et al., "The Physicians' Role in Health Promotion—A Survey of Primary-Care Practitioners," *NEJM*, 13 January 1983, p. 99, table 3. Only minuscule percentages felt they had actually been successful in helping patients in any of these areas. In England the percent of GPs who thought it appropriate for patients to seek help from them for family problems fell from 87 percent in 1964 to 67 percent in 1977. Cartwright, *General Practice Revisited*, p. 52.

59. Medical Committee for Human Rights, *Your Rights as a Hospital Patient* (Boston: Greater Boston Chapter MCHR), pp. 4–12, 41.

Chapter Nine: *Psychological Disease and Postmodern Medicine*

1. See, for example, John J. Schwab and Mary E. Schwab, "Psychiatric Epidemiology: Some Clinical Implications," *Psychosomatics*, 24 (1983), pp. 95–96.

2. Alan B. Raper, "The Incidence of Peptic Ulceration in Some African Tribal Groups," *Royal Society of Tropical Medicine and Hygiene, Transactions*, 52 (1958), pp. 535–546.

3. John F. Burnum, "What One Internist Does in His Practice," *Annals of Internal Medicine*, 78 (1973), p. 441.

4. Alexander Hilkevitch, "Psychiatric Disturbances in Outpatients of a General Medical Outpatient Clinic," *International Journal of Neuropsychiatry*, 1 (1965), pp. 373–374.

5. On Rochester, Ben Z. Locke and Elmer A. Gardner, "Psychiatric Disorders among the Patients of General Practitioners and Internists," [U.S.] *Public Health Reports*, 84 (1) (1969), p. 168. "British study 13 percent": Michael Shepherd et al., *Psychiatric Illness in General Practice*, 2d ed. (Oxford: Oxford University Press, 1981), p. 81, table 14, "total psychiatric morbidity" for 46 general practices in London, 1961–1962. The two studies estimating 20 percent: D. P. Goldberg, "Psychiatric Illness in General Practice," *BMJ*, 23 May 1970, p. 442. "Psychiatric disorders were present in about 20 percent. . . ." Michael A. Varnam, "Psychotropic Prescribing. What Am I Doing?" *Journal of the Royal College of General Practitioners*, 31 (1981), pp. 480–483, data on 1,543 patients seen in five weeks of practice.

6. "1979 survey": E. H. Uhlenhuth et al., "Symptom Checklist Syndromes in the General Population," *Archives of General Psychiatry*, 40 (1983), p. 1170, table 5. "Englishman nerves": Karen Dunnell and Ann Cartwright, *Medicine Takers, Prescribers and Hoarders* (London: Routledge, 1972), p. 16, table 7. "Florida sample": John J. Schwab et al., "Some Epidemiologic Aspects of Psychosomatic Medicine," *International Journal of Psychiatry in Medicine*, 9 (1978–1979), p. 148.

7. National Center for Health Statistics, Beulah K. Cypress, *Office Visits by Women: The National Ambulatory Medical Care Survey, United States, 1977*. Vital and Health Statistics, series 13, no. 45, DHEW pub. no. (PHS) 80-1796 (Washington: GPO, March 1980), p. 14, figure 12. Rates for women of other ages were all lower, and rates for men were still lower.

8. Bertram S. Brown, "Key Interactions among Psychiatric Disorders, Primary Care, and the Use of Psychotropic Drugs,"

in Brown, ed., *Clinical Anxiety: Tension in Primary Medicine* (Amsterdam: Excerpta Medica, 1979) International Congress Series, no. 448, pp. 3–13.

9. In 1971 Samuel B. Guze christened this *Briquet's syndrome*, after Pierre Briquet, a nineteenth-century Parisian physician who had written on hysteria. Guze et al., "Hysteria and Antisocial Behavior: Further Evidence of an Association," *American Journal of Psychiatry*, 127 (1971), pp. 957–960.

10. Jean Comaroff, "A Bitter Pill to Swallow: Placebo Therapy in General Practice," *Sociological Review*, 24 (1976) p. 86, "Dr. E."

11. David Wheatley, "Influence of Doctors' and Patients' Attitudes in the Treatment of Neurotic Illness," *Lancet*, 25 November 1967, pp. 1133–1135.

12. Remarks by Neil Kessel, in a symposium on "The Medical Use of Psychotropic Drugs," *Journal of the Royal College of General Practitioners*, 23, suppl. 2 (June 1973), p. 12.

13. See Glen D. Mellinger and Mitchell B. Balter, "Prevalence and Patterns of Use of Psychotherapeutic Drugs: Results from a 1979 Survey of American Adults," in G. Tognoni et al., eds., *Epidemiological Impact of Psychotropic Drugs* (New York: Elsevier, 1981), pp. 117–135. See also letter by D. Haskell, *NEJM*, 16 February 1984, p. 465.

14. A brief account of the history of these drugs may be found in Alfred G. Gilman et al., *Goodman and Gilman's The Pharmacological Basis of Therapeutics*, 6th ed. (New York: Macmillan, 1980), pp. 339, 418.

15. U.S. Bureau of the Census, *Statistical Abstract of the United States: 1982–83*, 103d ed. (Washington: GPO, 1982), p. 81, table 122, ages forty-five to fifty-four, white only. Rates for males below thirty-four by contrast, climbed sharply; those for females below 24 rose as well.

16. Symposium on "The Medical Use of Psychotropic Drugs," Dr. C. A. Watts from Ibstock in Leicestershire, p. 32.

17. Barry Blackwell and Ruth Cooperstock, "Benzodiazepine Use and the Biopsychosocial Model," *Journal of Family Practice*, 17 (1983), p. 453.

18. "California Clinic": Diane Stumbo et al., "Diagnostic Profile of a Family Practice Clinic: Patients with Psychosocial Diagnoses," *Journal of Family Practice*, 14 (1982), p. 284. "British GP": Varnam, "Psychotropic Prescribing," p. 481, table 2.

19. "46 London doctors": Shepherd, *Psychiatric Ill-*

ness in General Practice, p. 156, table 47. "American medical practice 1977": Roger A. Rosenblatt et al., "The Structure and Content of Family Practice: Current Status and Future Trends," *Journal of Family Practice,* 15 (1982), p. 713, table 21.

20. National Center for Health Statistics, B. K. Cypress, *Medication Therapy in Office Visits for Selected Diagnoses: The National Ambulatory Medical Care Survey, United States, 1980,* Vital and Health Statistics, series 13, no. 71, DHHS pub. no. (PHS) 83-1732 (Washington: GPO, January 1983), p. 20, table 15.

21. Kenneth E. Callen and David Davis, "What Medical Students Should Know about Psychiatry: The Results of a Survey of Rural General Practitioners," *American Journal of Psychiatry,* 135 (1978), pp. 243–244.

22. Ann Cartwright, "Prescribing and the Doctor-Patient Relationship," in David Pendleton and John Hasler, eds., *Doctor-Patient Communication* (London: Academic Press, 1983), p. 189.

23. Mark F. Longhurst, "Angry Patient, Angry Doctor," *Canadian Medical Association Journal,* 123 (1980), p. 598.

24. Peter Tate, "Doctors' Style," in Pendleton, *Doctor-Patient Communication,* p. 80.

25. Stewart Wolf et al., "Instruction in Medical History Taking," *Journal of Medical Education,* 27 (1952), p. 245.

26. Thomas E. Frothingham, *NEJM,* 15 July 1982, p. 194, letter.

27. W. Brouwer and F. Touw-Otten, "Van Klacht tot klagen: een analyse van de pre-medische periode," *Huisarts en Wetenschap,* 17 (1974), pp. 3–15. English summary, p. 15.

28. Pediatric clinic was Simon Yudkin's; see his "Six Children with Coughs: The Second Diagnosis," *Lancet,* 9 September 1961, pp. 561–563.

29. Patrick S. Byrne and Barrie E. L. Long, *Doctors Talking to Patients* (London: HMSO, 1976), p. 95.

30. J. P. Recordon, "Communication in the Doctor-Patient Relationship," *Journal of the Royal College of General Practitioners,* 22 (1972), p. 819.

31. Michael Balint, *The Doctor, His Patient and the Illness,* rev. ed. (New York: International Universities Press, 1972), especially pp. 228–229.

32. Robert Wood Johnson Foundation, *Special Report, Medical Practice in the United States* (Princeton: RWJF, 1981), p. 63. Of gastroenterologists' practice encounters, 6.1 percent were

chronic enteritis and ulcerative colitis, 5.0 percent "functional disorders of intestines," and so on.

33. Reviewed in Paul R. Latimer, *Functional Gastrointestinal Disorders: A Behavioral Medicine Approach* (New York: Springer, 1983), pp. 107–113.

34. Sheila L. Waller and J. J. Misiewicz, "Prognosis in the Irritable-Bowel Syndrome," *Lancet*, 11 October 1969, pp. 753–756.

35. Steven J. Young et al., "Psychiatric Illness and the Irritable Bowel Syndrome: Practical Implications for the Primary Physician," *Gastroenterology*, 70 (1976), p. 165.

36. Jan Svedlung et al., "Controlled Study of Psychotherapy in Irritable Bowel Syndrome," *Lancet*, 10 September 1983, pp. 589–591.

37. J. E. Lennard-Jones, "Functional Gastrointestinal Disorders," *NEJM*, 24 February 1983, pp. 433–434; my italics.

38. Latimer, *Functional Gastrointestinal Disorders*, p. 120.

39. Shaw, *The Doctor's Dilemma: A Tragedy* (Harmondsworth: Penguin, 1946), p. 26.

40. Figures in National Center for Health Statistics, *Health, United States, 1982*, DHHS pub. no. (PHS) 83-1232 (Washington: GPO, December 1982), p. 130, table 64.

SUGGESTIONS FOR FURTHER READING

I HAVE included only books that are still in print and that are accessible to the general reading public.

On the social history of medicine in America one might start with Richard H. Shryock's two classic works, *The Development of Modern Medicine* (rev. ed. 1947) (Madison: University of Wisconsin Press, 1979), and *Medicine and Society in America, 1660–1860* (1960) (Ithaca: Cornell University Press, 1972). For more detailed studies of the nineteenth century, try Charles E. Rosenberg, *The Cholera Years: The United States in 1832, 1849 and 1866* (Chicago: University of Chicago Press, 1962), which, despite its title, is actually a quite thorough account of the practice of medicine at that time. Also William Rothstein, *American Physicians of the Nineteenth Century* (Baltimore: Johns Hopkins Press, 1972), and J. Worth Estes, *Hall Jackson and the Purple Foxglove; Medical Practice and Research in Revolutionary America, 1760–1820* (Hanover: University Press of New England, 1979): again, despite its title, a wide-ranging account.

Among the extensive literature on the social history of medicine in Britain, I mention only M. Jeanne Peterson, *The Medical Profession in*

Mid-Victorian London (Berkeley: University of California Press, 1978).

On developments in specific areas of medicine, readers will find informative James Harvey Young's two works, *The Toadstool Millionaires: A Social History of Patent Medicines in America before Federal Regulation* (Princeton: Princeton University Press, 1961) and *The Medical Messiahs: A Social History of Health Quackery in Twentieth-Century America* (Princeton: Princeton University Press, 1967). George Frederick Drinka has written entertainingly of the history of psychiatry in *The Birth of Neurosis: Myth, Malady and the Victorians* (New York: Simon & Schuster, 1984).

For books that bring the history of American medicine up to date, making various political points, see Rosemary Stevens, *American Medicine and the Public Interest* (New Haven: Yale University Press, 1971), and Paul Starr's superb account, which I believe is the best social history of American medicine, *The Social Transformation of American Medicine* (New York: Basic Books, 1982). On the important question of new inventions and medicine, see Stanley Joel Reiser, *Medicine and the Reign of Technology* (Cambridge: Cambridge University Press, 1978).

Although doctors' memoirs abound, two that make especially lively reading are Michael J. Lepore, *Death of the Clinician: Requiem or Reveille?* (Springfield, Illinois: Charles C Thomas, 1982), and Lewis Thomas, *The Youngest Science: Notes of a Medicine-Watcher* (New York: Viking, 1983). Even though he comes across as a bit of a whiner, Charles LeBaron's account of the tribulations of a first-year medical student at Harvard still makes absorbing reading: *Gentle Vengeance* (Harmondsworth: Penguin, 1982).

On the doctor-patient relationship itself one might consult as an overview of the great body of technical literature, David Pendleton and John Hasler, eds., *Doctor-Patient Communication* (London: Academic Press, 1983). A nasty-tempered classic is Ivan Illich, *Limits to Medicine* (Harmondsworth: Penguin, 1977). Finally there is Norman Cousins's marvelously subjective account of the experience of being a patient, *Anatomy of an Illness as Perceived by the Patient* (New York: W. W. Norton, 1979).

INDEX

drug revolution, 180–94
  antibiotics in, 181–82
  health improvements after, 212
  impact of, 183–84
  internal medicine and, 194–95
  media response to, 181–82
  medical education and, 183–93
  postmodern patient and, 195, 212
  sulfa drugs in, 180–81
  see also medicines, postmodern
Dubois, Paul, 141, 147–48
  moral therapy of, 167–72, 177,
    229
Dunn, Charles, 103

ECG (electrocardiograph), 90–91
education, modern medical:
  competitive enrollment in, 102–3
  early, 29–30, 34–38, 69
  explosion in, 36–37
  postmodern vs., 185, 209
  scientific curriculum in, 78–81
education, postmodern medical, 36,
    183–93
  basic medical sciences in, 183–85
  biochemistry in, 184
  British, 191
  competitive pressures in, 191–92
  "crash" medicine and, 193
  drug revolution and, 183–93
  fact vs. principle in, 187–88
  lab facilities in, 186
  logic in, 184–85
  modern vs., 185, 209
  organic disease emphasized in, 185,
    190–93
  patient's expectations in, 235
  prerequisites for, 189
  psychiatry in, 249–50
  retention rate in, 188–90
  social sciences as secondary in,
    185–87
Ehrlich, Paul, 96
elderly:
  death rate and, 55–56
  as modern patient, 102, 110
  postmodern doctor and, 203
  traditional medicine and, 31
Eliot, Charles, 102–3

emergency departments, U.S., 216,
    239
emphysema, 76
epidemics:
  modern patient and, 119
  traditional medicine and, 56,
    182
ether, 95

family doctors, modern, 111
family doctors, postmodern, 202–7
  consultations with, 208
  "decline" of, 202
  "emotional" diseases seen by,
    242–43
  informal style of, 206–7
  internist as, 194–95, 203–4
  number of patients of, 203
  patriarchal style of, 204–6
family life, disintegration of, 218–
    19, 221, 228
Farquhar, John, 49–50
Feldman, Arnold, 192
Fenger, Christian, 86
fevers:
  sweating in, 65
  types of, 43
Fildes, Luke, 86
finances, fees:
  of modern doctor, 91, 98, 104,
    111–12, 126, 162–63
  of postmodern doctor, 202, 205–6,
    229
  of traditional doctor, 46, 51–53
Fishbein, Morris, 127–28
Fizes, Antoine, 41
Flexner, Abraham, 81, 186
Fox, Theodore Fortescue, 195, 203
foxglove plant, 51
FRCP (Fellow of the Royal College
    of Physicians), 27
"functional," 143

Gee, Ann, 59
Germany:
  drug industry in, 94, 96
  drug revolution in, 180
  pathology in, 79
  psychosomatic medicine in, 142–43

ABOUT THE AUTHOR

EDWARD SHORTER teaches history at the University of Toronto. Among other books he has written *Strikes in France, 1830–1968* (1974, with Charles Tilly), *The Making of the Modern Family* (1975), and *A History of Women's Bodies* (1982). He took time out to become a part-time "medical student" over a period of four years, and in preparation for writing this book also spent many months observing in various medical settings. He is married and has four children.